COSMOPOLITAN'S
HEALTH AND BEAUTY GUIDE

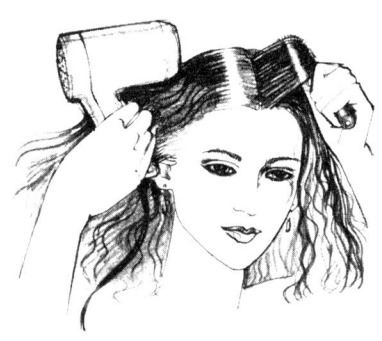

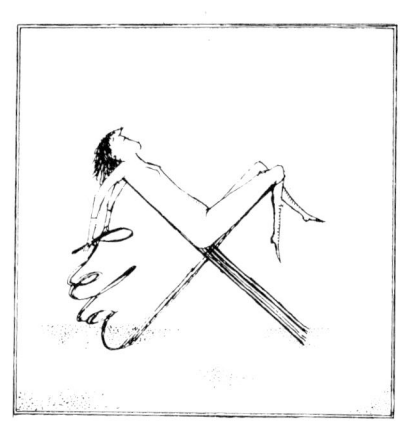

COSMOPOLITAN'S
HEALTH AND BEAUTY GUIDE

Edited by Pattie Barron

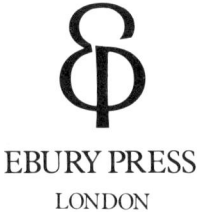

EBURY PRESS

LONDON

First published in 1980
by Cosmopolitan Magazine

This edition published by
Ebury Press
National Magazine House
72 Broadwick Street
London W1V 2BP

First impression 1980

ISBN 0 85223 178 4

ACKNOWLEDGEMENTS
Patricia Davis   Christine Doyle
Margaret Gaskin   Dinah Hall
Susan Jarzyk   Pandora Jeffreys
Joan Tinney

ILLUSTRATORS
Julia Butcher   Jan Griffin
McKinley Howell   Sara Midda
Pauline Rosenthal
Anny White

Printed and bound in Great Britain
at the
University Press, Cambridge

CONTENTS

INTRODUCTION   1

NUTRITION   3

SKIN CARE   15

SUN   29

SLIMMING   33

EXERCISE   67

THE BODY   95

HAIR   125

MAKE-UP   145

HEALTH   151

TEETH   165

COSMETIC SURGERY   171

REFERENCE SECTION   183

INDEX   189

INTRODUCTION

I dedicate this book to you, the reader, because I have learned more about my trade, the health and beauty business, from your letters than from any trip to a health hydro or cosmetics factory. A woman's attitude to herself conditions her appearance more than cosmetics or expensive surgery. There's nothing wrong — and everything positive and right — about wanting to look good. If you do, you are likely to function better both in your working life and in your private life.

In the years I have been health and beauty editor of *Cosmopolitan* I have read thousands of letters listing problems and asking advice. What everyone wants is not to be a mere Jane Fonda or Debbie Harry look-alike but to be herself, only more so. To have more vitality, more concentration, a more obedient body, healthier hair and skin, more peace of mind, a better way of life. The magazine is dedicated to helping all women achieve their goals in life. My function is to help every reader find the regime that suits her best. And this takes work, so we never promise the easy way.

Jane Fonda looks good at forty-plus because she works at it every day, with exercise, diet, a dance class as demanding as any ballet dancer's routine. Debbie Harry exudes glamour because she understands the exact technique of applying cosmetics. Both women are professionals who have learnt to assess their looks. That kind of assessment is open to us all.

On your account I have worked with experts in the fields of health and beauty: the trichologists, dermatologists, nutritionists and cosmetic surgeons. I have talked to dance teachers, make-up artists, hairdressers and the research scientists of cosmetic companies. I've asked the questions you most often ask me about your body, skin, hair, diet. And because I know almost every woman can achieve her full potential, I have selected the information that I hope will do most to help.

Cosmopolitan's Health And Beauty Guide is not a dream factory, nor a guide to glamour. The space usually given to fabulous colour pictures has been used to give more facts and practical advice. As a down-to-earth reference book, I hope you will use this guide often and keep it in your bag or desk drawer. In working on this book I have refined my ideas of beauty. I hope I shall do the same for you. **Pattie Barron**

NUTRITION

Your body is a complex piece of machinery and as such needs the right kind of fuel to function at optimum level. This section is designed to show you how, with the correct foods, you can keep your body at its healthiest — so you look and feel your best. With the help of the suggestions, diets and recipes outlined on the following pages, establish a sensible eating plan to suit your body and your life-style. Remember that the most important rule you can follow in the healthy eating stakes is to develop an awareness of every mouthful of food you take — and to enjoy it.

Re-assess your diet: A healthy eating plan to adopt/adapt

Below, you will find guidelines to a healthy diet you can follow for all time; you will discover that eating the best kind of foods does not mean inconveniencing yourself or others, shopping in specialised stores or being a bore at dinner parties or restaurants.

Breakfast

This is the most maligned meal of the day. Even if you are slimming you need the energy boost of food first thing to carry you through the morning, and the temptation to cheat on your diet with fattening snacks mid-morning will be less. Skip breakfast and you work at a lower rate of efficiency, feel famished at lunchtime and then probably overeat.

The well-balanced breakfast should consist of protein, vitamin C, and carbohydrate in the form of roughage. Protein could be a boiled egg (hard-boiled the night before if you want to save time), a couple of slices of lean meat or a wedge of cheese. Vitamin C content could be a glass of tomato, orange or grapefruit juice, or fresh citrus-fruit segments. For roughage, a slice or two of wholemeal toast spread lightly with vegetable margarine, or wholegrain cereal or muesli eaten with yogurt, milk or soaked in orange juice. Add a few raisins to the cereal for extra nutritional value, though not if you are weight watching. Slimmers should follow the breakfast "big three" ruling, too: a

slice of wholemeal toast, small glass of orange juice and an egg or small carton of cottage cheese. Limit yourself, slimming or not, to one cup of coffee or tea; if you have an insatiable sweet tooth, try substituting honey for sugar in tea, and raw cane sugar in coffee.

If you can't face food early in the morning, or have no time to prepare breakfast, drink your nutritional quota. You will need a blender (which is a sound investment as you can use it to prepare home-made soups, *pâtés*, dips and desserts); liquidise a mix of fruit, raw egg and yogurt or milk for several seconds to make a frothy fruit shake. My favourite combination is yogurt, a little orange juice, a banana, raw egg and spoonful of honey, with a sprinkling of wheatgerm and bran added afterwards. Try your own combinations: fresh peaches, figs and pears are particularly delicious. A word of warning: these energy-loaded drinks may take no time to prepare but need as much digesting as a solid meal; sip them slowly.

Snack foods

This heading should read snack drinks — coffee and tea are the "boosters" that so many people rely on to keep them going through the day, particularly if they are dieting. Keep a bottle of mineral water on your desk and drink some whenever you feel tempted to bolt for the instant drinks machine. It is easy to become dependent on the stimulative effects of the caffeine content of these drinks but they can make you feel jumpy and nervous; taken in excess, they can cause symptoms of anxiety and dizziness. If you are truly hooked on coffee, try the decaffeinated variety which has a pleasant, mild flavour. Develop a taste for the wide range of herbal teas with their varying properties: some energising, some calming; they have, of course, the advantage of needing less sugar and no milk. If you do not have a weight problem, you could eat a slice of fruit cake or couple of wholemeal biscuits for tea; if chocolate is your weakness, try a bar of carob, a chocolate substitute available from health stores which is just as delicious and far better for you. Nibble on a cereal and dried fruit bar or plain dried fruits such as apricots or peaches (try to buy the sun-dried, not sulphur-dried varieties), high in natural sugars; from health stores, too. At home, keep a supply of *crudités* in the fridge in a plastic bag: carrot and celery sticks, pepper slices and cauliflower florets.

Lunch

To maintain good health you should eat one large raw salad every day, and lunch is the ideal time for this. Avoid pre-packed salads, such as cole slaw in mayonnaise, from food counters: make your own. Even in winter, follow the same eating pattern accompanied by a mug of home-made soup from a Thermos. In 365 days of the year there is enough variety of fruits, nuts and vegetables never to repeat the same combination twice! Grate, chop or slice your choice and pack in a plastic container — or scrub the vegetables and leave them whole. With the salad, eat a carton of cottage cheese, natural yogurt or wedge of cheese, and a slice of wholemeal bread. A hard-boiled egg is fine, but not if you have eaten an egg at breakfast; one a day is the maximum. If you prefer sandwiches, use healthy spreads such as protein-rich peanut butter (for recipe, see page 6) or the vegetarian's favourite, Marmite, a yeast extract rich in vitamin B, and accompany them with fresh vegetables and fruit. Try wholemeal vegetable quiche or a slice of cold, sliced nut roast (for recipes, see pages 7 and 11) with a whole tomato and a piece of fresh fruit to follow.

Dinner

You *can* eat out healthily without sitting at a scrubbed pine table over a bowl of mung beans and sunflower seeds. Hamburger joints are fine: often the meat is mixed with texturised soybean, a very rich source of protein; opt for the jacket potato rather than the french fries, and choose oil and vinegar salad dressing instead of Thousand Island. Although the Oriental method of stir-frying vegetables preserves nutrients, Chinese food is not healthy eaten on a regular basis, as monosodium glutamate, used extensively in the Chinese method of cooking, can produce symptoms of dizziness and headaches; the full effects of this food additive are still not known.

A piece of grilled steak or fish served with crisp, fresh vegetables is a classic gourmet meal which is nutritionally well-balanced. Wine, in moderation, is good for you: many health farms include one glass of wine on their clients' daily diet sheet. Dilute with Perrier water for a delicious, less potent drink you can sip a lot more of! It serves as an attractively-coloured aperitif, too. Try Perrier water solo with a slice of lemon after the main course and you might feel less inclined to dip into a sweet. Avoid spirits, which contain no vitamins, are loaded with calories and dull the appetite, so food intake is replaced and nutritional value is reduced. Spirit alcohol tends to irritate the stomach lining and can lead to chronic indigestion; acute gastritis and cirrhosis of the liver are two of the more drastic symptoms of excess alcohol intake. Fresh fruit salad, crème caramel or a home-made sorbet are the wisest choices. Good restaurants are gradually adapting to basic wholefood principles, serving wholemeal bread instead of white rolls, Barbados brown sugar with coffee, and sub-stituting egg white or yogurt for cream, as in *cuisine minceur*.

When cooking at home, whether for one or for a dinner party, keep the meal well-balanced; serve home-made soup to start (simmered or steamed vegetables puréed in a blender), fish, meat or a savoury with vegetables, and fresh fruit for dessert; or follow a salad and light fish dish with a heavier fruit crumble (brown sugar, vegetable margarine and wholemeal flour topping). Home-made soup, fresh salad and slices of wholemeal bread are perfect fare for a simple winter supper. Serve wholemeal pasta with nutrition-rich toppings, such as tuna fish and black olives stirred in a little vegetable oil with tomatoes; for fun, adopt the macrobiotic way of cooking and serve stir-fried vegetables sliced lengthways, sprinkled with soy sauce and served with nutty brown rice, delicious with a dollop of yogurt on top. For more recipe ideas, see pages 6 and 7; for how to obtain maximum nutritional value from fresh foods, see opposite page.

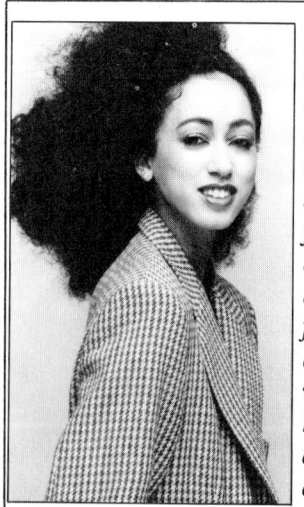

PAT CLEVELAND, *model: "I depend on my juice extractor: a lifesaver! My favourite drinks are a mix of carrot, celery and cucumber (if you like a sweet drink, add more carrots) or apple juice. For breakfast I have oat cereal; for lunch, fish and a salad; and for dinner, soup and a veal or fish course with salad. In the afternoon I love a cup of mint tea with honey and a snack of Swiss herbal candies or a piece of fruit. I don't add salt to food, as I think it can make you gain weight."*

Restock your larder

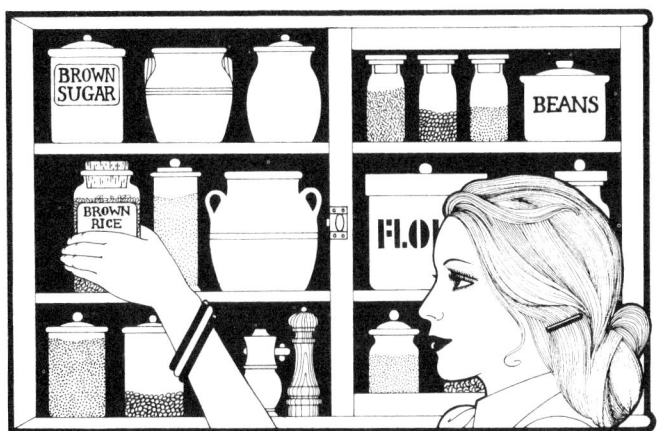

First steps to healthy eating habits are to exclude from your diet foods that are preserved, processed, refined and tinned. Below left, a list of the foods to remove from your kitchen shelves; on the right, substitutes are suggested.

THROW OUT	REPLACE WITH
Refined white flour	Stoneground wholemeal flour
Biscuits, cakes and all produce made with white flour	Biscuits and cakes made with wholemeal flour
White sugar	Barbados brown sugar or honey (ideally, cut out sugar totally)
Processed cheese, eg, ready-packed triangles and slices	Unprocessed cheeses, eg, Cheddar
White bread	Wholemeal bread: wholemeal rye bread
Refined cereals	Wholegrain cereals
Table salt	Sea salt
Animal fats for cooking, eg, lard	Vegetable oils, eg, corn, sunflower, olive
Butter	Soft vegetable margarine
White rice	Brown rice
Tinned fruit	Fresh fruit
Tinned vegetables	Fresh vegetables
Commercial peanut butter	Home-made (see page 4 or from health-food store)
Bottled mayonnaise	Freshly-made mayonnaise with vegetable oil and eggs
Malt vinegar	Cider or wine vinegar
Salted nuts, crisps etc	Dry roasted nuts, sunflower seeds, pistachio nuts

How to prepare and cook fresh food for maximum nutritional value

Although in certain cases cooking destroys potentially harmful organisms and bacteria, often it can destroy nutrients as well. Learn how to prepare and cook meals so you retain all the health-giving benefits — and you will find that food tastes much better, too.

Fruit and vegetables

Buy fruit and vegetables in their freshest state. Most fruit and vegetables can be eaten raw, in salads and as *crudités;* this is the healthiest way to eat them. However, root vegetables and onions may need a little cooking to break down their cellulose content and so make them more acceptable to the digestive system. Store root vegetables away from the light, which destroys much of the vitamin C content. All fruit and vegetables should be washed thoroughly under running water to remove possible chemical deposits as well as dirt. Where possible, do not peel vegetables and fruit; many of the mineral salts essential to good health are to be found just inside the skins; eg, potassium in potato skins and silicon in apple skins. Any fruit or vegetable that has to be peeled could be squeezed with a little lemon juice or vinegar: the acids help slow vitamin C breakdown. To remove ingrained dirt on skins, scrub vegetables thoroughly with a pot scourer (the non-detergent variety!).

Prepare and chop or slice vegetables immediately prior to cooking or eating. The leaves of vegetables such as celery and cauliflower can be used in the cooking pot, too; they provide goodness as well as flavour. Both vegetables and fruit can lose up to seventy per cent of vitamin C while cooking, so simmer them in a small amount of water for a minimum time and add a pinch of salt or drop of soy sauce after, not before, cooking. Better still, invest in a steamer; gourmet restaurants serve vegetables crisp and crunchy, never soggy. Keep the cooking water for stock, soups or juices as it contains many of the mineral salts from the vegetables. Try stir-frying finely sliced vegetables in a little oil as the Chinese do; not to be confused with deep frying, this three-minute method of cooking ensures few nutrients are lost and is a delicious way of serving food. Potatoes, onions and carrots are healthiest left whole, unpeeled and baked in the oven; the same applies to cooking apples.

Eggs

Eggs make perfect packages of nutrition kept in their shells and simmered slowly so the whites do not toughen; they are more easily digested soft than hard-boiled. Eggs retain their high vitamin and protein content however they are cooked, though they are better for you not fried.

Fish

Grilled with margarine or foil-baked in the oven and served with the juices are methods of cooking fish which are preferable to conventional deep-frying. Avoid pickled or smoked fish; tinned sardines, salmon and tuna are fine served as they are, and are a rich source of protein, iodine and vitamin D.

Meat

As a rule, the poorer the quality of the meat, the longer it should be cooked. The protein content is not decreased by long cooking, but the fat content (the kind that contributes to fatty deposits in the arteries) is. Where possible, cut out any visible streaks of fat before cooking. Quick-fry meat before roasting or casseroling, and seal juices before grilling by brushing them with a little oil to retain the high vitamin B content. Season with salt immediately before cooking as salt draws out the most valuable juices. Bacon, which should not be eaten often owing to its fat content — about sixty-five per cent — should be grilled; avoid the streaky variety. White meats, especially turkey, are rich in protein, niacin and low in cholesterol: they are best cooked in the oven. Try basting them with fruit juice to keep them moist and add flavour, or roast with a dab of margarine.

Know what to ask for

Terminology used to describe wholefoods is often confusing and can be misleading. Cast an eye on this glossary of the most common terms used and look for these food "labels" when you shop; they indicate that you are buying goods in their finest natural state.

ORGANICALLY GROWN fruit and vegetables have been cultivated on soil enriched only with natural fertilisers, and have not been sprayed with chemicals. Buy them from wholefood and health-food stores or, of course, ideally grow your own (far cheaper!). Remember that the label "organically grown" is not an indication that the fruit and vegetables are fresh; this is the most important criterion.

POLYUNSATURATED oils are extracted from nuts or vegetables and do not solidify at the lowest temperatures. These are the type to use for cooking and in salad dressings.

UNREFINED describes foods whose chemical composition is unaltered in the manufacturing process. Brown rice is the unrefined version of polished white rice; raw sugar is the unrefined version of white sugar.

WHOLEMEAL FLOUR is made from the whole of the wheat grain so that the germ and the bran, which contain most of the vitamins and minerals plus all the fibre content, are left intact. Always ask for wholemeal and not brown bread which could be white bread (mainly starch and far fewer nutrients) dyed brown.

Ten high-nutrition recipes to lure you to health foods

Wholefood dishes may evoke visions of nut cutlets but the following recipes will show you that the healthiest methods of cooking are the kind that gourmets approve of, too.

Lentil Soup

(Serves four)
175 g (6 oz) lentils
1 onion, finely chopped
1 carrot, grated
1 parsnip, grated or celery stick, chopped
400 ml (¾ pt) vegetable stock
bay leaf
pinch of mixed herbs
15 ml (1 tbsp) oil
25 g (1 oz) flour
150 ml (¼ pt) milk
5 ml (tsp) yeast extract, eg, Marmite
seasoning

Simmer lentils and vegetables in the stock with bay leaf and a pinch of herbs, until lentils are soft. Make a thin sauce with oil, flour and milk, and add yeast extract. Remove bay leaf from lentils and combine with sauce. Add seasoning and serve.

Walnut Pâté

25 g (1 oz) vegetable margarine
13 g (½ oz) green pepper and/or onion, finely chopped
25 g (1 oz) wholemeal flour
75 ml (3 fl oz) water
50 g (2 oz) walnuts
7 ml (1 tsp, heaped) tomato purée
5 ml (1 tsp) lemon juice
seasoning and herbs to taste

Melt the margarine and fry vegetables gently for a few minutes. Add the flour and mix well, then cook for 2 more minutes. Pour on the water and continue cooking until the mixture becomes paste-like. Add all the remaining ingredients, mix well and put into a dish to cool. Keep in the fridge until needed.

Peanut Butter

Shell monkey nuts (or buy shelled, unsalted peanuts). Place in a saucepan on low heat and stir; the nuts will cook in their own oil. Keep stirring until the nuts begin to brown. Remove from saucepan and grind to a coarse powder either with a wooden rolling pin or, if you have one, a grinder. Mash in a bowl with a little vegetable oil to moisten. If liked, sweeten peanut butter with a little honey. Pack in a pot and cover.

Cottage Cheese, Mushroom and Celery Quiche

Line a 20.5 cm (8 in) flan tin with wholemeal pastry. Boil three or four sticks of celery for five minutes; fry 50–100 g (2–4 oz) mushrooms until soft. Drain well. Beat two eggs with approx 200 g (8 oz) cottage cheese, add vegetables and seasoning. Pour into flan case and bake in a hot oven for 15 minutes, reduce heat to moderate and continue baking until the centre is firm to touch. Eat hot or cold.

Three-bean Salad

In a little water, simmer black-eyed beans and whole green lentils; cook aduki beans in a separate pan so that their red dye does not stain the others. Drain, then mix together with finely chopped onion and green pepper, and toss in an oil and vinegar dressing.

Baked Fish with Honey

(Serves four)
4 cod fillets or cutlets
4 tomatoes
1 medium onion
10 ml (2 tsp) lemon juice
30 ml (2 tbsp) vegetable oil
30 ml (2 tbsp) clear honey

Place fish in greased ovenproof dish. Thinly slice tomatoes and onion and arrange on top of fish. Heat together lemon juice, oil and honey until warm. Pour over fish, cover with greaseproof paper or greased foil and bake for 20 minutes at 190°C (375°F, gas mark 5).

Tarragon Chicken Brochettes

vegetable oil
salt and pepper
tarragon
bay leaf
a little freshly-made mustard
pieces of turkey or chicken, off the bone
red or green peppers, deseeded and cut into chunks
button mushrooms, stalks removed
tomatoes, cut in wedges
small onions, peeled

Marinade the meat in oil and seasonings for two to three hours, turning at least once. Cut turkey or chicken into small even-sized pieces. Thread alternate pieces of meat, pepper, mushrooms, tomatoes and onions on to skewers. Cook under a hot grill for 15 to 20 minutes, basting marinade over kebabs. Serve on a bed of brown rice.

Kate O'Mara's Blackberry Ice-cream

Stew blackberries with a little brown sugar until soft. Whisk together equal amounts of natural yogurt and cream cheese, plus a little honey to taste and some chopped nuts. Turn into a bowl and chill. Before serving, fold in blackberries. Other soft raw or stewed fruits can be substituted for blackberries.

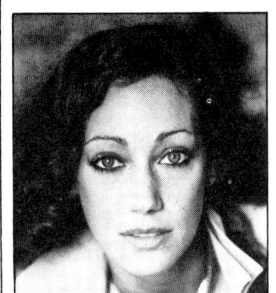

MARISA BERENSON, *actress:*
"I go on juice fasts for a week or so — nothing but juice I make myself. Or else I drink hot water for days at a time."

Hazelnut Shortbread

75 g (3 oz) vegetable margarine
75 g (3 oz) wholemeal self-raising flour
50 g (2 oz) sugar
50 g (2 oz) chopped or ground hazelnuts

Rub the margarine into the rest of the ingredients to make a crumble. Grease a shallow baking tin very well, then fill with mixture and press down lightly. Bake on the middle shelf of a slow oven for 30 minutes. Mark into portions, but leave in tin until cool.

Apricot Soufflé

(Serves four)
350 g (¾ lb) dried apricots, soaked overnight
5 egg whites
75 ml (5 tbsp) raw brown sugar

Drain and sieve apricots (or purée them in an electric blender with a little of the soaking water). Oil a 15 cm (6 in) soufflé dish. Whisk the egg whites until stiff, add the sugar a little at a time, then fold in the apricot purée. Pour into the soufflé dish and bake in a low oven for about an hour.

Are vitamin supplements necessary?

There is an increasingly popular belief that we do not receive enough vitamins from our diets to ensure good health and therefore artificial supplements are necessary; this belief holds particularly in America, where megadoses of assorted vitamins line bathroom shelves. Your doctor will inevitably tell you that supplementary vitamins are superfluous to a well-balanced diet. However, one multivitamin pill a day will certainly do no harm and can act as insurance against vitamin deficiency. Here, Professor John Yudkin, leading expert on nutrition, offers his opinions on the subject:

"Only a few minority groups need vitamin supplements:

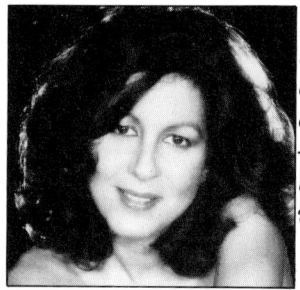

ELKIE BROOKS, *singer: "On the road I eat as much food as I can, but before a performance I can only take something very light — live yogurt, mixed with honey, banana and wheatgerm: I find it very energy-giving."*

infants are fed cod liver oil as a safeguard against rickets, because they do not get enough sunshine which is normally absorbed through the skin to be manufactured into vitamin D; old people sometimes need extra doses of vitamin D to strengthen weak bones. Supplementary vitamins are often prescribed , too, for pregnant women. Doctors suggest vitamin pills to certain patients as a psychological boost and on the basis that they will do no harm; extra vitamins cannot damage the system unless massive quantities of vitamins A and D are taken.

"For some reason, vitamins have an aura of being magical. The truth is, they will do nothing if you have already had enough. It is rather like filling a bath: whether you use two taps or four, the bath can only become so full, and then it overflows. In fact, the authorities who recommend daily vitamin intakes overestimate the amounts really needed so as to cover anti-health factors, eg, smoking, stress etc; thus in this country the recommended daily intake of vitamin C is thirty milligrams per day, whereas ten milligrams are quite sufficient.

"Many people believe that as a deficiency of vitamins can make them ill, so an enormous intake of vitamins will make them 'super-healthy'. This is untrue: if you do not take enough vitamin A you will not be able to see well in the dark — but if you take large doses of the same vitamin you will not be able to see any better than Nature intended! Because it has been proved that a lack of vitamin E in rats can make them miscarry, this research has been twisted into the belief than vitamin E will do wonders for the libido and fertility of human beings; this is not so. Taking large amounts of vitamin C will *not* guard against colds. But if a person includes no fruit or vegetables in his diet and becomes ill, then takes ten milligrams of vitamin C daily, the illness caused by the vitamin deficiency will be cured. And thirty milligrams will take care of any emergency need, too.

"There will always be people who eat badly, but their diet will be lacking in all kinds of nutrients; it is very unlikely that they will know which vitamins are missing, and what quantities they will need of each. The point to remember is that you can't turn a bad diet into a good one by sprinkling vitamins over it."

Yogurt: the high-value food

What's in it for you?
Yogurt is simply milk fermented by bacterial action, but that simple transition merits yogurt, to quote Gayelord Hauser, one of the world's leading nutrition experts, as a "wonder food". A rich source of protein, vitamins A and D, plus riboflavin and calcium, yogurt is a cheap, versatile food that can be eaten as a satisfying between-meal snack or mixed with other foods for added nutritional value.

The protein content is of a type that is easily digested, so making yogurt ideal for convalescents or those with "nervous" stomachs; it is recommended by doctors for patients suffering from ulcers and can sometimes even be substituted for antacid tablets. Eat yogurt to help reduce tension, fight insomnia, and when you are taking antibiotics, which kill off healthy bacteria in the intestines: yogurt recreates the necessary acid environment for the intestinal flora to flourish once more. Include substantial amounts of yogurt in your daily diet and your health will benefit.

How to make it
Many commercial yogurts contain rennet or commercial "thickeners"; though the best yogurt is obviously the kind you make yourself, the attraction of the bought variety to many is the words "low fat", which usually appear on the label. However, you can make your own slimmers' version by using low-fat dried milk and mixing it with water as directed on the tin; continue in the usual way. If you have never tried making yogurt because you believed the method to be too complicated, follow the rules below and you will find that, with a little practice, making yogurt will become as easy as boiling an egg.
1 You will need a "starter" — a teaspoon of fresh, unflavoured yogurt. Use the bought variety or, ideally, get some from a Middle East restaurant which makes its own.
2 Heat 568 ml (1 pint) of milk and remove from flame just as boiling point is reached. The milk must be cooled before the starter is introduced: yogurt bacteria live between temperatures of 30°C (90°F) and 50°C (120°F). The perfect temperature for successful yogurt making is 45°C (115°F). To check the temperature, use a kitchen thermometer or dip your elbow into the milk; if it feels just above body temperature, the milk is ready to be mixed with the starter.
3 Add the milk gradually to the starter, stirring well. Do not be tempted to use too much starter as the yogurt will not be thicker, but lumpier. Pour into a container and cover. If your starter is taken from "organic" yogurt, eg Loseley, which is inclined to be runnier, you can stir in 20 ml (4 tsp) of skimmed milk powder before fermenting to thicken.

4 Incubate the mixture in either of the following ways:

A wide-mouthed vacuum flask will keep the temperature constant; rinse in hot water first to warm it up.

Wrap towels around the container and place in the airing cupboard, near a radiator, on top of a warm stove, or any warm corner where the mix will not be disturbed.

The yogurt usually takes eight hours to ferment; but it may take as little as five hours in a vacuum flask, or as long as twenty-four. Your yogurt has not failed if there is a watery separation on top; this is just whey, and can be drained off.

Note There are yogurt kits on the market which cost a few pounds to buy. They consist of a vacuum container, instructions and thermometer; the method is basically the same but the time of fermentation is shorter, about five hours.

How to use yogurt

- Stir in fresh or dried fruit, cinnamon and wheatgerm for a nutritious snack; substitute for milk with cereals or muesli.
- Make blender "shakes" with fruit juice or fresh fruit and honey.
- Float on soups, add to sauces and use instead of cream on desserts.
- Make the Indian lassi drink by mixing three parts milk to one of yogurt (add black cinnamon for savoury version, sugar for a sweet one).
- Make cottage cheese by straining yogurt overnight through muslin to drain off the whey.
- Mix with vinegar and oil for a creamy salad dressing and blend with cottage cheese, garlic and cucumber to make a tasty dip.

The plus properties of fasting

Fasting may mean no more to you than a religious rite or pastime for health-food cranks but it is in fact an excellent way of "spring-cleaning" the system. While food passes through the body in the normal way, a certain amount is deposited on the colon walls where it accumulates to form toxic waste matter. By eating no food and drinking lots of liquids once in a while, not only are these waste poisons flushed out but the liver and digestive systems are given a well-earned rest and the stomach is prepared for smaller amounts of food. After a twenty-four hour fast, you should notice an improvement in your skin; the whites of your eyes will be clearer and your tongue a healthy pink.

The weekend is an ideal time to fast as your energy output is lower. The classic health farm fast is to drink only warm water with a little lemon juice, but mixing water with fruit juice will provide your body with vitamins and keep your blood sugar level up with the intake of natural sugars. Mix grape juice half and half with mineral water and drink throughout the day as often as you like; you could substitute orange juice, though the sugar content of grapes is slightly higher. Before retiring, drink a calming herbal tea such as camomile.

If you have a fast-acting metabolism and need the boost of frequent food intake, you can still benefit from a one-day fruit fast. One famous naturopath recommends a semi-fast of oranges and onions: oranges at breakfast and tea, steamed or baked onions, served in the liquor, at lunch and dinner.

Try this energy-boosting semi-fast passed on to me by Vidal Sassoon, a fasting enthusiast — his limit is thirty-six hours! "Enzymes in the papaya fruit," says Vidal, "act as a marvellous cleanser."

The papaya pick-up is specially suitable for semi-fasting, but any nutritious "food drink", such as the fruit shakes described in the breakfast section on page 1, would be acceptable, too.

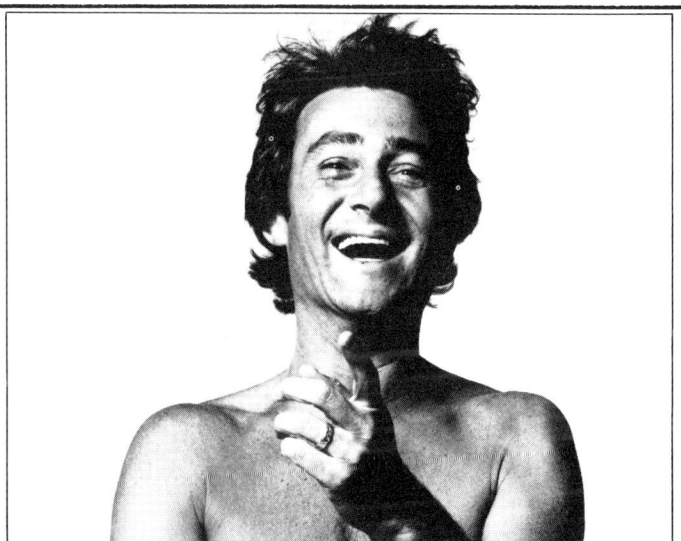

Vidal Sassoon's papaya pick-up

300 ml (½ pt) papaya juice, fresh or tinned
1 banana
2 fruit salad spoons of fresh fruit, chopped
30 ml (2 tbsp) wheatgerm
1 raw egg
15 ml (1 tbsp) soya lecithin

Blend ingredients throroughly. Drink one glass at midday and another glass mid-afternoon; sip hot water and lemon juice frequently throughout the day.

Note Limit fasts in winter to twelve hours, when the body uses more calories to generate heat. Find your own time level: a fast is not an endurance test. You will find that as you fast regularly, your body will gradually attune itself to longer periods without food. Fasts are not suited to migraine sufferers; if in any doubt, check with your doctor first.

Are vegetarians more healthy?

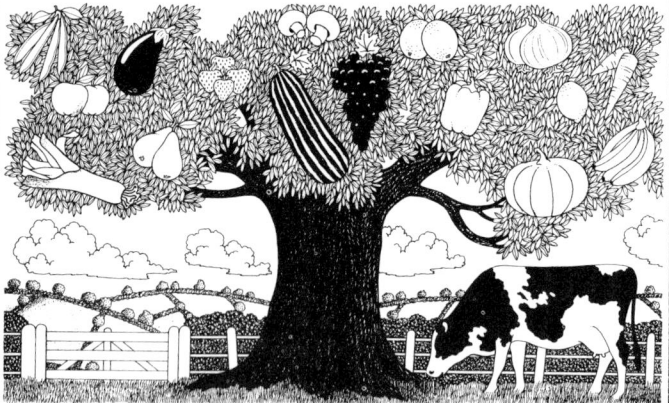

There is a strong nutritional argument in favour of vegetarianism, apart from ecologists' concern that animals consume ten tons of vegetable protein to produce just one ton of animal protein. The ideal vegetarian diet balances vegetables, grains and lentils with dairy foods. Fibre content is four times higher than that of the non-vegetarian diet; elimination is quicker and therefore healthier, and bowel diseases, such as diverticulosis (cul-de-sacs along the colon walls), are far fewer; the low consumption of animal fats cuts incidence of coronary heart disease in vegetarians by about thirty per cent. No nutrients are lacking in the well-balanced vegetarian diet: protein content normally obtained from meat can be found in wholemeal flour, nuts, cheese, lentils, bean, soya flour, skimmed milk powder and eggs, which are considered by some nutritionists to be superior sources of protein to meat. Dr Gordon Latto, President of The Vegetarian Society of the UK, points out that all vitamin groups necessary for good health are present in the vegetarian's diet:

Vitamin A: carrots, tomatoes
Vitamin B groups: wheatgerm, tomatoes
Vitamin C: fruits and vegetables
Vitamin D: manufactured by skin from sunlight; twenty-five minutes' exposure of the skin to light is all that is necessary for the skin to synthesise requisite amount of vitamin D
Vitamin E: sprouting grains, wheatgerm

Even if you are a confirmed meat-eater, try the following vegetarian eating plan and you will see how delicious, and simple to prepare, vegetarian foods can be. You will feel healthier and will probably lose a few pounds, too: vegetarians have a lower calorie intake than meat-eaters, as they consume fewer fats, and though brown rice and wholemeal flour are starchy, they are very filling so you will find you eat less of them than their refined versions.

The ten-day vegetarian eating plan

- All lunches can be prepared at home, and packed to be eaten at the office (or in the park!).
- For honey and fruit cakes, follow conventional recipes, substituting wholemeal flour for refined white flour and raw sugar for white.
- All recipes given serve two people.

Tomato and Leek Soup

225 g (8 oz) tinned tomatoes, roughly chopped
1 leek, finely chopped
15 ml (1 tbsp) oil
600 ml (1 pt) vegetable stock (buy in cube form from health-food shops)
seasoning and herbs to taste

Cook the tomatoes and leek in oil for a few minutes, then add the liquid and simmer for about 20 minutes. Add seasoning, herbs, and some soy sauce if you like a spicier taste. Can be served as it is, or liquidised for a smoother soup.

Stuffed Marrow

Cut marrow in half lengthways, scrape out pith and seeds, steam marrow until just tender. Drain, then pile each half with a mixture of cooked rice, chopped onion, pepper, celery, raisins and nuts. Cook in moderate oven until marrow is tender and stuffing is browned and crisp. You can cover the mixture with silver foil, then brown it under the grill if you prefer.

Peanut Soup

100 g (4 oz) smooth peanut butter (home-made or from a health-food shop)
600 ml (1 pt) vegetable stock
30 ml (2 tbsp) skimmed milk powder
salt and chilli powder to taste

Blend peanut butter with a little of the hot stock until it dissolves, then pour into a saucepan and add the remaining ingredients. Bring to the boil, stirring occasionally, then simmer for about 15 minutes. Serve hot with a dollop of whipped cream, or cold with slices of cucumber.

Molasses Biscuits

175 g (6 oz) self-raising wholemeal flour
5 ml (1 tsp) ground ginger
2.5 ml (½ tsp) ground cloves
100 g (4 oz) vegetable margarine
100 g (4 oz) brown sugar
1 egg, beaten
50 g (2 oz) molasses

BREAKFAST	LUNCH	DINNER	BREAKFAST	LUNCH	DINNER
Saturday			**Thursday**		
Glass grapefruit juice	Tomato & leek soup★	Marrow stuffed with rice, onion, pepper, celery, raisins, chopped walnuts★	Glass orange juice	Cold cottage cheese, mushroom & celery quiche★★	Moussaka (made with soya mince)
Egg baked in oiled dish in oven, with hot wholemeal roll	Raw cauliflower, celery with houmous & crispbread	Braised herbed carrots Jacket potato	Granola★ with added chopped nuts	Cabbage & carrot salad	Chicory & tomato salad
			Coffee or tea	Apple	Apricot soufflé★★
Coffee or tea	Grapes	Blackberry crumble made with wholemeal flour, raw brown sugar and vegetable margarine	**Friday**		
			Dried fruit compote★	Half an avocado sliced with raw chopped cauliflower, spinach and a few brazil nuts	Chick peas in cream sauce★ Jacket potato Cauliflower
Sunday			Wholemeal toast with peanut butter		
1 orange	Peanut soup★ Grated cabbage, carrot, chopped dried apricot Cheese (any kind)	Butterbean croquettes★ Spinach Mashed potatoes	Coffee or tea	Carton of natural yogurt	Chocolate jelly★
Porridge with skimmed milk & honey			**Saturday**		
Coffee or tea	Molasses biscuits★	Honey nut tart★	1 orange	Cheesey Scotch egg★ Tomato, celery, watercress	Seeded green beans★ Boiled millet
Monday			Grilled mushrooms & tomatoes on toast	Crispbread	
Apple & yogurt drink (glass of apple juice blended with half a carton natural yogurt, plus pinch cinnamon)	Melon Ratatouille Three-bean salad★★	Pea & cashew nut curry★ Sliced cucumber in yogurt Brown rice	Coffee or tea	Wholemeal fruit cake	Gooseberry snow★
			Sunday		
			Prune juice	Lentil soup★★	Pancake with leeks in cheese sauce★
Bran muffin★			Scrambled eggs with added wheatgerm	Lettuce, chopped prune, apple, banana slices, almonds	Endive salad
Coffee or tea	Cheese and biscuits	Banana cream★			
Tuesday			Coffee or tea	Honey cake	Melon and orange segments
Orange & grapefruit juice	Walnut pâté★★	Hot spinach & cheese flan★			
Muesli with added bran	Celery Wholemeal roll	Brussels sprouts tossed with lightly fried peanuts	**Monday**		
			Lemon & apricot juice	Gazpacho soup★ Hard-boiled egg, chopped leeks & tomatoes with oil & vinegar dressing	Herb & nut roast★ Braised leeks Jacket potatoes
Coffee or tea	Wholemeal date scone★	Stuffed apple★	Wholewheat toast with honey or raw-sugar marmalade		
Wednesday					
Half grapefruit	Sweetcorn salad★ Watercress, tomato Cheese	Lentil and mushroom pie★ Stir-fried vegetables	Coffee or tea	Fresh fruit	Cottage cheese dessert★
Baked egg Wholemeal toast					
Coffee or tea	Hazelnut shortbread★★	Fruit salad & natural yogurt	★ Recipe, pages 10–14 ★★ Recipe, pages 6 & 7		

Mix the flour, ginger and cloves together. Rub in margarine until the mixture is the consistency of breadcrumbs. Stir in the brown sugar and then mix in the egg and molasses. Roll pieces of dough into balls the size of walnuts and place well apart on a greased baking sheet. Cook in a hot oven for 10–12 minutes.

Butterbean Croquettes

Soak butterbeans overnight, then simmer in water until soft. Fry chopped onion and a small stick of celery in oil until soft and transparent. Add the vegetables to the butterbeans and mash them together to form a thick paste. Add lemon juice, a beaten egg, fresh breadcrumbs and seasoning. Shape into individual croquettes, coat with wholemeal flour or toasted breadcrumbs, and shallow fry them until golden brown.

Honey Nut Tart

Line flan tin with sweet wholemeal pastry (half the weight of fat to wholemeal flour, with a little brown sugar to sweeten) and bake blind

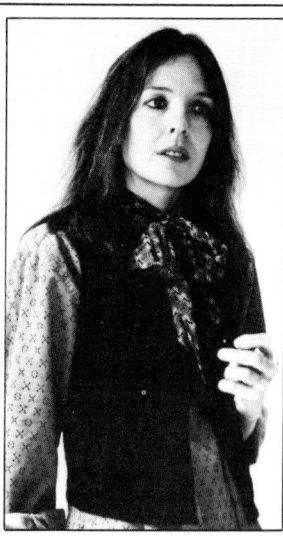

DIANE KEATON, *actress: "I used to be hooked on candy and junk food, but these days my vice is honeyed oats."*

for 15 minutes. Melt 30 ml (2 tbsp) honey over a low heat, then stir in whatever fruit you choose — chopped apples, dried peaches or apricots, pear slices etc. Make sure the fruit is well coated in honey, then remove from heat, and when cool use to fill the flan. Sprinkle chopped, roasted hazelnuts generously over the top, and eat as it is, or heat in an oven for 10–15 minutes.

Bran Muffins

(Makes 12)
175 g (6 oz) plain wholemeal flour
22.5 ml (4½ tsp) baking powder
2.5 ml (½ tsp) salt
75 g (3 oz) sugar
175 g (6 oz) All-Bran
350 ml (12 fl oz) milk, preferably skimmed
40 g (1½ oz) vegetable margarine, melted
2 eggs, beaten
50 g (2 oz) broken walnuts (optional)

Sift the flour with the salt and baking powder; add the sugar. Cover All-Bran with milk and leave to soak for 10 minutes. Add melted margarine and eggs to bran mixture, stir it all into the flour and beat thoroughly. Add nuts. Fill ready-greased patty tins to the top and bake in a hot oven for 20–25 minutes.

Pea and Cashew Nut Curry

Make your favourite curry sauce (or follow one from a recipe book). About half an hour before it is ready, add about 100 g (4 oz) whole cashew nuts and about 200 g (8 oz) of fresh peas (if using frozen peas, cook them a few minutes first and drain off excess liquid).

Banana Cream

Mash ripe bananas to form a smooth consistency, add a little honey to sweeten if desired. Then stir in enough sour cream to turn mixture a pale beige colour, chill, and sprinkle with toasted coconut strands.

Wholemeal Date Scones

(Makes 8)
225 g (8 oz) wholemeal flour
2.5 ml (½ tsp) salt
5 ml (1 tsp) baking powder
25 g (1 oz) vegetable margarine
25 g (1 oz) raw brown sugar
milk to mix
50 g (2 oz) dates, chopped

Sieve flour, salt and baking powder into a bowl. Rub in the margarine, add sugar and finely chopped dates. Mix to a soft rolling consistency with the milk, knead the dough, then roll out to 1 cm thickness and cut into rounds. Place on greased baking sheet and bake at the top of a very hot oven for about 20 minutes. When firm to the touch, the scones are cooked.

Spinach and Cheese Flan

Line flan tin with wholemeal pastry, and bake blind for 15 minutes. Mix about 225 g (8 oz) cooked spinach with 2 eggs, a little margarine, milk and about 100 g (4 oz) grated cheese. Beat mixture well, then turn into a flan case. Top with extra grated cheese and cook for about 30 minutes in a moderate oven.

Stuffed Apple

Choose a large apple and core it, leaving a little of the apple in place to form a base at the bottom. Fill the hole with a mixture of nuts, dried fruit and oats — bind them with tahini (sesame paste, available from health-food shops). Bake in a moderate oven gently till apple is cooked.

Sweetcorn Salad

Drain a tin of sweetcorn, add finely chopped green and/or red pepper, a few chopped nuts, and oil and vinegar dressing.

Lentil and Mushroom Pie

Soak and then simmer lentils until soft and mushy. Add herbs, seasoning, cooked mushrooms and soy sauce, then pile into a dish and cover with a pastry topping. Bake in a fairly hot oven until pastry is crisp and golden.

Granola

45 ml (3 tbsp) oil
225 g (8 oz) thin honey
450 g (1 lb) rolled oats
100 g (4 oz) mixed, chopped nuts
100 g (4 oz) sunflower seeds
100 g (4 oz) wheatgerm
dried fruits

Heat the oil and honey gently in a large pan, then add the oats, stirring them until all are covered with the honey mixture. When oats turn light gold, add the nuts and seeds, stir well and continue cooking for 10 minutes. Add the wheatgerm, and cook until the granola is a rich brown. Remove from heat and add dried fruit of your choice.

Note This makes enough granola to last for ages, so store it in an airtight tin or jar, and use sparingly — it's very satisfying and full of good things! Can also be cooked in the oven.

Dried Fruit Compote

Soak dried apricots or prunes in water for a few days; drain off liquid and use for apricot and prune juice.

Chick Peas in Cream Sauce

Soak chick peas overnight, then simmer in water until tender. Set aside vegetable water. Make a sauce by heating a little oil in a saucepan, then add at least 15 ml (a good tablespoonful) of wholewheat flour and brown it. Dissolve some skimmed milk powder in the vegetable juice (the more you add the creamier it will be) and add mixture to the pan. Stir. Pour over chick peas, cook in a moderate oven for about 20 minutes, serve topped with lightly fried onion rings.

Chocolate Jelly

568 ml (1 pt) milk
7 ml (1 heaped tsp) agar agar (a gelling agent for vegetarians, available from health-food shops)
30 ml (2 tbsp) sugar
18 ml (1 heaped tbsp) cocoa

Bring milk to boil; sprinkle agar agar on to it a little at a time and stir until agar agar dissolves completely, then bring back to boil and simmer for a few minutes. Add sugar and cocoa, whisk well, leave to set. Sprinkle with flaked nuts.

Cheesey Scotch Egg

Boil two eggs until hard; then shell. Mix just under 25 g (1 oz) wholemeal flour with 50 g (2 oz) finely grated cheese, seasoning, a few drops Worcestershire or soy sauce, pinch Cayenne pepper, 1 egg, and enough milk to bind. Divide mixture into two and roll each portion round the egg. Coat in crisp breadcrumbs, fry, eat hot or cold.

Seeded Green Beans

Cook either fresh or frozen green beans. Drain them. Heat a little vegetable margarine in a frying pan, add raw sunflower seeds and cook gently until they turn light brown. Add drained green beans and stir them well so they are well mixed with the seeds. Season and serve with millet (available from health-food stores). Top with grated cheese for added protein.

Gooseberry Snow

Purée gooseberries, fold in stiffly-beaten egg white and sweeten with honey. Chill for a few hours.

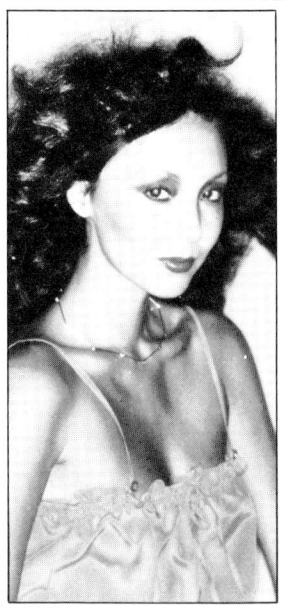

MARIE HELVIN, *model: "I eat lots of fruit, fish, grains, soya, couscous, tofu (bean curd) — and, most important, I drink a glass of champagne every day."*

Pancake with Leeks in Cheese Sauce

Make pancakes to the usual recipe, substituting wholemeal for white flour. Cook well on one side. On the other side arrange a mixture of cooked leeks that have been chopped into bite-size pieces, and covered in a creamy cheese sauce. Fold pancake in half, top with a sprinkling of nuts and/or fried onions.

Gazpacho Soup

(Made with an electric blender)
450 g (1 lb) tomatoes, skinned and finely chopped
1 medium cucumber
1 small green pepper, de-seeded and finely chopped
1 clove of garlic, crushed
1 small onion, or several spring onions, finely chopped
a little oil
seasoning
lemon juice

Put all ingredients, except seasoning and lemon juice, into an electric blender, and combine well. You may need to add a little water to make soup the right consistency. Serve well chilled with lemon juice and seasoning added, plus a sprinkling of diced cucumber.

Herb and Nut Roast

30 ml (2 tbsp) oil
1 medium onion, chopped
1 medium pepper, chopped
3 medium tomatoes, skinned
50 g (2 oz) mushrooms, sliced
225 g (8 oz) grated nuts, any variety

100 g (4 oz) wholemeal breadcrumbs
1 egg, beaten
15 ml (1 tbsp) soy sauce
vegetable stock
mixed herbs and seasoning

Cook onion and pepper gently in oil for five minutes, add tomatoes and mushrooms and cook for a further two minutes. Meanwhile mix together nuts and breadcrumbs, then bind with beaten egg. Add the mixture to cooked vegetables. Add soy sauce to the stock, pour enough over vegetable mixture to moisten; season. Place in oiled loaf tin. Cover with foil and cook for about an hour in a hot oven. Serve hot with a white or cheese sauce, or cold with salad.

Cottage Cheese Dessert

To a small carton of cottage cheese, add some finely grated orange peel (or lemon), 5 ml (1 tsp) honey, chopped nuts and a little black pepper. Pile into a glass, top with fresh orange segments. (The cottage cheese tastes best if it has had time to absorb all the flavours, so this dessert is best prepared the night before.)

Twenty sensible eating habits to cultivate now

1 On average, every person in Great Britain eats his own weight of white sugar every year. White sugar has little nutritional value and absorbs calcium which is needed to build healthy bones and teeth. Cut it out of your diet.
2 Decrease your consumption of high-cholesterol sources, eg, butter, whole milk, eggs and red meats; chicken and turkey are both rich in protein but low in cholesterol.
3 Saturated fats collect in the arteries like fur in a kettle and are thought to contribute to heart disease. Reduce your intake of animal fats and always use vegetable oils for cooking.
4 Try to buy organically grown vegetables and fruit. Do not be put off if the skins are marked or they are smaller in size than other fruits and vegetables: these factors do not affect the quality. Make sure they are fresh.
5 Eat more fish, a highly nutritious food with a protein content that is easier for the body to assimilate than the complex proteins in meat. Herring, for example, is a much ignored but tasty fish: it contains phosphorus, vitamins A, D, E, B_1 and B_2 — and it's cheap.
6 A certain amount of roughage per day is necessary for healthy elimination. The amount you need daily: 2 tablespoons bran, or three slices of wholemeal bread — alternatively, 121 slices of refined white bread!
7 Recognise the high nutritional value of yogurt and increase your consumption of this easily digestible food in your diet by using it in sweet and savoury dishes. If you cannot make your own, try to buy yogurt — eg, Loseley — from health stores, and avoid the commercial fruit-flavoured variety: always add your own fruit.
8 Eat fresh fruit and vegetables, not tinned: you can then better control your intake of sugar and salt, two additions to processed foods.
9 Eat wholemeal bread; at only eighty calories a slice, slimmers can include it in their daily regime. As well as adding roughage to the diet, wholemeal flour contains valuable B and E vitamins.
10 Sprinkle wheatgerm, the untreated variety, over salads, yogurt and desserts; renowned for its high vitamin E content, wheatgerm is also a source of protein, A and B group vitamins, calcium, magnesium, phosphorus and iron.
11 The "apple-a-day" maxim is worth observing: apples are rich in vitamin C and have excellent cleansing properties. They make an ideal natural snack food.
12 Make salads with fresh, raw spinach. Spinach is richer in nutrients than lettuce, contains vitamins A, C, B_2 and K, and a high level of iron.
13 Try to drink before and after, rather than during, a meal, as liquids dilute the gastric juices and impair healthy digestion.
14 Tap water is fine to drink; minimum intake daily should be about six glassfuls which will help to flush kidneys and clear a problem skin. Bottled mineral waters contain valuable mineral salts; each has different properties, for example, Vichy water aids digestion. Check on the labels.
15 The caffeine content of coffee, tea and cola drinks upsets the nervous system; try to substitute with decaffeinated coffee, herbal teas and fruit juices.
16 Try curbing a taste for sweets and chocolates with a glass of warm water into which a large slice of lemon has been squeezed; it also helps cleanse the system and improves the skin.
17 The Chinese philosophy of chewing every grain of rice slowly is nutritionally sound: chewing food well gives the saliva a chance to mix thoroughly with the food and therefore aids the digestive process.
18 Avoid reheating food: its nutritional value will be far less then when first cooked. It may be uneconomical to throw away leftovers but it is certainly healthier.
19 Combine proteins to obtain the highest nutritional value. Chicken, fish or peanut butter in a sandwich of wholemeal bread is an ideally balanced meal.
20 Don't lose friends along with your new set of eating habits. Social situations may necessitate straying from these nutritional guidelines — occasional lapses won't harm you!

SKIN CARE

Skin is the biggest health giveaway: poor diet, little exercise and lack of sleep are all reflected in the skin's condition. Skin is the display case for our emotions, too; just as embarrassment causes the skin to flush, so tension causes blemishes. In this section you are shown not only appropriate products and techniques, but all the other factors that affect your skin — so you can use them to make the very best of your complexion.

A dozen skin-care myths

How much do you know — or think you know — about what is good for your skin? Here are some popular misconceptions:

1 *Vitamin E is marvellous for the skin; the oil of a vitamin E capsule makes a good moisturising treatment, and helps heal scars.*
Vitamin E oil, applied topically (ie, to the skin's surface), is too rich for most skins. It is known to cause skin allergies and to worsen acne conditions. Laboratory tests have been carried out to test the healing properties of vitamin E and there have been no positive results.

2 *Foundation protects skin from the environment.*
If you use foundation most of the time, your skin may suffer; the less you wear, the better. Some foundations clog the skin and cause break-outs; always choose a light base that allows the skin to "breathe", and only apply where you need it.

3 *Moisturiser is a barrier to stop foundation sinking into pores.*
Foundation can clog pores just as readily with or without moisturiser.

4 *Chocolate causes spots.*
The good news is that chocolate has been proved not to cause pimples, though a diet high in sugar is not beneficial. In America, this test, typical of many, was carried out on a group of people who had mild acne: half the group were given special chocolate bars that contained massive amounts of chocolate; the other half were given chocolate bars which tasted the same, but in fact had no chocolate content. There was no difference in the skin conditions of either group over a considerable length of time.

5 *Health foods are good for the skin.*
There is growing evidence that certain health foods can in-

crease oil production of greasy skins and aggravate acne conditions: among them are seaweed (taken as kelp in pill form), sea salt, wheatgerm and peanuts. Multivitamin supplements *can* create more trouble for the skin than a vitamin deficiency; it is far better for your health, and your skin, to take your vitamins by eating natural foods.

6 *Certain skin-care creams can penetrate the skin to combat wrinkles and dryness.*
No cosmetic product penetrates below the epidermis, the outer layer of skin; any cream that is able to do this contains hormones, which reach the bloodstream, and are prescription-only medications which can have adverse side-effects. Moisturising creams merely serve to "plump up" cells in the top layer of skin.

7 *Creams that contain collagen, a protein, strengthen the collagen in skin to increase suppleness and slow the ageing process.*
The sad truth is that once collagen fibres — the connective tissues that give skin its resilience — have slackened, nothing can help the skin regain its elasticity. Protein content (derived from cowhide) in a cream cannot be absorbed into the dermis, where the collagen fibres are situated. However, protein can condition and improve texture of *surface* skin.

8 *"Pure and natural" skin-care products are best for the skin.*
Wholesome-sounding ingredients — for example, honey, strawberries or apple — are no guarantee that a product is good for your skin. The most important criterion is whether a skin product is suited to your type of skin — and that can mean either a simple home-made cream, or a sophisticated commercial cosmetic.

9 *Soap and water are bad for the skin.*
Many of the facial soaps now manufactured are specially formulated to have an affinity with the skin's acid mantle, the

natural oil-and-water protective covering of the skin, and therefore do not have the drying effects often associated with soap. However, all dermatologists agree that excessive use of soap, whatever kind, can be harmful to the skin.

10 *Facial saunas are bad for the skin, and can cause thread veins.*
A facial sauna — holding the head over a bowl of hot water — is an effective way of cleansing the skin and does not cause thread veins: these are an inherited condition.

11 *Open pores can be shrunk with corrective cosmetics.*
Open pores are sebaceous glands that are often clogged with dirt. Deep-cleansing the skin would help lift out dirt and thus make them appear smaller. Astringents and lotions that are often claimed to minimise pore size can, in fact, have the reverse effect by temporarily stretching the skin. Moisturiser makes the pores appear smaller because it increases the water content of the outer layer of skin; the cells around pores expand and make pores appear smaller by comparison.

12 *All skins need moisturiser to protect and nourish.*
No moisturising cream is able to protect or nourish skin, and in fact moisturiser has been proved to be the largest single contributory factor to spots. Use only if, and where, you need it: on patches of skin that feel dry to the touch. Be careful, too, that you do not use too strong a moisturiser; while dry skins benefit from a rich oil-in-water emulsion, normal skins need only a light water-in-oil emulsion.

What factors influence the condition of your skin?

There are many factors which have a temporary or more lasting effect on the skin, advantageous or otherwise. Have you ever considered that any of the following could affect the condition of your skin?

Stress
Stress is one of the skin's worst enemies. Tension can cause lines around the eyes and forehead which can become permanent wrinkles; if skin conditions are not initially caused by stress, all are aggravated by it. Skin tends to be oilier in the working week than at weekends because of stressful situations, which is why oily skin often corrects itself on holidays, even if the sun is not shining! Many dermatologists now prescribe tranquillizers as an indirect method of improving skin ailments; perhaps meditation, yoga or a similar calming occupation would prove a healthier, if not as immediate, aid.

Diet
A balanced diet with vitamins taken in their natural state is essential for the reproduction of healthy new skin cells, and subsequently a fresh-toned complexion. Drinking a minimum of 1 litre (2 pints) of water per day (this amount can be taken in the form of herbal teas) helps flush out toxic substances in the body which surface as blemishes on the skin. Oils and fats in the diet have no effect on oil secretion, and in fact skin specialists recommend taking a spoonful of vegetable oil per day to keep skin in good condition.

● See page 19 for the seven-day-diet for a healthy skin.

Sleep
Sleep is the most important beauty treatment you can give yourself. However much care you take of your skin, if you do not have your adequate quota of sleep (and the amount varies with the individual: only you can judge) your skin will suffer by losing its resilience and healthy tone.

Pollution
Pollution contaminates the skin's natural protective film with paraffin hydrocarbons from factory chimneys, exhaust fumes; living in cities means extra cleansing of the skin to avoid skin problems caused by bacteria and pores clogged with grime. Rather than protecting the skin with make-up, wear as little as possible, and remember that a fine film of moisturiser is more effective than a thick layer.

Humidity
The greasiest skin can develop a condition known as "surface dryness" in winter; overheated rooms and cold winds are responsible for chapped lips and dry skin with temporary wrinkling. Counteract by turning down the central-heating thermostat, placing large pans of water by radiators to humidify the air and keeping windows open a little. Alter skin regime temporarily by stepping up use of moisturiser; dampen skin before application.

Weight loss
Rapid weight loss, as the result of an illness or excessive dieting, causes the skin to dehydrate. As well as proteins, vitamins and minerals, adequate calories are vital for the skin to function normally. Crash or fad diets rarely encompass all the nutrients necessary to good health, and should be avoided: sufferers of *anorexia nervosa*, for example, experience dry, scaly skin and hair loss as early symptoms.

Cosmetics
Indiscriminate use of cosmetics can have a disastrous effect on the skin. Occlusive foundations (those that don't allow the skin to "breathe") can clog pores and cause acne. Excess use of moisturiser can aggravate acne, particularly the pre-menstrual type, and can upset the balance of organisms on skin so bacteria flourish on the moist, humid surface. Alternatively, if skin loses more than ten per cent of its water content and this is not replaced by adequate moisture, skin will crack and chap. Drying soaps and harsh skin lotions are among other prime causes of skin disorders.

The pill

The pill can have advantageous or adverse effects on the skin. For some, the pill causes brown pigmentation on the face, simulating a symptom of pregnancy. The mixed pill, containing progesterone and oestrogen, can delay ageing effects of the skin; some acne sufferers have been prescribed this pill instead of antibiotics, by dermatologists, with promising results.

Alcohol

Alcohol can have a dehydrating effect on the skin, especially if skin is normally dry. Excess consumption of alcohol causes blood vessels to dilate and can result in permanently enlarged capillaries; an excess of caffeine can have the same effect.

Ultra-violet rays

Though sun lamps, and the sun, can help decrease excess oil secretion and improve acne, too much exposure to sunlight results in slackening of the skin's connective tissue, the collagen fibres which provide tone and elasticity to the skin. The effect is irreversible, and is not immediately obvious as the damage is worked on the dermis, the bottom layer of skin where collagen fibres are situated. However, temporary wrinkling from minimal exposure to sun can be remedied with application of an after-sun moisturising agent.

Smoking

Apart from obvious health hazards, the heavy smoker may experience skin discoloration, a result of constant exposure to burning tobacco. Crows' feet — fine lines around the eyes — are often a direct result of the smoker wrinkling up her eyes to avoid cigarette smoke.

Skin-care products:
Know what to ask for

Before you can devise an effective skin-care regime, you should know exactly what each type of cosmetic can do for your skin.

Soap

Soap should be used as a facial cleanser, and not as a make-up remover, unless the soap is specially formulated for this purpose. Many facial soaps are now called "cleansing bars" which provide the psychological satisfaction of a soap-and-water lather without the drying effects associated with soap. They contain emulsifying agents similar to those in cleansers and most are pH balanced, which means they have an affinity with the acid mantle, the skin's protective oil and water covering. The importance of this is explained by Dr Ron Harris, lecturer in anatomy, physiology and endocrinology at the University of California and Co-ordinator of Biological Research at Redken laboratories, pioneers of the acid-balanced "cleansing-bar":

"Some alkaline soaps can have a pH as high as 8 or 9 (healthy

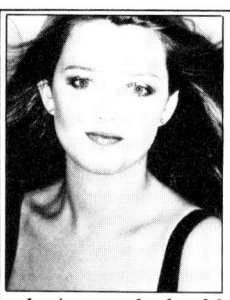

FIONA KENNEDY, *an actress, works in Glasgow but lives in the country near by. Although she attributes her good skin largely to inheritance, she is aware of the damage that can be caused by climate and environment. "Up north, where weather conditions are more extreme, you see many girls with dry skin and broken veins, though on the whole, girls in the Highlands have clearer complexions and a healthier colour than city girls. I feel this is due to the fresh air and the fact that they tend to wear less make-up. I notice the difference in my skin on visits to London: I look so pasty and find the hard water terribly drying after the lovely soft water we have up here in Scotland.*

"My most important skin-care task is cleansing — particularly so because of my profession: a facial sauna once a week is invaluable for really deep-cleansing the skin. I always wear lipstick and moisturiser as protection against the weather, though the 'damp cold' we have here does not cause the same extent of dryness and chapping as 'dry cold'. Also, because there is not so much central heating and air conditioning in the north, extremes of temperature are rarely a problem — it's as cold inside as it is outside! A friend of mine had lovely skin until she took a job at the airport: now she's living proof of the damage that can be caused by a succession of late nights, rushed snacks, and working in an artificially heated environment."

skin has a pH of around 5.5) which temporarily destroys the skin's acid mantle. Within twelve hours, the body produces a new acid mantle to return the skin to its natural pH, but in that time micro-organisms can flourish on the skin's surface; even flu germs can penetrate."

These soaps are ideal for cleansing the skin without drying, but if you have very greasy skin or acne, you could try a medicated soap which contains drying agents — eg, sulphur — to help the condition; if in doubt, check with your doctor. Avoid so-called deodorant soaps which contain hexachlorophene, a drying chemical that can irritate the skin. Super-fatted soaps contain moisturising emollients and are designed for dry skins. *Note* The decision to use soap rests simply on whether you like a soap-and-water rinse; if a cleanser and toner suit your skin there is no need to change the regime.

Cleansers

Cleansers contain emulsifiers and agents which dissolve foundation. Most need the use of a skin toner afterwards to remove any residue; you may prefer a soap-and-water rinse. CLEANSING MILKS leave lipids on the skin which replace natural oils that have been removed by the detergent part of

How to identify your skin type

Your daily skin-care regime, if you have no serious problems, should be very simple; the difficult element is to be your own skin diagnostician, so you can treat your skin accordingly. It is important to realise that few people have simple dry, normal or oily skins; most have a combination, which can be affected by many factors.

Dermatologists recommend the following method of defining your skin's natural condition: in the morning, before washing, tear up small pieces of brown paper (the kind paper bags are made of) and smear them over parts of your face. The skin's oil secretion will darken the paper, which is normal, but if the paper becomes translucent, that area is excessively oily. Try this operation frequently; use your clean fingers and a magnifying mirror, daily, to spot minor alterations. Be flexible in your regime, varying it as your skin varies. On the following pages you will discover techniques, equipment and explanations of the products available to you — so you can evolve your own, individual skin-care plan.

the product; with correct application, no after-tonic is necessary, unless skin is excessively greasy. Many milks are formulated into dry, oily, normal skin type variants; check on the bottle.
LIQUEFYING CREAMS are greasy in texture, but dissolve on contact with the skin, and are therefore suitable for the oiliest skin.
COLD CREAMS make excellent make-up removers but are best suited to dry skins.
CLEANSING OILS can be used for oily skins, provided the oil is the non-penetrating kind that rests on the surface of the skin; this variety of cleanser is ideal for sensitive skins.
RINSABLE CLEANSERS are suited to all skin types, but be sure the one you choose is designed to remove make-up as well as clean the skin.

Tonic

A mild lotion for all skin types, a skin tonic refreshes and stimulates skin, as well as removing any traces of make-up remover after cleansing: the simplest toners for the skin are distilled water or rosewater. Skin tonic should be applied to clean skin before the application of moisturiser.

Astringent

These stronger skin tonics are more suited to greasy skins; many are alcohol-based and applied after cleansing and whenever excess oil needs to be mopped up. A frequent error is to use an astringent that is too drying for the skin, so creating temporary excessive surface dryness, trapping oils underneath.
Note For morning cleansing, a wipe with a cotton-wool pad

soaked in the appropriate toner or astringent is all that is necessary to remove skin debris, unless you prefer soap and water, or a specialised treatment is required.

Moisturiser

There are two types of skin moisturisers: the occlusives (Vaseline is the simplest example of this) which form an oil barrier on the skin to prevent water loss through evaporation, and the humectants, which pull molecules of water from the air into the skin. The best moisturisers contain urea, which prevents water evaporation *and* attracts water. Greasy skins do not need moisturiser as the layer of sebum in the skin acts as a natural occlusive, although temporary dryness can be alleviated by a light water-in-oil emulsion. Dry skins should use a heavier oil-in-water emulsion, a richer cream.

Nourishing cream

This word is a misnomer as no cosmetic cream can "nourish" or feed the skin; all have a surface action only. The term refers to the heavier type of moisturiser which is an oil-in-water emulsion, often with added emollients; it is suited to very dry skins and can be used as a night cream.

Night cream

According to Dr Peter Thackray, research dermatologist, laboratory tests have proved that the rate of skin's water loss at night is lower than the rate lost in the day. Night creams are more occlusive and tend to be less cosmetically pleasing because their function is to retain more moisture arising from within the skin, whereas a daytime moisturiser has a formulation which is more acceptable for daytime use.

Mask

A face mask that is suited to the skin and applied correctly will have a beneficial result, although it is important to note that no mask will alleviate any serious skin problems. Most masks have only a temporary action on the skin. They may be divided into the following basic categories:
CLARIFYING MASK for oily skins. These are often clay-based, to help draw out impurities and de-grease; the mask dries on the skin and is rinsed off with warm water.
STIMULATING MASK for all skin types. Acts as a mini-shock treatment to the skin, enlarging blood vessels temporarily and bringing oxygen to the skin's surface, resulting in a fresh, pink skin tone. Usually in a brush-on, peel-off form.
MOISTURISING MASK for normal/dry skins. Firms tissues of skin and plumps up topmost layer of skin cells; results last up to eight hours only. In a cream form, moisturising masks are non-drying and are required to be left on the skin for a minimum of ten minutes, after which they are rinsed off.
EXFOLIATING MASK for all types. A cream which, when left to dry on the skin, can be rubbed off with the fingers; surface grime and skin debris are removed with the mask.

The seven-day diet for a healthy skin

Health farms specialise in diets which de-toxify the system; one of the first apparent effects is a clearer, fresher complexion. Try this seven-day regime devised by the dietician at Champneys Health Resort of Tring, and follow the diet's guidelines — fresh fruits and vegetables, simply cooked proteins and lots of water — on a permanent basis. In this way, you will provide your skin with the best possible conditions to keep it healthy.

Daily

○ First thing, drink a glass of hot water to which a slice of lemon has been added.
○ Drinks should be restricted to water and herbal teas; minimum intake should be 1 litre (2 pints).
○ For all vegetable salads, make a dressing of olive oil and lemon juice, lightly seasoned.
○ Non-slimmers can eat one slice of lightly buttered wholemeal bread at lunch.

Day One

Breakfast	Half grapefruit and honey
	Muesli with sliced banana and milk
Lunch	Two slices of ham, rolled and filled with cottage cheese and pineapple
	Courgette, tomato and mushroom salad
	Small carton natural yogurt with honey and chopped nuts
Dinner	Poached haddock and fresh tomato sauce
	Steamed spinach
	Jacket potato
	Fresh fruit salad

Day Two

Breakfast	Glass fresh orange juice
	Poached egg on wholemeal toast, lightly buttered
Lunch	Half avocado filled with cottage cheese and fresh grapefruit
	Mixed green salad
	Baked apple stuffed with dried fruit and honey
Dinner	Casseroled chicken
	Boiled brown rice
	Steamed courgettes
	Small carton natural yogurt with orange segments

Day Three

Breakfast	Half grapefruit
	Stewed apple sweetened with honey
	Small carton natural yogurt
Lunch	Smoked mackerel fillet
	Carrot, white cabbage and green pepper salad
	One banana

Dinner	Mushroom omelette
	Baked tomatoes
	Jacket potato
	Fresh fruit salad

Day Four

Breakfast	Orange juice
	Muesli with chopped nuts, dried apricots and milk
Lunch	Large carton cottage cheese and pineapple
	Cucumber, tomato and celery salad
	One orange
Dinner	Baked green pepper, stuffed with savoury mince
	Boiled brown rice
	Small carton natural yogurt and honey

Day Five

Breakfast	Half grapefruit
	Small carton natural yogurt and 3 or 4 stewed prunes
	Wholemeal toast, lightly buttered, with honey
Lunch	Grilled chicken
	Red cabbage, onion and banana salad
	Baked pear with nuts and honey
Dinner	Cauliflower Mornay (coated with a light cheese sauce)
	Jacket potato
	Sliced steamed carrots
	Grapefruit and orange cocktail

Day Six

Breakfast	Glass fresh orange juice
	One boiled egg
	Wholemeal toast, lightly buttered, with honey
Lunch	Tomato filled with cooked brown rice, tuna fish and mushrooms
	Celery, apple and carrot salad
	Small carton natural yogurt and chopped, dried apricots
Dinner	Grilled gammon and pineapple
	Steamed Brussels sprouts
	Jacket potato
	One orange

Day Seven

Breakfast	Half grapefruit
	Muesli with grated apple and milk
Lunch	Large carton cottage cheese with chopped peppers
	Avocado, tomato and watercress salad
	Small carton natural yogurt with chopped banana and nuts
Dinner	Grilled plaice with lemon and parsley
	Poached mushrooms
	Broccoli
	Jacket potato
	Fresh fruit salad and honey

Basic techniques

Did you realise there is a right — and a wrong — way to wash your face? There are methods the professionals favour in performing the simplest of skin treatments. Adopt the following for optimum results from your skin-care products.

How to wash your face

1 Wet skin with lukewarm, not hot water; extremes of temperature can cause spider veins and blotchy skin.
2 Work up a soapy lather with your clean hands and apply to face in light, circular movements; use a complexion brush for a more stimulating treatment. Avoid using too much soap; the cleanliness of skin is not dependent on amount of lather used!
3 Rinse face thoroughly with lukewarm water from running tap for at least thirty seconds, as some soaps can leave a deposit of insoluble salts which can irritate sensitive skins.
4 Pat face dry with tissues.
5 If skin feels tight, apply moisturiser.

How to moisturise your face

Re-assess skin before every application of moisturiser as condition of skin can vary from day to day.
1 With clean fingers, feel skin for dry patches; apply moisturiser only on these areas.
2 Splash skin with cool water and pat near-dry.
3 Smooth moisturiser evenly over required areas with fingertips using upward and outward movements and being careful not to drag the skin.
4 Pat moisturiser around delicate eye area with the little finger.
5 After five minutes, if there is any visible residue, wipe off excess with cotton wool. In cold weather, it may be necessary to re-apply moisturiser before applying foundation.

How to remove make-up

1 Blot off surplus lipstick.
2 Remove eye make-up gently with cotton wool soaked in specialised remover, or use eye make-up remover pads.
3 Using fingertips for cream cleanser, and cotton wool for milk or oil removers, apply with circular massage movements. Start at bridge of nose and graduate to around the eye area, working out from centre of face. Concentrate on nose and chin, where dirt tends to become ingrained. Finally, massage around jaw and neck, using upward strokes.
4 Remove cleanser with cotton wool, or cotton wool soaked in a tonic lotion.

How to abrade your face

In the same way as the texture of wood is smoothed and refined with sandpaper, so your skin benefits from a planing or thinning of the surface. The purpose of abrading is to slough off the surface skin cells which are technically dead, and so expose the newer, finer-textured skin underneath. Exfoliation, or flaking of dead skin, occurs naturally, but abrasion speeds the process to promote fresher-toned, healthier skin. Frequency of abrasion depends on skin condition, but most skins will benefit from this thinning exercise, especially oily skins which are inclined to acne. If you have delicate, sensitive skin, take the treatment slowly and desist if skin becomes aggravated. Directly after abrasion, the skin is at its most receptive for moisturiser.
1 Scrub the skin with a flannel, loofah or similar abrasive material, and soap. To start with, scrub the face for one minute only, and build up treatment gradually with every session.
2 Washing grains are small granules which, when worked into the skin with a little water, have an abrasive action on the skin. Facial scrubs are creams which contain these grains, and are rubbed into the skin before rinsing off.
3 Clarifying lotions are stong astringents which are designed to exfoliate skin. They can be drying, and are suitable for greasy skins only.
4 Try an excellent natural sloughing agent: rub the inside of a papaya skin on your face, rinse.

Equipment for super skin

All of the following can improve the condition of the skin, are fun to use and, most important, you might find that using specialised equipment gives you the extra discipline you need to follow a skin-care regime.

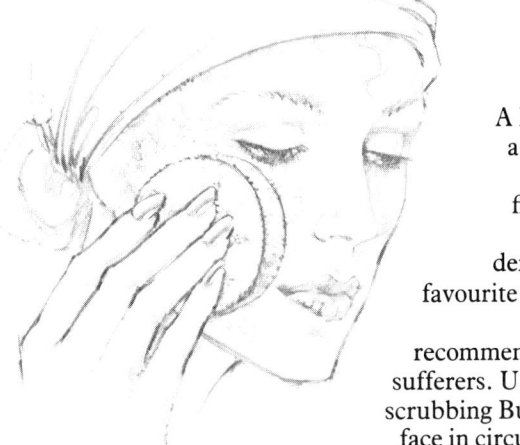

A BUF-PUF is a circular wad of polyester fibre. It is the American dermatologists' favourite skin abrader and is often recommended for acne sufferers. Use with soap, scrubbing Buf-Puf on the face in circular motions.

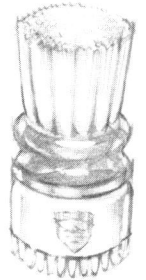

A COMPLEXION BRUSH stimulates circulation and deep-cleanses skin. Whip up lather with soap and loosen oil plugs with the bristle brush; massage skin with the rubber tips.
This complexion brush (left) by Kent.

A COMEDON EXTRACTOR lifts out blackheads. At either end is a small spoon-shaped disc, with a tiny hole in the middle. When the hole is centred on the blackhead, and pressure is exerted, the blackhead should pop out. Use only after steaming or softening skin with hot water, and do not persist with stubborn blackheads; leave till next time.

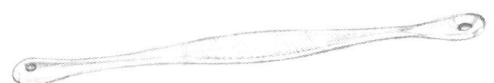

A SHAVING BRUSH is a gentler alternative to the complexion brush. In France, a popular treatment to refine the texture of open pores is to work a little borax powder on to the affected areas with a shaving brush dipped in warm water. Rinse off immediately.

Give yourself a salon treatment—at home

Treat yourself to a relaxing, self-indulgent facial. Both the following treatments are used by professional beauty therapists in salons, and have been adapted for you to use at home; with care you can achieve the same beneficial results. The skin-clearing facial is especially for oily, blemished skin; the Payot facial incorporates massage and exercise movements and is suitable for all skin types. Both facials should be used once-weekly. Professional salons advise keeping face clear of make-up for at least twelve hours after treatment.

The skin-clearing facial

The skin-clearing facial de-greases oily skin and, if a special kaolin mask is used, will help draw out impurities. Initially your skin may look worse than before the facial: this is because the toxins under the skin have been pulled to the surface. Gauge the effect after forty-eight hours, when your skin should look clearer and fresher.
Note This skin-clearing facial is used by many salons, but if you think you have a severe skin problem professional advice should be sought.
1 Cleanse skin thoroughly.
2 Apply skin tonic with cotton wool to remove residue.
3 Give yourself a facial sauna; salons use a machine called Vapozone, which has the same effect, but you have the advantage of using fresh or dried herbs in your sauna which are beneficial to the skin. Fill a bowl with boiling water, and make a herbal infusion by adding a handful of any, or all, of the following, choosing them according to their properties.
   Camomile — soothing
   Rosemary — stimulates circulation
   Lavendar — purifying
   Comfrey — healing
Place head over bowl and cover both with a towel; do not hold head any closer than 45 cm (18 in) from water, and finish sauna after maximum of five minutes.
Alternatively, make an infusion of your chosen herbs in hot water, soak a clean face flannel in the lotion and keep on face for same amount of time; the effect is the same, but you might prefer this method of "relaxing" pores.
4 Remove any visible blackheads with clean cotton wool and your fingers, using a gentle rolling movement to dislodge them; the professional salons use a comedon extractor, which is effective but needs to be used with care. For instructions, see above. Do not force stubborn blackheads, but leave till next time. Never attempt to squeeze blackheads without first softening skin with hot water or steam, as scarring may result.
5 Apply clarifying mask to face and neck (see page 24). Leave on for a minimum of ten minutes, placing cucumber slices on the eyes to freshen.
6 Remove mask with cotton wool wrung out in warm water.
7 If skin feels dry or tight, apply a thin film of moisturiser.

The Payot facial

Practised at many French beauty salons, this facial was evolved by Dr N G Payot, founder of the cosmetics firm, at the request of Anna Pavlova, the prima ballerina. Dr Payot reasoned that the ballerina developed a firm body through exercise, therefore the muscles of the face could be toned in the same way. The massage actions are based on the lymph drainage system, which carries body toxins to the lymph glands to be filtered, and then into the blood system to the heart and lungs where they are eliminated through the process of breathing. The aim of the Payot massage is to increase this flow, and thus help improve the condition of the skin. Further to assist the elimination of toxins, it is advisable to drink one pint of water a day. The exercise and massage movements may look time-consuming but in fact they take only a few minutes each; both may be practised at any time, so long as the skin is supple and moisturised.

1 Apply cleanser with fingertips in light, circular movements.

2 Remove with water-dampened cotton wool and skin tonic.

3 Follow massage movements outlined below, using a moisturising cream or light oil.

4 Follow exercise movements outlined below.

5 Remove cream or oil by blotting with tissue.

6 Loosen any blackheads by soap cleansing. The driest skin can suffer from blackheads; scrutinise your skin with a magnifying mirror in a strong light. If skin is spotty, omit soap cleansing stage as blemishes could be aggravated. Apply a thin film of moisturiser or soothing cream; with non-alkaline soap and a complexion brush, work up lather in rotary action on affected areas. Rinse off well with warm water.

7 Apply appropriate mask (see below for recipes for home-made masks), placing cooling agents — tonic-soaked cotton-wool pads or chilled damp tea bags — on eyes.

8 Remove mask after stipulated time with warm water.

9 Apply moisturiser, then remove excess by blotting lightly with tissue.

Payot massage

These massage movements help stimulate blood circulation, prevent skin blemishes and remove dead skin cells; use light, firm pressure of the fingertips and be careful not to pull skin around the delicate eye area. If you use a night cream, adopt the movements shown here to apply.

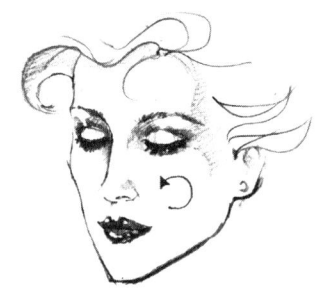

Form continuous circular mostions on cheeks, in an upwards and inwards direction.

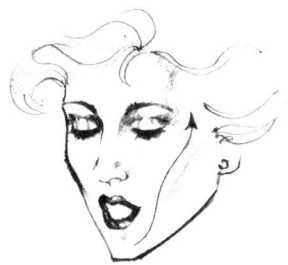

Make a yawning shape with mouth; stroke skin in upward/outward direction from chin to temple.

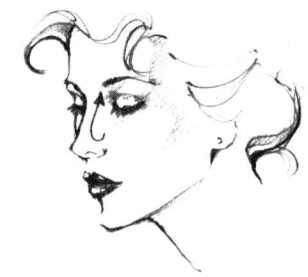

As if deep cleansing skin with cream, make a circular motion at side of nose and continue upward.

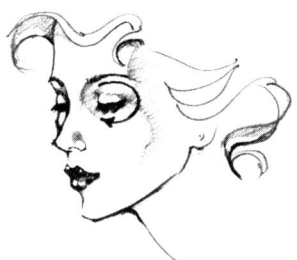

Stroke fingers outwards from inner brow and inward under lower lid.

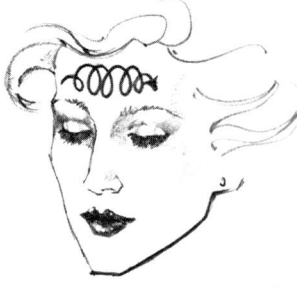

Make circular motions across forehead with fingers forming a spiral.

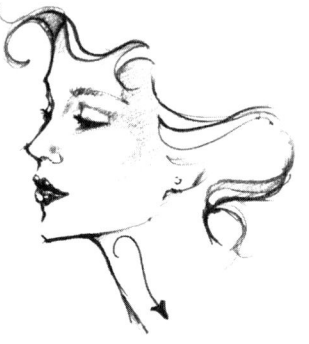

With light fingers, stroke neck in downward direction in a single movement.

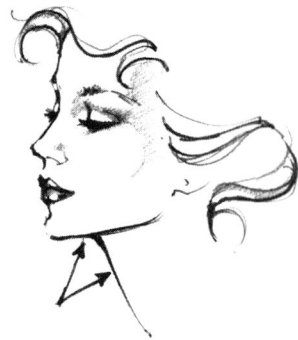

To firm chin, use a vigorous patting motion under jawline.

Payot exercises

These facial exercises help firm and strengthen supportive muscles of the face and neck.

1 Make sounds *oo* and *icks*, moving jaw vigorously; repeat ten times. Firms cheek muscles.

2 Press two fingers against each temple to hold the skin, then open and close eyes vigorously; repeat ten times. Exercises muscles around eyes, which tend to lose elasticity most.

3 With backs of both hands, push chin upwards using neck muscles to counteract this action; repeat ten times. Prevents sagging chin muscles.

4 Push head backwards, resisting this action by pulling forward with hands placed at nape of neck, repeat ten times. Firms neck and back of neck.

Make your own skin-care treatments

Home-made skin-care products are fun to make and pleasant to use; the concept of using herbs, fruits and flowers in the manufacturing process is an attractive one. However, there are significant advantages for the skin. Clare Maxwell-Hudson, author of *The Natural Beauty Book* and practising beautician who devised the following recipes, has been marketing her own skin-care products for the last ten years, and claims:

"Cosmetic preparations you make yourself are good for the skin as, like making your own bread, you can afford to use the best ingredients; commercial manufacturers have such large advertising and packaging costs that they are forced to economise on quality. Cosmetic companies often use mineral oil; you can use finer almond and avocado oils — and still make cheaper skin-care products than you can buy. Some of the most popular synthetic constituents in shop-bought cosmetics are derived from herbs and plants. Allantoin, for example, a widely-used ingredient which encourages healthy skin cell growth, is extracted from the comfrey root. If you are allergic to many cosmetics, you can make products that are free of synthetic fragrance, a frequent cause of adverse skin reactions."

Basic ingredients for these home-made products can be bought or ordered from any good chemist; vegetable oils, from health stores. For a list of herbs and essential oils available by mail order, write to Culpeper, Hadstock Road, Luton, Cambridge, enclosing an sae. As no preservatives are used, these skin-care products do not last as long as commercial brands; expect a shelf life of approximately two months, and try to store creams and lotions in the fridge. For fragrance, add a few drops of your favourite oil to the creams.

Facial scrub

These washing grains slough off dead surface cells and loosen ingrained dirt. Greasy skin will benefit greatly from using the grains every day; fine, dry skins should use them once a week only. Elderflowers are renowned for their skin-clearing properties; they are available dried from herbalists and health stores, and can be found growing wild in spring and summer all over the countryside. To make a facial scrub, you'll need:

1 cup medium oatmeal
1 tbsp dried elderflowers
Method Crush elderflowers and mix both ingredients together. Store in a jar. To use, pour about a teaspoon into the palm of your hand. Mix into a paste with a little water or milk and use to wash face.

Light moisturiser

Almond and avocado oils penetrate the skin readily and make this moisturiser suitable for day. It provides a good base for foundation.
Oil phase
15 ml (1 tbsp) beeswax
15 ml (1 tbsp) emulsifying wax

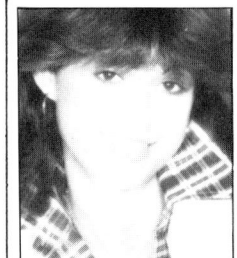

LESLEY JACOBSON *is a secretary working in London. She is aware of the skin-damaging factors of city life and protects herself accordingly.*

"*My skin dries very easily in the extremes of temperature in London, particularly going from a centrally-heated office to the cold outside. I never use soap or even ordinary cleansers because I find they dry my skin. I cleanse with a mixture of half witch-hazel, half rosewater — and in London I need to do this at least three times a day. The only time I use water on my face is after a bath when I splash my skin with cold water to close the pores. Occasionally I give my face a steam treatment (under a towel 'tent' over a basin of hot water) to thoroughly cleanse my skin of London grime, but the best skin treat of all for me is simply fresh air — and you really can get plenty of this in the city.*

As often as possible I go for walks in the parks, as being cooped up all day in an office can give the skin a dull tone. I never wear foundation — pores get blocked up enough with dirt: there's no point in adding to the problem! I really do believe that diet is reflected in the skin: the only time I ever get spots or blemishes is when I've eaten junk foods — one of the pitfalls of a busy office life when you've only time to dash to the café over the road. As a rule, though, I try to eat only healthy foods — lots of vegetables and fresh fruit — and I'm convinced this is the reason for my normally clear complexion."

15 ml (1 tbsp) avocado oil
75 ml (5 tbsp) almond oil
Water phase
225 ml (15 tbsp) rosewater
5 ml (1 tsp) glycerine
2.5 ml (½ tsp) borax
Method Melt the oil and water ingredients separately in double boilers or over water baths, ensuring borax is completely dissolved. Keeping the oils on the heat, add waters slowly, stirring well. After two minutes remove from heat. Beat with a wooden spoon or use the lowest speed on kitchen mixer, adding essential oil, if liked, after one minute. The cream will become thick and fluffy in texture.

Rich moisturiser

Suitable for dry skins and as a night cream; wheatgerm and honey soften skin.
Oil phase
15 ml (1 tbsp) lanolin
15 ml (1 tbsp) beeswax
15 ml (1 tbsp) honey

45 ml (3 tbsp) wheatgerm
45 ml (3 tbsp) sunflower oil
(Some or all of these ingredients can be replaced with home-made aromatic oil: for recipe, see The Body chapter).
Water phase
90 ml (6 tbsp) distilled water
2.5 ml (½ tsp) borax
Method Follow method for light moisturiser but when oils have melted, remove from heat before slowly adding the distilled water and borax.

Cleansing cream

Effectively removes make-up and lifts surface grime; slightly greasy in texture, the cream liquefies on contact with the skin. Suitable for all skin types. Baby oil is used in this recipe as it rests on the surface of the skin and does not penetrate.
Oil phase
15 ml (1 tbsp) beeswax
60 ml (4 tbsp) baby oil
30 ml (2 tbsp) coconut oil
Water phase
30 ml (2 tbsp) distilled water
15 ml (1 tbsp) witch-hazel
2.5 ml (½ tsp) borax
Method Melt oil ingredients in a double boiler or over water bath. In a separate bowl, dissolve borax in hot water, then add witch-hazel. When oils are melted, remove from heat and slowly mix water into oils, beating all the time. Add essential oil when cream begins to cool. Beat until mixture cools and thickens, using either a wooden spoon or lowest speed on kitchen mixer. To use, rub into skin with fingers and remove with tonic-soaked cotton wool.

Elderflower skin tonic

A fragrant lotion suited to normal and dry skins. You'll need:
30 ml (2 tbsp) dried elderflowers
300 ml (½ pt) boiling water
Method Pour boiling water over elderflowers. Let the infusion stand in a covered pot overnight, and then strain. If liked, for added astringency stir in 25 ml (1 fl oz) witch-hazel.

Cucumber skin tonic

Refrigerate and use chilled to refresh as well as tone skin; soak cotton-wool pads in the lotion for a tingling eye mask that de-puffs eyelids and surrounding eye area. This treatment is especially beneficial to oily skins, as cucumber has slightly astringent qualities.
Method Cut a cucumber into chunks; liquidise. If you do not have a blender, mash and sieve cucumber.

Masks

All of the following masks should be applied to face and neck, left on for at least ten minutes, then rinsed off with warm water. Keep skin free of make-up afterwards for as long as possible; if skin feels tight after treatment, apply a thin film of moisturiser.
CLARIFYING MASK
For a greasy skin inclined to blemish: kaolin and fuller's earth share the property of drawing out impurities. Immediately after treatment, your skin may look blotchy; assess the improvement after twelve hours.
Method Make a paste of 30 ml (2 tbsp) kaolin or fuller's earth (available from good chemists), 15 ml (1 tbsp) milk, 5 ml (1 tsp) honey and 4 cloves, ground.
MOISTURISING MASK
For normal and dry skins.
Method Mash a ripe banana, and mix with 15 ml (1 tbsp) honey and one beaten egg. Sieve. The remainder will keep in the fridge for several days.
MINI FACE-LIFT MASK
For all skin types. This mask has a temporary tightening effect on the skin and is ideal to use before a party.
Method Beat the white of one egg and add 15 ml (1 tbsp) of honey. If your skin is dry, add a few drops of almond or peach kernel oil.

Dermatologist or beauty therapist — which to consult?

The condition of the skin is not merely a question of beauty; it is also an indication of health. This may cause some confusion for anyone suffering from a skin ailment, who may feel guilty approaching their GP with what they consider a minor complaint, but on the other hand may worry that beauty therapists are limited to purely cosmetic treatments.

Katherine Corbett, a licensed beauty therapist at 21 South Molton St, London W1D Y1D (01-493 5905), explains the function of her profession: "A beauty therapist treats skin complaints which do not actually indicate a physical condition, but can nevertheless damage a woman's morale: thus I am a therapist in the true sense of the word."

A top dermatologist warns against non-medical treatment of seemingly superficial conditions: "It is often difficult to distinguish between a slight developmental abnormality, such as a mole, and a manifestation of some more serious internal disorder; where there is any doubt, you should always consult a doctor who will, if the condition warrants, send you either to a hospital skin consultant or to a private dermatologist. In some cases, he will send the patient to a beauty therapist. Skin conditions which involve rashes, flaking, inflamed or irritated skin cannot possibly be mistaken for the cosmetic and complexion problems which are exclusively the beauty therapist's concern."

Several of the more common skin complaints listed below may be treated either by a dermatologist or a beauty therapist. For a list of qualified beauty therapists in your area, send an sae to The Secretary, British Association of Beauty Therapy and Cosmetology Ltd, Flat 5, 27 Denmark Avenue, Wimbledon, London SW19 4HQ. Dermatologists may be consulted only with a letter of referral from your GP.

Whiteheads are tiny waxy sacs of excess sebum situated just below the surface of the skin; beauty therapists remove them with the aid of a small scalpel, but it is inadvisable to attempt any form of home treatment.

Red veins, spider-like formations, are caused by burst capillaries. Katherine Corbett uses sclerotherapy to treat this condition: a chemical is injected into the area which dries up the traces of blood, leaving bruise marks; these soon fade. A tracery of fine red veins over the face is due to varying factors: they are often hereditary and common in those leading an outdoor life, but may also signal an internal disorder, such as liver disease. A doctor should be consulted before treatment is given by a beauty therapist. Single veins resembling a piece of red cotton are comparatively easy to remove, but camouflage make-up is the only solution for a general high colour.

Skin tags, flesh-coloured moles attached by a short stalk to the skin, are harmless, but if felt to be disfiguring can be removed by a beauty therapist.

Warts are viral growths that can occur anywhere on the body but are prevalent on the hands. They are generally harmless, though unsightly. In rare cases, however, they may constitute more serious disorders and though diagnosis is usually simple, treatment should not be attempted by a non-medical person. A qualified beauty therapist will not remove a wart without prior medical approval. Some GPs will treat warts, but if they prove resistant, will refer the patient to a hospital skin consultant or a private dermatologist. The warts are then removed by appropriate treatment; they are most commonly scooped or burnt out, though some specialists use cyrosurgery — freezing with carbon dioxide.

Pigmented moles: dermatologists feel that pigmented moles should be removed if they are constantly irritated by clothing or are aesthetically embarrassing. If they are removed by a beauty therapist, a doctor should first be consulted; in some cases he might recommend treatment by a dermatologist.

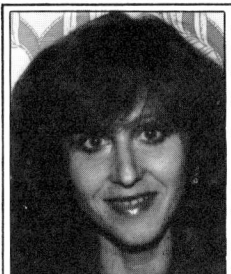

JUDY ABRAHAMS *is a freelance PR consultant, writer and lecturer. Having lived in London, she can feel justified in defending Newcastle.*

"Surprisingly, the skin's enemy is not the smoky atmosphere for which the North East is renowned — London air is far more pore-clogging — but the biting east winds blowing inland from the coast, which attack the skin with a vengeance. I use a bran wash cream because it is less drying than soap, and moisturise my face day and night; I also use a moisturising bath oil. Lip gloss is another necessity and if my lips do become chapped I find that zinc ointment is an excellent remedy. A common problem in this area is what we call 'keens', when the fingers become cracked through dryness and cold. I avoid chapped hands by drying them well after washing and using a hand cream: Boots Glycerine And Rosewater is particularly effective.

"My skin probably suffers more from my life-style than from environment: busy, stressful days and snatched meals, for example. But I do get plenty of fresh air, walking the dog in the countryside outside Newcastle. I try to keep make-up to a minimum but find I need to wear more in winter when my complexion takes on a greyish tinge. If my skin is looking particularly dingy I apply a home-made honey-and-oatmeal mask when I'm having a bath, so that the warmth opens pores and stimulates circulation. In the summer we do not get much respite from the east wind, so my regime remains very much the same throughout the year: the weather does have its good side, though — a dermatologist told me the skin ages less quickly here owing to lack of exposure to the sun!"

Moles should be carefully watched, and any change in their appearance reported to a GP.

Liver spots, commonly found on the hands and faces of older people, are caused by years of exposure to sun and wind. Though beauty therapists can bleach them, dermatologists prefer the use of camouflage make-up. In rare cases they may indicate a more serious skin condition and may need removal.

Freckles are a conglomeration of pigment, fortunately considered attractive, as their removal is not recommended. Some beauty therapists use bleach or skin-peel to remove freckles but any such treatment should be approached with great caution — and medical approval. Raised freckles and brown patches which show a tendency to growth should not be treated by a non-medical person as they may be caused by a fungal infection, hormonal changes or, in some cases, more serious complaints.

Birthmarks: the most common remaining after childhood is the "port wine" mark: composed of blood vessels, it is flat and

Skin peeling

Surgical skin peeling, performed by plastic surgeons, is often the only way to improve the condition of skin badly scarred by acne or chicken-pox; it has also been used with some success on superficial wrinkling. The damaged surface layers of skin are removed by one of two methods: chemosurgery, which involves the application of strong chemicals to induce skin peeling, and dermabrasion, which is a "Sanding down" of the skin with a rotating wire brush. After a few weeks, during which time the skin is red, raw and swollen, a new, less blemished skin grows. Peeling is most successful on fair complexions, as darker skins are more likely to develop pigmentation problems. Many surgeons will operate only on the most severe cases of scarring, because results on slight blemishes rarely justify the cost. Chemosurgery permanently reduces the melanin-producing cells so that a tan can never be acquired, and although dermabrasion does not affect the melanin, new skin is extremely sensitive to the sun.

Some beauty salons offer a skin-peeling treatment, which usually involves the application of exfoliating masks or lotions. These remove dead cells that give the skin a dingy appearance, but can have a drying effect. A few salons perform a service called "deep peeling", which removes faint blemishes and freckles: the methods used are similar to chemosurgery and, in the hands of non-medical operators, should be approached with great caution.

purple in colour. There is no satisfactory treatment available. Plastic surgery may help in some cases, but where this is not possible, camouflage make-up is recommended.

Cold sores are blister-like lesions which occur mainly on the mouth. They are caused by a virus which is believed to lie dormant in the body until triggered off: the virus attacks when the body's resistance is low, which is why cold sores often accompany minor illnesses such as the common cold. Other trigger mechanisms are extremes of weather, a traumatic shock, general stress and the lowered oestrogen level that occurs just before the menstrual period. Doctors can prescribe lotions, but many believe that the cold sore heals faster if dried out with some form of alcohol — cologne, for example.

Boils are painful, pus-filled lumps which start as an inflammation in the hair follicle. They should be seen by a GP, particularly if recurring, as they can indicate internal ailments.

Hives (Urticaria) are reddish, raised bumps, surrounded by a white ring. They may be an allergic reaction to a food or medication: aspirin, penicillin and the pill are common precipitants. Nerves and stress are other causes. Anti-

histamine is usually prescribed but it is advisable to find the allergenic factor if possible when hives are a recurring complaint.

Xanthomas, fatty white pimples on the eyelid, may indicate high blood cholesterol; though they can be removed by a beauty therapist, they should first be seen by a doctor.

Eczema tends to be inherited and is sometimes related to an allergy, though there is no accepted medical cause. It appears as a group of skin eruptions, characterised by redness and small blisters. Chronic itching invariably leads to scratching which causes a scaly, thickened surface layer. Eczema usually affects hands, face or the backs of knees and elbows. Often eczema disappears spontaneously, and then recurs for no apparent reason. The complaint may be alleviated by salt baths and exposure to the sun, but medical advice must be sought.

Psoriasis is a chronic disease which causes much unhappiness owing to the discomfort it causes and its unsightly appearance — round, red patches covered with a thick silvery scale, which may affect any part of the body. In its advanced state, nails may become pitted or ridged. The disease is hereditary and tends to attack when health is poor or at a time of serious stress. Its course is erratic: sudden reprieves are followed by a worse attack. Like eczema, psoriasis may improve with salt baths and exposure to the sun, but specialist medication is imperative.

Shingles, an often painful condition, is caused by a virus which attacks nerve endings; most adults who suffer from the disease will have had chicken-pox in childhood, because the virus of the two diseases is the same. Small yellow blisters erupt on one side of the mid-line anywhere on the body and gradually dry into a thick crust. There is a possibility of scarring; early treatment by a doctor is essential.

Acne: Causes and cures

Acne is not confined to adolescents; practising dermatologists treat as many as ten women with acne conditions, daily. Oily skin that suffers from occasional spots can be kept clear with preventive measures, but it must be realised that acne is a medical condition which can last a lifetime if left untreated.

Dermatologists cannot always pinpoint causes, but it is known that hormone levels in the blood are related to acne conditions. When the hormone balance of the body is altered, the oil glands become over-stimulated and produce too much oil, which gathers under the skin's surface and clogs pore openings. Oil becomes trapped, and irritates surrounding skin; inflammation results. The condition is generally most frequent on the face and back, where oil glands are concentrated.

Hormones which over-stimulate the oil glands are triggered into action for several reasons. The chief offender, dermatologists believe, is stress: women with high-tension jobs are often at risk. The progesterone-based pill can sometimes induce acne in skins that are sensitive to hormone levels, or can worsen existing acne. Diet, though not a cause of acne, can aggravate the condition; it has been proved that the foods once believed to increase oil production most in the skin and therefore promote acne — ie, chocolate, sugar and fats — have no influence on the skin's condition. Occlusive cosmetics and over-moisturising the skin can also contribute to acne.

How you can help the condition

Acne is a medical complaint and should be treated professionally, either by your doctor, or a dermatologist your doctor will refer you to. However, these are steps you can take to improve the condition.

• Adopt a skin regime that de-greases the skin; this involves clearing out pimples, and then drying out the area. It is essential to squeeze spots and blackheads, but this exercise should be performed by a qualified beauty therapist; amateur treatment could worsen the condition, and possibly scar skin tissue. Be scrupulous about cleansing, and never touch your face with dirty fingers, or pick at spots. Abrade the skin regularly, with cleansing grains or a loofah and medicated soap that will strip off excess grease and release oil. Using a sun lamp, in moderation, will have a beneficial peeling effect on the skin and will kill harmful bacteria, but note that ultraviolet rays can cause sunburn! Mop up surface oils with an astringent; you might have to do this as much as three or four times daily. Keep skin clear of make-up, using light medicated foundation when you feel you really have to cover affected areas. Avoid greasy blushers, occlusive Erace sticks, moisturisers and face powders.

• Keep your hair scrupulously clean; oily hair always accompanies an oily skin and can worsen acne considerably.

• Adopt your diet: Dr Jonathan Zizmor, Chief of Dermatology at St Vincent's Hospital, New York, cites food rich in iodides and androgen — one of the hormones that increase sebum production — as those which aggravate acne. These include kelp (or seaweed), wheatgerm, shellfish, sea salt, spinach, peanuts and multivitamins in pill form, which often contain iodide additives.

• Avoid wearing polo-neck sweaters, or any scratchy fabric that is likely to irritate the skin, especially if your back is acne-prone.

• Try to follow a less stressful life-style: the above suggestions may ease an acne condition; learning to relax may cure it!

How your doctor can help the condition

Depending on the severity of the acne, your doctor will adopt one or more of the following treatments:

TOPICAL DRYING AGENTS, which can be effective, but may ultimately cause flaking and scaling through excess drying of the skin; it can be argued that the latter is a less serious

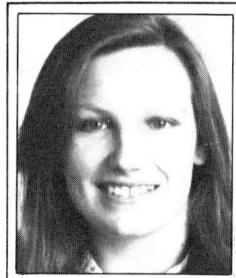

CAROL BUTLER *went to art college in Brighton in 1971 and loved it so much that she stayed on to work as a teacher.*

"The sea air is wonderfully bracing and makes you feel really healthy, but the salt in the atmosphere can be extremely drying for the skin. I find in winter, when the wind from the sea is especially cold, that I develop patches of dry skin on my forehead and chin. I use a lot of moisturiser to counteract this and, throughout the year, wear Nivea on my lips to prevent them from chapping. I rinse my face very thoroughly after cleansing because I don't think that cream alone is adequate for removing all the salt deposits left on my skin. My hands need extra protection, too, so I moisturise them in summer and wear gloves in winter.

"I have a naturally pale complexion, and after a day's teaching look really drained, but a walk along the seafront soon brings a colour to my face. That's one of the benefits of my job; I'm not cooped up in an office from nine to five and so can take advantage of the daylight. I avoid school stodge, which can be ruinous for the skin as well as the figure, and take fresh fruit and wholemeal bread for my lunch.

The best bonus of all here in Brighton is the sun: in summer I race back from school and put in a couple of hours' sunbathing on the beach. Although I smother myself in moisturiser and suntan lotion, I know my skin will suffer eventually — but right now, it makes me fell sixty million times better!"

complaint than acne! The other hazard of a topically-applied medication is that often oil plugs remain trapped underneath.

ANTIBIOTICS. Tetracycline is the drug most frequently prescribed; after six weeks a great improvement should be noted, but the patient with severe acne might have to take antibiotics indefinitely. Possible side-effects are yeast infections, such as thrush.

HORMONE THERAPY simply involves changing to a different brand of the pill; an increased oestrogen level is often all that is necessary to arrest acne in many cases.

TRANQUILLIZERS are occasionally prescribed when it is felt that relieving stress may alleviate acne, but should not be considered as a long-term panacea.

The best of the cheapest

All the skin-care products that follow cost very little yet are just as effective as their pricier counterparts. Buy in large sizes — for instance witch-hazel and rosewater can be ordered from chemists in two-litre containers — and you can save even more.

LIQUID PARAFFIN makes an excellent moisturiser for all skin types; apply a very fine film.

NIVEA, based on petroleum jelly and water, is a slightly richer moisturising cream for normal to dry skin types, and can be used as a night cream, too.

ROSEWATER makes a mild skin tonic for normal or dry skins. Apply with cotton wool after cleansing to remove every last trace of make-up, and to tone skin.

WITCH-HAZEL on cotton-wool pads refreshes tired eyes and reduces puffiness: a perfect astringent for greasy skins, witch-hazel can be diluted with a little rosewater if too drying.

VASELINE acts as an occlusive moisturiser for chapped lips. It is the cheapest and most efficient make-up eye remover (try it on waterproof mascara!) and conditions brittle lashes.

ALMOND OIL patted lightly around the delicate eye area is a good substitute for an eye cream.

COLD CREAM, any make, removes foundation quickly and easily and is more suited to dry skins. Be sure to remove any residue with a skin tonic, or with soap and water, afterwards.

MINERAL OIL and BABY OIL are two cleansing agents especially good for sensitive skins.

CALAMINE LOTION soothes itching, inflamed skin.

BOOTS E45 cream, a favourite of dermatologists, can be bought over the counter; it is an emollient cream which is excellent for chapped skin and eczema.

TCP Liquid Antiseptic, dabbed on spots, prevents spreading of bacteria and promotes healing.

Further economies

- Keep white toilet paper by your skin-care kit instead of more expensive tissues.
- Buy surgical cotton wool — the kind that is layered, Swiss-

Seven speedy skin treatments

Try any of the following; their effectiveness lies in the fact that women have been using these natural remedies for centuries!

1 Persian women apply yogurt to the face to help erase wrinkles; rinse off after ten minutes with water.

2 Rinse face with lemon or orange juice after using soap, to help degrease an oily skin.

3 Ancient Greeks used almond meal to soothe and soften skin; mix ground almonds with milk for a facial scrub.

4 The juice of an onion has long been believed to prevent blemishes. Mash and sieve an onion: apply the juice nightly to the skin.

5 Strawberries are renowned for their astringent qualities. Mash them, leave to dry on the face and rinse off.

6 Rub orange peel over the skin to soften.

7 A mix of watercress and honey was favoured by the ancient Medical School of Salerno for its skin-clearing properties; apply to blemishes with a cotton-wool pad.

roll style, in blue paper — to remove creams and apply skin tonics. It is the cheapest variety, is 100 per cent cotton which makes it non-irritant for sensitive skins, and is more absorbent than synthetic mixes. Unroll and cut into 6 cm squares; store in a pot for easy availability. To make skin tonics go further, soak a pad in the lotion, separate pad in two and you have four surfaces of lotion to apply to skin, instead of one.

Note See page 22 for money-savers you can make yourself.

SUN

A tan achieved after a holiday in the sun can be beneficial for the skin as well as the psyche — but you should look to the long-term, too, for the effect ultra-violet rays can have on your skin. Excessive and careless sunsoaking causes irreparable damage; sensible sunbathing can do wonders for the skin.

Positive properties of the sun on your skin

- Heliotherapy — healing by means of the sun — has been practised since the times of ancient Egypt. The sun helps heal wounds, strengthens bones; it is not just for a rest that doctors advise convalescents to take to the sun!
- The tanning process provokes the lower skin cells into producing extra pigment — melanin — as a natural defence against skin burns. When melanin combines with the skin's protein, and sensible sunning precautions are observed (follow the advice given in this chapter!), the skin is actually strengthened and becomes more resilient.
- Sunlight is an important source of vitamin D, essential to help the body assimilate calcium and phosphorus. No amount of synthetic form of vitamin D has proved as effective as this natural method of intake.
- Just as dermatologists recommend the use of sun lamps in clearing certain skin conditions, so they advocate the sun as an excellent treatment for eczema, psoriasis, boils etc; ultra-violet rays act as a drying agent for excessively greasy skins, and are especially beneficial for most forms of acne by encouraging drying and peeling of the skin.
- The sun is claimed to be the greatest natural antiseptic agent, combating many kinds of skin bacteria that might otherwise flourish.
- The sun's infra-red rays are actually drawn into the skin and used beneficially by the blood corpuscles of the body. (The infra-red rays are the ones you can feel warming your body; they have the added benefit of reducing stress and fatigue.)

Negative properties of the sun on your skin

- Dermatologists agree that the sun is *the* greatest skin ager. In the tanning process, the skin thickens and coarsens which, within limits, is beneficial. However, after continuous exposure — and many "thickenings" later — the skin stays that way, and cannot be altered.
- The sun is known to heal, and help skin problems occasionally, but certain skin ailments can be worsened by exposure to sunlight. In rare cases, acne can be triggered by ultra-violet (UV) rays.
- Excessive sun-soaking can and does result in the breakdown of the skin's collagen fibres, the connective tissues under the skin that give the skin its elasticity and resiliency; once these fibres have slackened, the effect is irreversible.
- Brown spots — darker blotches on the skin — were once considered by dermatologists to be a sign of ageing, but are now appearing on women in their twenties, all of whom have spent considerable lengths of time in the sun.
- Temporary wrinkling — fine lines on the skin — is common after sunbathing and can be erased by correct after-sun care, but frequent over-exposure to the sun results in permanent dryness and wrinkles; when this happens, no amount of moisturising can correct the damage.
- Skin cancer is more frequent among those who work outdoors or who have emigrated from a temperate to a tropical climate; it must be stressed that skin cancer is not a serious cancer, and is likely to occur only when the skin is constantly exposed to the sun.

Tanning preparations – how they work

It is sad but true that the most sophisticated tanning products will not turn you a golden brown if your skin naturally remains pink in the sun. Your degree of tan is dependent on the amount of melanin your body produces and this cannot be changed.

Sunscreens

All commercial sunscreens contain chemicals that filter UV rays to a lesser or greater degree, plus moisturisers; some include cooling agents and insect repellents in the formulations. Beware of suntan mixes suggested by the locals when on holiday; you may have heard these are very effective, but remember that the natives have a different skin tolerance to the sun! The most effective sunscreens contain PABA — para-amino-benzoic acid; look for the ingredient on the pack. Watch-point: PABA can stain synthetic fabrics.

If you have sensitive skin, you should use a sunscreen in milk, lotion or cream form; with olive-toned skin that tans readily, you can use an oil. To simplify choice, many brands carry a sun-protection factor: the higher numbers are suited to skins that burn easily, while lower numbers are for skin types that tan readily or have already been exposed to the sun or UV lamp. If you are in doubt as to which strength is suited to your skin, choose the higher number. You will not tan less slowly, but chances of burning will be minimised. Note that you might need to use a different suntan preparation for your face than for your body; it may work out more expensive but remember, the skin on your face is rarely the same type as that of your body and therefore needs different treatment.

Sunblocks

These are suited to skins that need total protection from the sun. Designed to block out *all* the sun's rays, effective sunblocks contain zinc oxide, which forms a barrier between skin and sun. If you need a sunblock for the face only, you can use a heavy, occlusive foundation which, a leading dermatologist points out, will have the same effect.

The sun and drinks

Lime juice is a known photosensitiser (causes adverse reaction to sunlight). Avoid drinking lime juice, and don't be tempted to squeeze the juice from a lime wedge in your poolside cocktail on to your skin — it can cause burning.

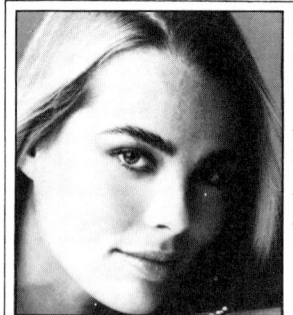

MARGAUX HEMINGWAY, *model and actress:* "*I never wear make-up in the sun; I get so freckled and brown I don't need it. I don't lie in the sun, I play in it, but I always use a sunscreen.*"

How to brown and not burn

1 Apply suntan agent *before* you leave for the beach: you can burn in the time it takes to apply it in the sun.

2 Golden rule for golden skins: build up gradually. The best defence against the sun is a suntan: one that builds up slowly and progressively. If you have had no sun, sunlamp or solarium pre-conditioning, start with no longer than fifteen minutes sun-soaking a day on either "side". If you have a couple of weeks' holiday in the sun, you can afford to keep moving for the first few days or so — thus allowing your body to become acclimatised to the sun's rays. When you start serious suntanning, your skin will brown more readily.

3 Protect vulnerable areas with extra sunscreen: forehead, nose, ears, neck, knees; use a lip balm or gloss with built-in sunscreen.

4 You may not want sunglasses marks — but you should always protect eyelids, which are extra sensitive to sunlight. Cover lids with eyeshadow which will occlude the sun's rays — or use seashells. In St Tropez they use wedges of wet cotton wool on eyelids; go one better and soak cotton wool in soothing cold, herbal tea.

5 Re-apply sunscreen after every dip in the pool or sea. Most sunscreens are water-soluble, though a few *are* resistant to water; check on the pack.

6 The Continentals may make you laugh with their disciplined tanning regimes: five minutes on either side with an alarm bell to mark strict time — but they do not burn, nor, biggest sunburn danger of all, do they fall asleep!

7 You are not exempt from the sun's rays when you are in the water; UV rays actually penetrate water so you can burn even when you are swimming! Beware, too, of sunning yourself dry in wet swimming gear after a dip — wet clothes, too, transmit UV rays.

8 It is worth noting that the closer you are to the equator, the more powerful the sun.

9 *Never* use a sun reflector: you will be asking for trouble.

10 Like the natives, make midday your siesta time. Restrict tanning sessions to early morning or late afternoon when the sun is low in the sky; these are times when the longer UV rays, the safer rays, are more prominent and will provide a longer-lasting tan; the shorter UV rays, at midday, tan skin more quickly but results are more temporary and peeling often results.

11 Cloudy days may indicate a lack of sun, but don't be fooled; clouds are full of water, and transmit the sun's rays even if the sun is not visible. A windy day, too, can be deceptive; the wind cools the body, but the sun is as strong!

12 If, after a few minutes of sunbathing, you notice small white lumps or blisters, move into the shade fast — and stay there.

The sun and medications

If you are taking any medications, such as antibiotics, check with your doctor first whether you can lie in the sun; an allergic skin reaction could develop. Some users of the pill find their skin more sensitive, and brown patches might develop on the face owing to hormonal skin reaction to the sun. Use a sunblock! Even aspirin is a hazard: it eliminates redness in pigmentation, so it is not possible to assess degree of tan while in the sun.

After sun treatment

There are many specialised after-sun skin care preparations on the market; few will alleviate sunburn but all will at least moisturise the skin, and prevent surface wrinkling. Always apply a moisturising agent after sunbathing; it will not prevent long-term damage from the sun, but will ease out tiny surface temporary wrinkles which often appear after a short time in the sun. Norman Orentreich, a top American dermatologist, advocates the use of water on the skin before a thin layer of oil is applied for maximum moisturising benefits. Take a shower or bath, pat skin nearly dry with a towel and apply oil or oil-based moisturiser. The oil will seal the moisture in the top layer of skin and make it less likely to evaporate.

The sun and fragrance

Certain scents trigger off allergic skin reactions when exposed to sunlight; bergamot oil is the biggest offender. It is found in many perfumes, and can cause severe burns.

The sun and fluid retention

Your body needs more fluids when you are soaking up the sun: excess perspiration can dehydrate. It is not necessary to take salt pills; simply drink lots of water.

Sunburn soothers

Severe sunburn or sunstroke should, of course, be medically treated but minor sunburn can be eased by the following methods. Sufferers should stay out of the sun until skin is back to normal and wear loose, cotton clothes; synthetics restrict skin "breathing" and tight garments will irritate inflamed skin.

● Israelis use eshel — their form of yogurt — to relieve smarting, red skin. Apply natural yogurt to affected areas and leave to dry, which takes about ten minutes. Gently remove with damp cotton-wool pads.

● In the same way that chilled tea bags, potato and cucumber make good natural cooling agents for inflamed eyes, so can they cool an overheated body. Mash cucumber to a pulp, finely grate raw potato or use cold, strong tea; apply directly to the skin without massaging. Leave on for as long as is felt to be of benefit.

● Dermatologists and doctors recommend Boots' Calamine and Glycerine cream, and Calamine Lotion to soothe inflamed skin.

Artificial tanning

Solariums and sun lamps

The greatest benefit of using a solarium or sun lamp is that your skin is prepared for the sun; used as a pre-sunning conditioning treatment, you will find you can stay in the sun for longer periods and skin will brown more readily. Whether or not a tan is achieved from a course of "sunbathing" with artificial UV rays varies with the individual; after a course of twelve sessions, I remained as white as before! It is advisable to undertake UV sessions under supervision at a solarium in a gym or beauty salon, where your distance from the rays can be accurately gauged, and timing can be checked. The possible pitfalls of using your own sun lamp are: a) you will fall asleep; b) you will over-time your sessions; c) the lamp will be too close to you. Severe burns can be the result of injudicious use of home suntan lamps. Always follow instructions accurately. Moisturise skin after every session and wear special goggles provided; ordinary sunglasses do not offer the same degree of protection.

Cosmetic creams and lotions

If you cannot acquire a natural tan, don't worry. Many models fake their tans with creams that tint the skin about four hours after they have been applied. Fake tanning creams can be applied professionally at beauty salons, but if you follow the pointers below you should achieve equally good results.

● Patch-test fake tanner first; some turn yellow/orange on certain skins, and look browner on others. It is worth trying two or three to find the one most suited to you. Avoid the mousse variety; it tends to be messy and difficult to apply.

● Moisturise elbows, knees, ankles and any skin areas where tanning agent is likely to settle and cause uneven marks.

● Apply cream or lotion with a damp make-up sponge in long, light strokes. Ask a friend to cover difficult-to-reach areas, eg your back, and backs of legs. Remember that the insides of arms never naturally tan as much as backs of arms. You can use fake tanner on your face, though the tint is inclined to emphasise large pores; in this case, you might prefer a temporary staining gel or lotion.

The sun and black skins

It is possible for black skins to burn in the sun, but very unlikely as dark skins have a natural resistance to the harmful effects of sunlight. Also, the skin wrinkles less and loses elasticity slower in the long term. However, precautions should still be observed.

● Wait five minutes before re-applying tanning agent. Do not attempt to fake a colour much darker than you would normally tan; make three shades deeper than your normal skin tone the maximum.

● Be sure to wash — even scrub — hands after application to be sure they do not stain.

● If you find results are less than perfect, slough off "tanned" surface skin in the bath with a loofah or friction mitt; moisturise and re-apply. Do not attempt to correct small areas as blend marks will show.

SLIMMING

Am I slimming for the right reasons? Does water retention affect my weight? Which is the best way for me to lose weight? What is cellulite? If you have ever asked yourself these questions, and hundreds more like them, you will find this chapter compulsive reading. You will find no short cuts to losing weight because sensible, *healthy* dieting is the only method that works, but you will find plenty of encouragement from fellow readers' slimming experiences, plus lots of sound advice from the experts. And when all the facts and fallacies of slimming have been laid bare to you, you can delve into the second section of this chapter: Cosmo's collection of enjoyable, hard-working diets.

Why slim?

If you turned to this chapter with more than a passing interest, you probably already know why you want to be slimmer. Still, it is worth taking a long, hard look at your motives before you start: firstly, because accurate knowledge of *why* you want to slim is the first essential of successful dieting and secondly, because you might find that you are looking to dieting to solve problems that do not have anything to do with your weight.

All of us are insecure to some extent; women especially tend to focus all their insecurities on their looks. How many times have you thought, "Everything would be all right if I were thin", just as, for some girls, it's "Life would be wonderful if I didn't have a big nose" or, "my hands weren't so ugly"? It is not just unhelpful but dangerous to think like this about slimming and expect too much from a diet. The most successful diet in the world will make you thinner but it will not necessarily make your job less boring or your man come back to you. If you expect it to, and it fails to deliver the goods, there is always a danger that you will think it is because you haven't slimmed *enough*. Then dieting becomes an end in itself, irrespective of what weight you have reached, and that is one way to slip into the slimmers' disease, anorexia nervosa.

You can also overestimate what a diet can do for your physical shape. You cannot be Twiggy, any more than you can be Einstein or Beethoven, unless Nature provided you with the basic equipment to work on. That means firstly your build:

if you are large-framed, reducing the fat on your bones won't make you petite. It also means metabolism: just because your friend, who seems to exist on nervous energy and huge gooey cakes, keeps wonderfully thin, it doesn't follow that you, with a slower rate of burning up calories, can have the same figure

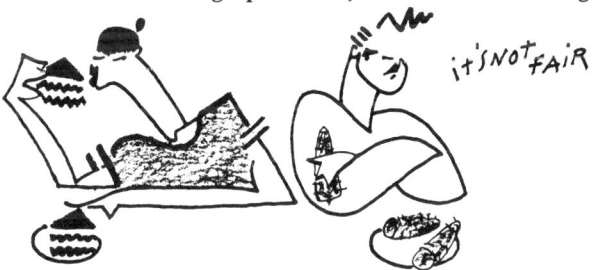

it's NOT FAIR

eating the same foods. This is cause for great bitterness among the fat but it is no use complaining about it. Mould your expectations on reality and on people with your own build and own body shape who look good.

Having made all the reservations about what slimming can do for you, it is worth stressing why you *should* still try to keep your weight down to a reasonable level. Most importantly, it affects your general health. Life assurance companies, who have a professional interest in knowing how long we are likely to last, have come to the conclusion that overweight tends to earlier death, especially if the excess weight first appears in early life, say before thirty-five. Fat people are more likely to suffer from heart and circulatory diseases, diabetes and postoperative complications. General fitness also suffers — if you are fat, you do not feel like running around or playing games, partly through self-consciousness and partly because it is hard work dragging your bulk through strenuous exercise.

Dieting and exercise should proceed together as you go along. The danger of dieting, especially if you lose weight quickly, without exercising at the same time, is that you can get flabby and look *worse* than you did before.

Is fat hereditary?

"It's my glands/genes/cells," is the common cry of the fat girl who likes to blame her overweight on something substantial — other than her desire for food! Of course there are sound medical reasons that make some people unable to lose weight, but more often than not blame is unjustly attributed to heredity. Can fat be inherited? Scientifically controlled tests have indicated that overweight tends to run consistently in families, so that if your parents are overweight, you have a greater chance of being overweight than your friend who has slim parents. But don't sit back and think, "Fine, it's inherited, I'm destined to be fat," because you *can* still lose weight and become slim. Scientists have in fact not fully determined whether overweight parents beget overweight children because of their genes; Professor John Yudkin puts forward the theory that it may be unhealthy *eating patterns* that are inherited!

One thing is clear: your overall body shape is likely to be determined by your predecessors. Wide hips and narrow shoulders may be the shape of every woman in your family, and it is a fact that whichever basic shape you inherit, there is not a great deal you can do to change it.

Should you be on a diet?

If you and the world about you are in general agreement about whether you should be on a diet, there is no real problem. But often, although *you* feel you should lose weight, other people think you are about the right size. This is a problem because you cannot wholly trust other people to be right about the way you are! There are reasons why some people prefer to see you fatter than you would like to be: perhaps slimmer you would threaten *them*. On the other hand, they could be right: we all know at least one girl who looks stunning, worries endlessly about her extra two or three pounds and drives everyone crazy with her pointless diets. With the dangers of complacency on one side and perhaps even anorexia on the other, how can you tell who is right?

The opposite problem occurs when you are getting nagged to lose weight but you do not believe you need to diet. Again, there are all sorts of reasons why some people might want you to diet: an insecure man might think a model-thin girlfriend

will improve *his* image; some people might want to undermine your confidence. On the other side, you might be unwilling to see how fat you are because that involves you in the effort of dieting and guilt for having let yourself get out of hand. So once again, how can you tell who is right?

Here are some checkpoints:

1 Do most weight-charts make you overweight or not? If you cling to just *one* that indicates you should lose weight or one which says, if you allow for large build, heavy bones, water retention etc, you are only a *few* pounds overweight, you are fooling yourself and you should listen to someone else.

2 Can you think of any reason why the people advising you should be lying or mistaken? To balance against this, could you be fooling yourself? Do you deny you are fat but choose not to do things that you would do if you were thinner? Or are you hoping a diet will solve some sort of problem which has nothing to do with your weight? Get some insight into your own and other people's motives and then make up your mind whose judgement to trust.

3 Finally, does your doctor think you are overweight? This is the acid test because the doctor's concern is not with your beauty but with your health. If the doctor says you are too fat, you are. If he says you are not, you should think *very* carefully before dismissing him as an old fuddy-duddy who just doesn't understand about fashion.

Feel slimmer, be slimmer, stay slimmer

It is now widely recognised that obese people do not eat in response to hunger but in response to the way they feel, to habits of eating, to triggers like the sight of food or simply situations which remind them of eating. Such people can put themselves on a diet and lose a great deal of weight. However, if they have not broken the basic pattern of the way they respond to food, the weight will pile back on as soon as the diet ends.

What we are talking about is the difference between appetite and *appestat*. Your appestat controls how much you eat when you are eating normally. When you feel really hungry, that is your appestat "switching on". Your appetite is *how much*

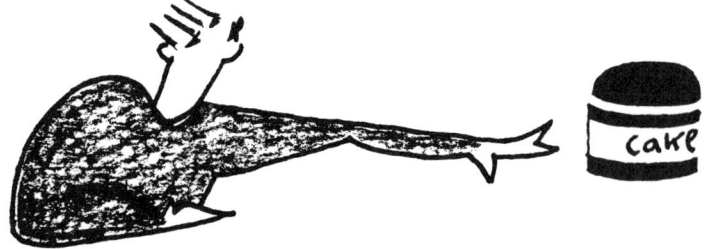

you want to eat, for whatever reason, hunger does not enter into it. Think of what we mean when we say that food is appetising — it looks good, is nicely presented, tickles the tastebuds — it is all about tempting us to eat food that hunger would not prompt us to want. That sort of eating has to be cut out on a diet.

Think about your responses to food, watch yourself when you are eating normally: when your hand reaches out for a slice of bread, what trigger is it responding to? When you have had enough, do you still feel compelled to finish the plate? Why? To avoid waste? Analyse your behaviour to understand it and fight it. Refuse to be manipulated by old habits and taboos. Work out new eating patterns which form a rational response to your real needs. Do not use food as a substitute for any form of comfort.

There is an especially dangerous circle of despair in which we eat for comfort. We need comfort because we feel fat and ugly, we feel fat and ugly because we have been eating for comfort . . . and so on. One way to break out of this vicious circle is to recognise your other strong physical points which do not relate to weight: good hair, good teeth, good skin, good posture are things you can work on *now*. You do not have to wait till you are thin. Try to dress for your gradually diminishing bulk — even if it means swapping clothes with friends. You will not look attractive in baggy, ill-fitting clothes even if you have lost half a stone, and you need the compliments to start rolling in to keep you motivated.

Rules of thumb

Everyone has their own strategy for avoiding the worst temptations, so take your pick from these:

1 Keep out of the kitchen if you do not have to be there.
2 Pamper yourself in non-food ways — there is no need to be a puritan! Long luxurious baths, little pick-me-up presents to yourself, whatever turns you on.
3 Make a point of eating from a smaller plate so that a smaller dinner still looks a "proper" dinner.
4 Do not eat when you are doing something else, like watching TV or reading a book.
5 Get plenty of sleep.
6 Avoid your "danger" emotions — be it nervousness, stress or boredom.
7 Do not have forbidden foods in the house — what is not there cannot tempt.
8 Plan meals in advance: throwing something together may tempt you to throw in something extra.
9 With any processed food, check the ingredients: they should be listed in order, largest proportion first. Avoid anything canned in oil or syrup.

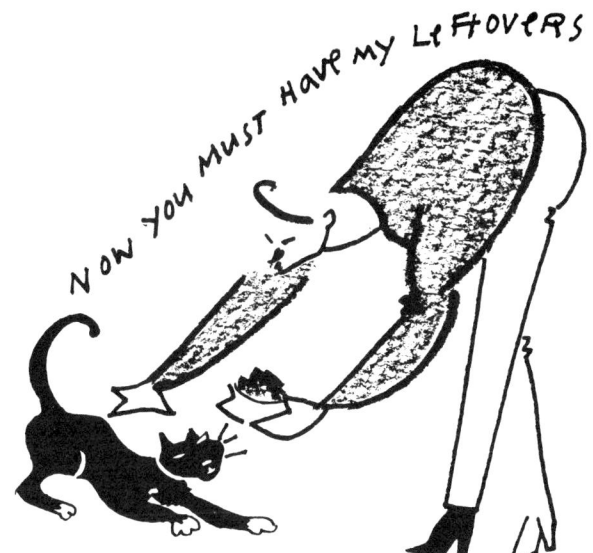

NOW YOU MUST HAVE MY LEFTOVERS

10 If you feel you have had enough to eat, do not be afraid to leave food on your plate, and throw out *all* leftovers. Yes, waste is terrible but if you feel guilty about the Third World, send a donation to Oxfam — eating other people's crusts helps no one. Make sure the throw-outs stay thrown out.

11 Make every meal into an event: eat slowly, sip water with your meal; if you are having a dessert, wait a while before serving it. And, if you can bear it, eat in front of a mirror — the sight of yourself *shovelling* in food will slow you down.

12 Do not wait till you are ravenous to eat or you will lose the ability to control the amount you consume.

13 Do not skip a meal. You will probable resort to little staving-off hunger snacks instead which will tot up calories without your noticing.

14 Substitute skimmed milk for ordinary. You will hardly notice the difference (watch out, though, not all powdered milk is skimmed — avoid those that say they have fat added).

15 Most people *do* notice the difference with butter and sugar substitutes so it might be easier to do without them altogether. Herbal or lemon tea is a refreshing alternative to ordinary tea and coffee and does not use milk or sugar.

16 Cut down on your meat portions, too. Just because meat is full of protein does not mean it has no calories (especially fat meat). In the average meal, meat makes up more calories than bread or potatoes.

17 Bread is often not as bad as what you put on it. Cheese, jam or even butter can double the calories you are taking in with your snack, so stick to savoury spreads like Marmite.

18 If you need to nibble, make it vegetables rather than fruit. Ounce for ounce, fruit has two or three times the calorie content of vegetables.

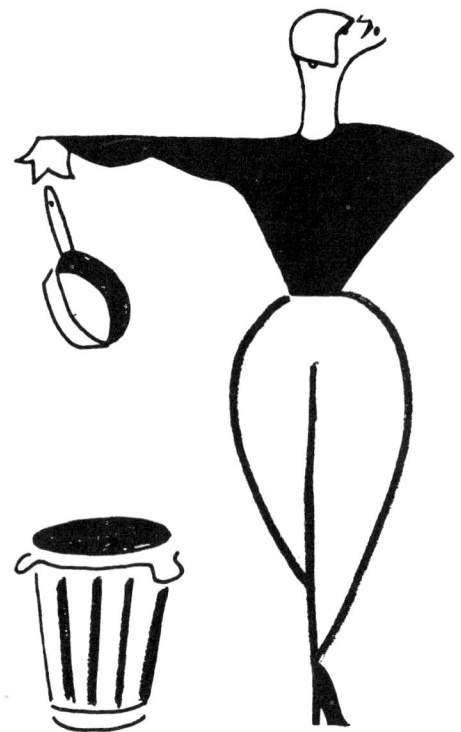

19 Don't eat fried *anything*. Banish the frying-pan from your kitchen.

20 When putting food away, wrap it securely so that it is harder to nibble absent-mindedly.

21 Never sit if you can stand, never stand when you can walk, never walk when you can run. It all helps burn calories.

22 Stay *out* of fast food restaurants. Hamburgers may not be fattening if you discard the bun, but there are always the French fries to be discarded, too. . .

23 Never let the waiter in a restaurant put a basket of rolls on the table; he will not be offended if you ask him to remove them.

24 Wait a little after your main course before you decide if you still need a dessert. Give food a chance to tell your brain — via your stomach — whether you are hungry or not. Five minutes can make all the difference.

25 When you order your low-calorie side salad at a restaurant, ask for it to be served without dressing: do not kid yourself you can shake it off the lettuce leaves!

26 Use herbs and spices instead of sugar, salt, alcohol and artificial flavourings in food. They are more slimming and you will find your cooking will liven up, too.

27 Buy a pair of blue jeans, a sexy slit skirt or skinny silk shirt

— one size too small. Keep it in your wardrobe where you will see it, constantly, for the best slimming incentive you could have.

28 Chew your food slowly and thoroughly: you will better appreciate it and, by not bolting it down, less will seem like more.

Emergency–"I must eat something in the next few minutes or go crazy"-tips

1 Have a hot drink — something savoury like *bouillon*, Bovril or consommé.

2 Eat vegetable nibbles that are ready prepared in the fridge.

3 Tackle a fiddly, intricate job, like mending a plug, which occupies your hands *and* brain.

4 Ring someone or write a letter.

5 Clean your teeth.

6 Drink a glass of iced water.

Shopping for a diet

In an ideal world, the slimmer would avoid supermarkets altogether — the consumer psychology and seductive "come-buy" siren song is fatal to any diet. Still, for most of us, it is something to be faced, so how best to tackle it?

1 Do not shop when you are hungry and more likely to fancy things that are not really necessary.

2 Take a shopping list with you, and stick to it.

3 One major danger point is when you have finished the bulk of your shopping at the far end of the store and your path back to the check-outs is booby-trapped with crisps, fruit cordials, tinned fruit and sweets. Fortunately there is usually one escape route via the washing powder, bleach and dog biscuits. Take that one.

4 The other major danger point is when you are waiting in the queue beside the racks of sweets laid out to catch last-minute waverers: if possible, use the six-item-or-less check-outs which do not have them. Otherwise, if there's a long queue and you can't resist, buy one of the magazines which are also sold at the check-outs, turn to the short story or the knitting (not the cookery pages) and lose yourself in it till it is your turn to be served.

Slimming foods

While some people have lost weight by using special slimming foods and aids, there is reason to doubt their usefulness to the average dieter. Apart from the expense, there is the question of building up healthy eating patterns: milk shakes, chocolate bars and biscuits, even with vitamins and nutrients added, do not make a good basis for long-term dieting. That is not to say that you should not use them, as long as they suit you, and as

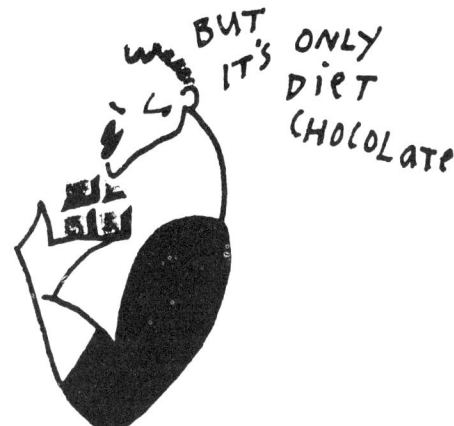

long as you only use them occasionally. (Most of them carry a warning that you should only replace three meals a day under supervision from your doctor.)

Do make sure you know how many calories they contain; the average serving is designed to make up about a third of your daily allowance. We all know the story of the fat girl who was eating diet chocolate as *well* as her meals — it won't work.

Cellulite

Just mention cellulite (pronounced cell-u-leet) these days and you are up to your ears in controversy. For one set of experts, it describes the lumpy fat that accumulates on thighs and buttocks and which, when pinched, dimples like orange skin (the French, who first identified it, also call it *peau d'orange*). For another set of experts, it is simply a fancy name for fat!

The case for

It is a fact that even malnutrition victims have been found to have fat deposits around the cellulite-prone areas. If this fat cannot be dieted away, it is as well to recognise it, rather than go below your healthy weight just because you have large thighs or a big backside. Also, the fact that this puckering fat only occurs in women seems to suggest a hormonal cause rather than simple overeating.

The case against

The sceptics argue that cellulite is not very different from other fat and does not need special treatment. They point out that many of the experts who say it does often also offer their own patent remedies — at a price!

If you are normal weight but are troubled by isolated problem areas, try the hydrotherapy treatments in the Body section and spot-reducing exercises described in the Exercise section. You should find they help firm up flab, but do not expect drastic reduction: you cannot radically alter your basic body shape.

It's (almost) all in the mind

First the bald, bad news: if you want to get thinner, you have to eat less. Next, the good news: eating less is not hard, at least, not *physically* hard. You are standing in front of an open packet of biscuits. Looking at it objectively, it requires no hard physical effort to simply close the packet and put it away in the cupboard. Still you cannot do it, or at least not until you have eaten just one, and perhaps kept a second one out for later.

Why is it so difficult? Because it is in the mind that the diet battle is won or lost. You will never get far with your diet if you regard it as something you do primarily with or to your *body*. In many ways, the dieter is still like the child, obeying all sorts of impulses to eat other than just plain hunger. To stop you doing this, try to find out *why* you eat. For a day or two before your diet, observe yourself eating normally. Carry a notebook and jot down what you eat, when and *why* you have eaten it. Do not just write "hungry" every time — that may be right for your evening meal but you cannot then put it for your sweet course or the after-dinner glass of wine.

Soon you should be able to see that, if this Mars Bar is boredom and that gin and tonic is nervousness, by cutting out boredom and nervousness you could cut down calories without ever having to fight real hunger.

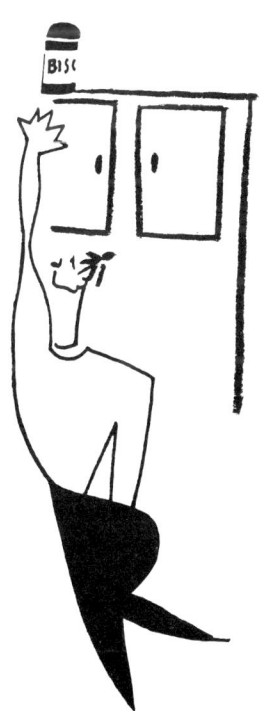

Water retention: Does it affect your weight?

Water retention is one of those old, old excuses for people who put off dieting with the "It's not that I'm fat, it's just . . ." routine. "It's just water retention, it's just heavy bones, it's just these particular scales."

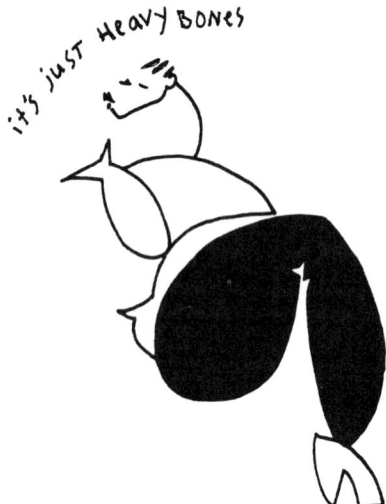

it's just Heavy Bones

Water makes up about 60 per cent of your body weight and the amount of water will fluctuate relatively little from day today: it will account for perhaps a pound or two in normal circumstances. Sometimes women retain too much water just before a period and the doctor may prescribe a mild diuretic to help eliminate it. You should not prescribe water reducing tablets for yourself or take them for long periods of time: if they do make you lose weight, it is only because they interfere with your normal bodily functions. The body needs water so that the kidneys can process the sodium in our bodies; the amount of sodium determines how much water the body retains. Fasts, high-protein and low-carbohydrate diets are all marked by rapid weight loss at the very early stages. This is because they interfere with the kidneys' ability to retain sodium, therefore bringing down the body's water level. The water level will re-establish itself fairly quickly, so that this loss will only be temporary unless it is followed up with a steady calorie-reduced diet. Both high-protein and low-carbohydrate diets can do this successfully in the long term, so it is fine to use them just as long as you are not fooled by your apparently "miraculous" early success.

Be careful not to accumulate extra water when there is no need: over-salting food, for example, is unnecessary and leads to extra water retention. Drinking too much alcohol also increases water retention, giving a bloated feeling over and above those extra calories it gives you. *Note:* To save confusion over what is water — and what isn't — always weigh yourself first thing in the morning, after you have been to the lavatory, and before you have eaten anything. This will probably be your lowest weight for the day!

How they lost weight–and how you could too

Follow the case histories of five Cosmo readers who all lost considerable amounts of weight through lesser-known regimes. Their methods may not necessarily work for you — and please check with your doctor if you decide to copy — but at least they will spur you on to higher goals!

Caroline Neal, a nineteen-year-old Cambridge student, is 1.74 m (5 ft 8½ in), and once weighed 84 kg (12½ stone). She had tried many diets, but always put back any weight she had lost as soon as she started to eat normally again. Doctors only told her the obvious: eat less. Finally, she consulted a homeopathic doctor who diagnosed that the hormonal glands which affect weight control were not functioning properly in her case. The diet he devised, based on the celebrated Dr Bircher-Benner's theories on the value of raw food, was aimed to correct this problem: for reasons not fully understood, the hormonal glands are stimulated by roughage together with vitamin C, so the diet consisted of limitless quantities of fruit and raw vegetables.

For breakfast, Caroline had one cup of raspberry leaf tea, bran and fruit; for lunch and supper, a salad. She was allowed a piece of fruit mid-morning and mid-afternoon, but could not have any liquid apart from the tea at breakfast, as the fruit and vegetables supplied sufficient water for the body's needs. Caroline was instructed to eat lots of watercress daily due to its high iodine content, necessary for the proper functioning of the thyroid gland.

Initially, Caroline was put on the diet for one week only, but she felt so healthy and active on it that she continued for two months, during which time she lost 13 kg (two stone). One of the main benefits of the diet was that it had results beyond a temporary weight loss: on a two-week holiday she made no attempt to diet, and only gained half a kilogram (one pound). This would seem to substantiate the doctors' theories on sluggish glands, and could be good news for despondent dieters who have resigned themselves to a size 16 future with a sigh of, "It's my glands"!

After the birth of her second child, journalist Frankie McGowan was shocked to be told by her doctor that the surplus 4.5 kg (10 lb) around her stomach and legs was nothing to do with "post-baby flab" as she had thought —it was *fat*. Horrified at the thought of following a strict diet, Frankie decided to devise her own eating plan around general nutritional guidelines. If breakfast is good for you, then two breakfasts must be twice as good, was the philosophy behind a bowl of Special K for breakfast, and another bowl for lunch.

Frankie's second ruling — no eating between meals — was an easy rule to follow, because she found that the high protein content in Special K meant she felt no hunger pangs throughout the day. In the evening she would have a balanced meal, cutting out starchy foods like bread, potatoes and pasta. She had an average portion of meat or fish, plus a salad with French dressing, and a glass of wine. In addition, Frankie allowed herself *one* treat each day, such as a small portion of apple pie, or ice cream. Frankie combined her diet with special postnatal exercises to strengthen stomach muscles, and within six weeks was down to her usual weight of 52.5 kg (8 st 4 lb). Her brief experience of dieting seems to have taught her a lot more than most "seasoned" dieters: she continues to exercise (in the evening while her bath is running) and is now a confirmed believer in the value of breakfast, finding that it leads to a much more balanced diet as a whole.

"I've discovered that I don't like food and never have done really," claims a girl who used to eat more than her father and brother together and who weighed 84 kg (12½ stone) at 1.60 m (5 ft 3 in) on leaving boarding school! Gillian Kemp, now a twenty-five-year-old estate agent, tried all the usual diets from starvation to Weight Watchers and though she managed to reduce to 77.5 kg (11½ stone), mainly as a result of leaving behind boarding school stodge, felt that she was not getting to the root of her problems.

Depression over her weight only led Gillian to eat more, until she met a physiotherapist who has had great success in treating overweight people. His treatment consists of diet, figure-shaping exercises and a hard, and at first painful, massage to help break down cellulite deposits. Guided by the physiotherapist, for three months Gillian ate only fruit, vegetables and one meat meal per day: an average portion of grilled chicken or steak. Liquid intake was kept to a minimum. After one month, she had lost 6 kg (1 stone) and now, after a year of supervised treatment, Gillian weighs 54.5 kg (8 st 8lb) and can eat normally, although food is still psychologically something of a problem. Gillian is aware of what she eats almost to the extent of being frightened of food, as she remembers the power it once had over her!

Exercise was obviously a vital part of success: her figure is firm and trim, and shows no sign of the flabbiness that can accompany weight loss by diet alone. She exercises for several minutes each morning, and believes that fitness enables you to cope with anything.

Gillian has a strong philosophical attitude which she has developed towards dieting. She believes that losing weight is essentially a very long process, just as it takes a long time to put on weight. Ultimately, dieting is something you have to want to do, and to do by yourself; it's no use being told by other people not to eat something, because that only makes you resentful, which throws you back on to your oldest friend and comforter, food. Most important of all is mental discipline and putting food and yourself into perspective: "Most people live to eat: it should be the other way round".

Sue Young suffered badly from water retention. When in desperation she went to see a homeopathic doctor, her body was swollen and she looked six months pregnant. She was told that her problem was linked to her lifestyle: a photographic agent and mother of a six-year-old child, she suffered from constipation as well as water retention — both conditions which can be linked to stress. The regime prescribed for her was thus aimed at reducing both water retention and stress.

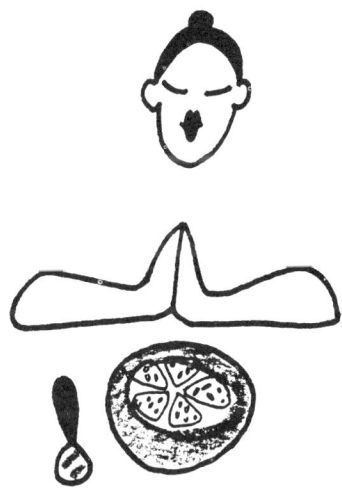

For one week Sue was put on a very strict fast: the first day, nothing *at all* to eat or drink; the second and third day, half a grapefruit three times a day; the fourth and fifth day, a whole grapefruit three times a day, and the sixth and seventh day, a small bunch of grapes three times a day. After this, she followed a basic diet of muesli with yogurt for breakfast, fruit and cheese for lunch and in the evening a "normal" meal, with certain foods forbidden: animal fats, bread, potatoes, spinach, tomatoes, spirits and coffee. The basic ruling was never to leave a meal feeling bloated, and to have the last meal of the day before 9 pm.

The diet meant adapting her lifestyle: she only allows herself the occasional "social" glass of wine, and has to avoid late-night restaurant meals. Meat is not forbidden, but is not recommended, and after a while Sue found she could easily forego it.

After eight weeks, Sue's weight dropped from 65 kg (10 st 3 lb) to 58 kg (9 st 2 lb), quite average for her height of 1.65 m (5 ft 5 in), and she lost 50 mm (2 in) from her hips and 40 mm (1½ in) from her waist. She had spots for the first time in years, but they do, she feels, testify to the effectiveness of the diet, as they are the body's way of ridding itself of impurities; an added bonus was the improved condition of her hair and nails.

Sue was advised to follow the diet for a further two months, but was so happy with the results — and felt so much healthier than before — that she feels she might adopt the diet as a life-time regime.

Lynn Bednash gradually and steadily increased her weight to nearly 108 kg (17 stone); the more she looked at herself, the more she ate. When she heard of a cousin in America who lost forty pounds in three months at a clinic, Lynn decided that drastic action, with no expense spared, was called for. "I made a reservation and told everybody I was going so I *had* to achieve what I set out to." On her return four months later, Lynn had lost 32 kg (5 stone), and felt marvellous.

The "clinic" is called The Rice House, and is part of a university medical centre in Carolina. The diet Lynn followed was originally evolved for patients suffering from high blood pressure, kidney trouble and diabetes, but it was discovered that it was a healthy and successful way for obese people to lose weight. The Rice Diet is based on a totally salt-free, fat-free regime; no dairy goods at all are permitted. The protein content in the diet is derived from rice, is high quality and of the type easily assimilated by the body. Daily liquid allowance: 910 ml (32 fl oz) of tea, water, decaffeinated coffee or fresh lemonade made with artificial sweetener.

Initially the patient is given a total medical check-up — three days of intensive tests — so that the diet can be tailored to suit individual requirements. Lynn's high cholesterol count meant she could have no red meat or eggs. For breakfast she was allowed half a grapefruit and a cup of black coffee; lunch and supper (the latter at 4.30 — the doctors at The Rice House believe food is not metabolised after 6 pm) a small bowl of steamed white rice and two pieces of fruit, or any two helpings of different canned fruit. The fruit could be any variety, but as the potassium level of the body drops when salt content is removed from the diet, Lynn was encouraged to eat a banana at least twice a week as they are rich in potassium. After three weeks, Lynn was permitted to substitute vegetables for fruit; celery, spinach and parsley were not allowed, as they are high

in salt. Daily workouts in the gym ensured Lynn firmed up her body as the weight came off.

Lynn still adheres to a salt-free diet, seasoning foods with black pepper, and whenever she wants to crash diet she returns to the rice and fruit bowls for two to three days. "I'm not embarrassed to take my own slimming meal — perhaps a piece of plain boiled chicken — to dinner parties. I've kept my largest pair of jeans, so whenever I'm tempted to slip back into my old ways, I just pull them out of the wardrobe. It always works!"

Food myths

Dieters are always being bombarded with so-called "miracle foods" or "wonder diets". Newer and more bizarre ones are popping up all the time but perhaps we should scotch a few of the old faithfuls once and for all.

1 *No* food "burns up" calories. There is the story that boiled eggs take more calories to digest than they contain, but that is nonsense. So is the claim that grapefruit dissolves fat. That does not mean, of course, that both grapefruit and boiled eggs cannot contribute to a calorie-controlled diet.

2 There are always new fad diets coming along which offer amazing weight loss if you eat nothing but oranges or peanuts or bananas and spinach three times a day. Sometimes they can produce a weight loss, sometimes they cannot, but the important point is that a diet of a single food or kind of food can be extremely dangerous if continued beyond twenty-four or forty-eight hours. Dieters need a balanced diet like anyone else (see chapter on Nutrition) and faddish diets can result in serious deficiencies of vitamins, minerals and other essential elements of a healthy diet. On top of this, two days of eating lettuce, say, does not give you any basis for reforming your long-term eating patterns, which is the only way to permanent weight loss.

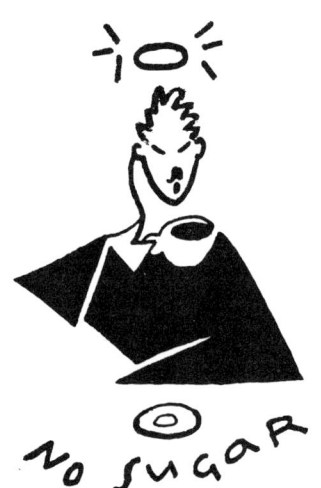

NO SUGAR

3 Do not believe people who say sugar is an essential part of your diet because it gives you energy. Energy is measured in calories and any food which contains calories gives you energy. The trouble with sugar is that it does not give you anything else: proteins, vitamins, etc. Nutritionists argue about all foods but they are fairly unanimous in condemning sugar as dangerous. Do not think of glucose as an alternative to sugar; it tastes less sweet than normal sugar (sucrose) but is barely less fattening.

4 You may be a glutton for many foods but it is unlikely that you can become addicted to them in the way a smoker, say, is addicted to cigarettes. The only exceptions are alcohol and, according to some experts, sugar. Your irresistible craving for peanuts is therefore purely psychological, not physical!

5 There is *no* point in trying to diet by eating diabetic foods. These are designed to cut out sugar, not calories and are, for the most part, just as fattening as their sugary counterparts (and usually much more expensive).

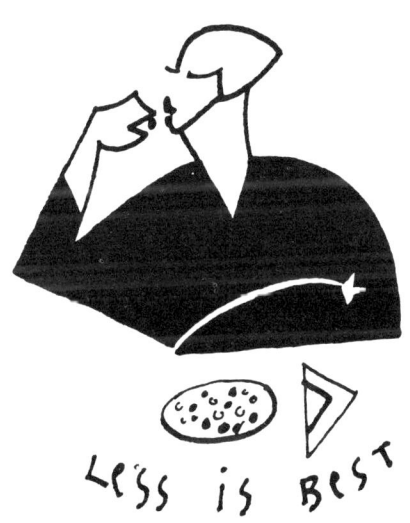

6 Health foods are health foods and *not* slimming foods. Wholemeal bread, free-range eggs and home-baked biscuits have a lot going for them but less calories than their mass-produced counterparts isn't one of them! Vegetarians tend to have fewer weight problems but this is less to do with the simple fact of cutting out meat than their general attitude toward food: they take note of and are concerned about what they are eating, an attitude would-be successful slimmers have to acquire. It is worthwhile noting that the high roughage content in the vegetarian's diet allows him to feel satisfied on less. If you are in doubt, eat wholemeal bread for breakfast one morning, and processed bread the next. You will find you eat far less of the wholemeal variety, as the high fibre content makes it more filling, yet does not add any calories. Lots of roughage in a diet — and that includes raw fruits and vegetables — keeps the digestive system in good working order: regular elimination helps keep weight down, too!

Slimming clubs: could they work for you?

If your dieting will-power levels off at around zero — and you like sharing your desperation — you might find that a slimming club, where you pool your problems and confess your lapses — is the answer. Slimming clubs work on the principle of Alcoholics Anonymous: you confess you are hooked, and you are with people who are, joy, as addicted as you. You encourage one another to kick the habit, in this case, eating too much of the wrong foods. You are given a target weight, the club's diet plan is explained to you and you meet once a week to be weighed, and report progress.

Many weak-willed slimmers who have tried all diets and failed, achieve success with slimming clubs because they have the strength and support of the others in the club: rather than be humiliated by confessing to eating ten biscuits which accounts for those extra two pounds (yes you *are* weighed in front of everyone) they don't eat those ten biscuits. If they lose two pounds they are made to feel so good about it that they are encouraged to continue.

Sounds like the system could work for you? Contact one of the two biggest and most successful slimming organisations in the country for your nearest branches: Weight Watchers, Group Therapy Classes, 635 Ajax Avenue, Slough, Berks, Slough 70711; Slimming Magazine Slimming Clubs, 4 Clareville Grove, London SW7, 01-370 4411.

Fasting

It cannot be stressed enough that continuous fasting is not a satisfactory or healthy way to lose weight. The dieter who lives on cups of black coffee for days lives on her nerves alone, and though she will suffer drastic weight loss at first, will be in poor health. There is little point in being thin if you feel — and look — awful! However, the occasional fast — to cleanse and purify the system — makes an ideal introduction to a healthy and balanced diet plan, or can be used as a weight-loss regime on a weekend where you will be fairly sedentary, and will burn less calories than on a working weekday — when you *need* greater food intake. For more on the right way to fast, see **The Plus Properties of Fasting** on p 9 of the Nutrition chapter.

How much should you weigh?

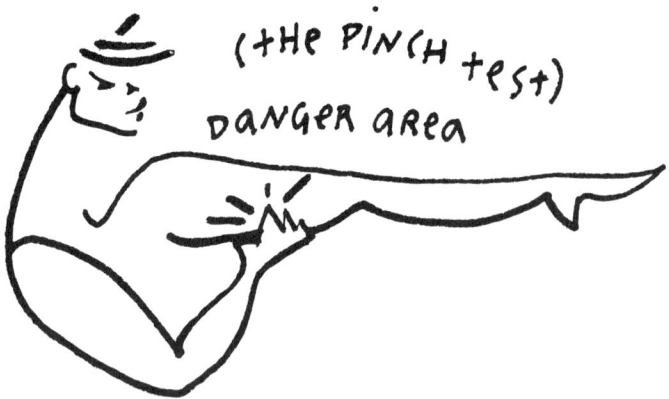

(the PINCH test)
DANGER area

If you feel you are too fat, try the pinch test. Grab a "danger area" — tops of thighs, upper arms or stomach — between finger and thumb. If you can grab a substantial fold of flesh, you should be without it!

For a more accurate guide on the correct *healthy* body size for your height and frame, consult the Weight and Height Chart on p 152 of the Health chapter.

Anorexia nervosa: The slimmer's disease

Anorexia describes the mental and physical condition where a slimmer has become totally obsessive about dieting, to the extent that she worries about how much one grape can add to her weight. It is an alarming, self-deceptive disease that distorts the sufferer's brain — and eye — so that she sincerely believes she is enormously fat when she is in fact so thin that in some cases she is suffering from malnutrition. Consequences are severe and can involve long periods of hospital internment and/or permanent internal malfunctions.

The causes of anorexia are complex but the classic example is the emotionally disturbed slimmer who believes that if she becomes slim and svelte her problems will be at an end. Anorexia is mostly confined to adolescents, although women experiencing menopause are sometimes affected. This frightening disease should prove to *you*, whatever your age, that being obsessive about your weight is not only boring but dangerous, and that only slow and steady dieting will bring about a healthy weight loss. For advice or help on anorexia, go to your doctor.

Drugs: Can they help you lose weight?

Ten or fifteen years ago drugs such as amphetamines and barbiturates were commonly prescribed by doctors as an aid to dieters: amphetamines to suppress the appetite, barbiturates to calm the nerves. It is now recognised that these drugs are not only dangerously addictive, but of very temporary value in a diet, and no doctor will prescribe them for dieters.

Emphasis now is on weight loss by controlled, or in some cases crash, diet. Even extreme cases who are hospitalised to cut them off from temptation will find that drugs play next to no part in the treatment. If they are prescribed anything besides their stringent calorie-controlled diet, it may be the drug Fenfluramine, which although related to the amphetamines, is not addictive.

Diuretics

A diuretic makes you lose water, not fat. As soon as you stop taking it the water, and hence the weight of the water, is once again retained by your body. The effect of rapidly losing weight but then putting most of it back on again can be such a disappointment that the patient abandons the accompanying diet which is the real basis of long-term weight loss.

Slimming foods

Diet rolls and biscuits contain the compound methyl cellulose. This expands in the stomach to give a feeling of fullness so that you eat less at mealtimes. These products certainly do no harm and can train you to need less food, but the moment of truth comes when you give them up.

The value of exercise in a diet

1 High weight loss accompanied by no exercise results in folds of flab settling on your new slimmer silhouette.
2 Exercise burns up fat.

The above two facts should convince you of the merits of exercising during a weight-loss plan, as should the opinions of this doctor who is medical adviser to Weight Watchers: "To have energy you must expend energy. After ten minutes of exercise, circulation increases, more oxygen is carried to all parts of the body, and you feel good, whereas if you try to reduce merely by not eating, you're running your body machine on low power and will feel sluggish. Some women won't lose a single pound on a diet of two thousand calories per day. The reason of course is that they're not exercising. Their calorie intake is low enough to keep them from gaining further weight, but not low enough to cause their bodies to burn fat already there."

Remember that the more vigorous the exercise, the more fat will be consumed. If you want to know just how much weight you are losing — while you are shaping up your body — consult our chart of the most popular sports, and approximately how many calories each of them burns in an hour:

Jogging	600
Swimming	600
Disco dancing	600

Tennis (singles)	500
Cycling	450
Tennis (doubles)	400
Walking (vigorously)	350
Golf	300
Walking (moderately)	200

Slow, slow, quick, quick, slow...

The best way to lose weight is gradually. Everyone is agreed on that: it allows the skin to shrink back while still retaining good tone; it involves the restructuring of long-term eating patterns, which is the best path to permanent weight loss; it allows the dieter, by exercising regularly during gentle weight loss, to avoid any ghastly post-diet flabbiness. Yes, everyone is agreed . . . except the dieter. Never mind today, she wants to be thin *yesterday*. So how can we reconcile desire with reality?

It is really up to you to decide what you, as a dieter, need, and what you can stand. If you know you need a short sharp weight loss to get you going, try one of the three-day or one-week diets we have given you. You can also try them in the middle of a long-term regime if you seem to be flagging. On the other hand, if you are forever losing weight quickly then putting it all back on again as soon as you come off the diet, in a compensatory binge, the only thing to do, sad to say, is to put all short-term diets behind you and plan for at least three months of sensible eating.

The three-month diet is fundamentally different from the three-day diet and should be approached differently if it is to work. On a three-day diet, you say "no" to an eclair with the subconscious reassurance that you're only *putting off* the day when you can safely eat that eclair. If you are three-month dieting, you must say no to eclairs for the foreseeable future. You have to learn to see it as a no-no rather than the prize you will award yourself if you lose a few pounds. You have to learn not to want the forbidden.

You *have* to say goodbye to certain foods for three months. Can you bear it? In a lot of cases you can without martyring yourself. We tend to eat a lot of foods because they are there rather than because we really relish them. Those foods you really cannot resist must just be avoided. Do not have them in the house if you are in charge of the shopping. If your danger-point is when the tea-lady comes round with the tea and biscuits, don't try to resist the chocolate digestives, *avoid* them. For example, take to drinking orange juice instead of tea — it might have more calories than black tea but if you are likely to be tempted into having milk and just one sugar, orange is your best bet, the added bonus is that you will not be tempted by biscuits because there is something particularly *un*appetising about orange juice and biscuits.

If you are tempted to buy chocolate every morning when you go into the newsagent's for a paper, switch to a news-stand, away from temptation. If it is usual to hand sweets round the office, there is no need to make a fuss about refusing — just explain that you will not be *buying* them in future so it would not be fair to take one — most people will not press you after that.

The better prepared you are each day, the better chance you have of a successful day's dieting. It is all very well to *try* to keep to something light at lunchtime but if you have actually prepared a lunch-box of filling, low-calorie salad, you will more likely than not eat it, and then you are less likely to be tempted to have beefburger and French fries.

Are you a lion or a donkey dieter?

You know about crash diets, faddy diets, long-term diets, diets that let you eat fat, diets that let you eat anything but. . . It seems that there are different diets for every circumstance. If you have gone all through the various kinds of diets but have not found anything that works, it could be that you don't need a different diet — but to recognise that you are a different kind of dieter.

Are you a donkey dieter?
Most of us are. Dieting donkeys are ordinary folk who want to be slimmer, do not really want to diet and so have to be beaten, dragged, cajoled or pushed until they finally reach their goal and can relax. Most slimming clubs work on the donkey dieter, as do most diets. Their major weapon is guilt. You must feel guilty if you overeat. At most slimming clubs, weight-gain is announced to the multitude so that you can be properly ashamed of yourself; weight loss wins congratulations and fuss. That is the way they train chimpanzees, performing dogs and donkeys and that is the way they train dieters. It works. You can see how it works over and over again as people lose phenomenal amounts of weight. But it does not work for everybody. If you tend to eat for comfort anyway, anything that makes you feel miserable and guilty has great dangers. If you have ever eaten an illicit chocolate biscuit and felt so much guilt and self-disgust that you have to finish the whole packet to cheer yourself up again, you might consider the possibility that you are not cut out to be a donkey dieter.

Could you be a lion dieter?
Being a lion dieter is both easier and harder than being a donkey. It is easier because you do not have to feel miserable on your diet, even after an occasional backslide. It is harder because you have to make every step along the way by yourself. It means you have to have more will-power (rather than the donkey dieter who is powered less by will-power than by guilt that she has none). The lion dieter has to be prepared to say,

"I'm overweight, I've eaten too much, I'll have to eat less in the future," and then *stick to it*. The donkey dieter, if offered a chocolate biscuit, will say "Don't tempt me," the lion will say,

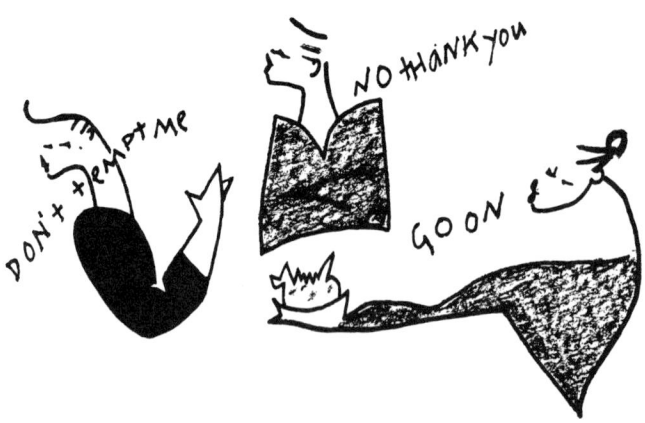

"No thank you". Once she has made up her mind not to overeat, she is too proud to let her will be overcome by something as silly and unnecessary as a chocolate biscuit.

The lion's testament
The lion's diet is more likely to be a long, slow, steady one than a crash diet. Something is needed to sustain her through the months and she will carry her testament in her head at all times:

1 A diet is a private contract between my mind and my body. I do not owe it to anyone else to get slim; I do not cheat anyone else if I give in.

2 Fat is bad for me but it is not immoral. If I sneak an extra bar of chocolate on top of my allowance, I am not wicked, just weak and silly.

3 If I do backslide, that is no excuse for giving up; I will just have to diet that much longer, which is annoying, but not the end of the world.

4 I am an intelligent human being; I refuse to be deflected from my chosen course by anything as trivial as unnecessary food.

Number 4 contains the key to the different kinds of dieters — only a lion could possibly think of food as trivial. A donkey dieter always thinks of food as important and, in general, the longer she diets, the more important it will seem.

Pick the kind of diet that suits *you*. If a donkey tried to stick to a lion's diet, she would not lose any weight at all. If a lion tried to stick to a donkey's diet she might make a little headway, then grow so fed up that she would put back twice as much weight in defiance. If you have tried several diets unsuccessfully as a donkey, think about trying one as a lion . . . or vice versa!

DIETS

For Diet read Discipline. Whichever diet plan you follow, you must be prepared to sacrifice favourite foods, forego lifelong eating habits. Be comforted that by adhering to a sound slimming diet, you are breaking those bad habits and developing good ones, eg, increasing water intake, cutting out snacks between meals.

Any successful diet *reduces calorie intake*. Good diets do this while offering you a healthy and varied eating plan; the fad diets may instruct you to cut out protein, eat only carrots or gorge on fats alone, but they are all based on the calorie-reduction principle. You will find no fad diets on these pages; the emphasis, whether the diet is a two-day semi-fast or a five-day eating plan, is on a balanced regime with a sensible weight-loss limit that will leave you feeling healthy — possibly healthier than when you began the diet!

Some of the diets will be more suited to you than others: there are diets designed for those who can't resist sweet foods, for those who crave snacks, for those who don't need strict discipline but can have the freedom to select from food groups.

Read through a diet carefully from beginning to end before you decide if it feels "right" for you. Many of these diets you will have heard of or read before on the pages of Cosmo; you see them again on these pages because we know they *work*.

The importance of following an exercise regime while dieting cannot be emphasised too strongly. Hanging folds of slack skin are a too-familiar sight after a heavy weight-loss regime and can be avoided if a regular exercise plan is developed; see Exercise chapter for inspiration!

Only while you are on a semi-fast or fast should you adopt a *temporarily* more sedentary regime.

IMPORTANT If you are under medical supervision, or feel for any reason that you are not in sound health, you *must* consult your doctor before embarking on any new diet. If you feel faint or dizzy at any time during a diet, stop immediately. Remember that a diet is not an endurance test — it should be enjoyed!

To count or not to count calories?

Perhaps the most classic way of losing weight is to count calories. The dedicated calorie counter knows, either by heart or her chart which she is never without, how many calories are in a pretzel, large steak, three acid drops or a large helping of Dutch chocolate ice-cream. Calorie counting can be a sound way of losing weight *provided* you are not tempted to eat by calories alone, and lose awareness of nutritional values; you may only eat 900 calories if you consume apple pie and ice-cream for one day, but you will hardly be doing your body a

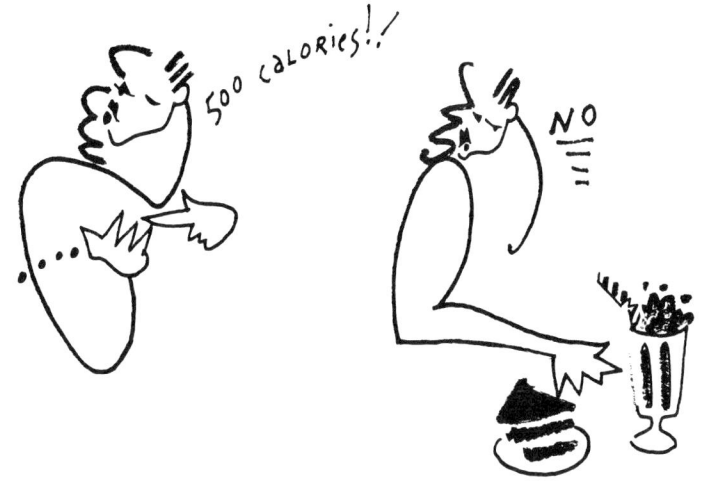

favour. Beware the other danger: becoming a Calorie Bore, regaling others with "Did you know those carrots/sprouts/breadsticks etc you are eating contain 100/200/300 calories?" Keep your calorie counts to yourself — and be aware of your nutritional intake as well as your calorie intake — and the counting-calorie theory of losing weight could work for you.

Average daily calorie count for the cautious dieter? 1000 calories. Less than that, and you are on the way to a semi-fast diet; if you choose a diet of 500 calories a day, you should follow it on a sedentary day when you are relaxed and not working. Below, you will find Cosmo's comprehensive calorie count chart to study!

Calorie chart

The dieter cannot live by calorie counting alone, for she knows the importance of a balanced regime. But it is helpful to know just how fattening (or slimming) a food is. Here we cover all the foods you are likely to eat or want to eat with their calorie content listed alongside, plus warning symbols that denote which foods you can eat plentifully (G), which foods you may eat in moderation (P) and which foods you should cut out completely (R).

PRODUCT	MEASURE	CALORIES	
Anchovy paste	5 ml (1 tsp)	14	G
Apples	1 medium, raw 125 g (4 oz)	40	G
Apricots	125 g (4 oz)	48	G
	dried 125 g (4 oz)	208	R
Artichoke	125 g (4 oz)	20	G
Asparagus	125 g (4 oz)	20	G
Aubergine	125 g (4 oz)	20	G
Avocado	half (without dressing)	125	P
Bacon	lean, grilled, 50 g (2 oz)		
	(2 rashers)	185	P
	fat, grilled, 50 g (2 oz)	350	R
Baked beans	125 g (4 oz) tinned in tomato sauce	100	P
Beans	125 g (4 oz) broad, boiled	48	G
	125 g (4 oz) runner, boiled	8	G
Beef	125 g (4 oz) corned	264	P
	125 g (4 oz) silverside, boiled	344	P
	125 g (4 oz) sirloin, lean, roast	256	P
Beef steak	125 g (4 oz) grilled	330	P
Biscuits	Cream cracker (one)	40	R
	Digestive (one large)	60	R
	Water biscuit (one)	30	R
Bovril	10 ml (2 tsp)	12	G
Bread	brown (1 slice)	52	R
	white (1 slice)	52	R
	Slimcea, white/brown (1 slice)	32	P
Broccoli	125 g (4 oz) boiled	16	G
Butter	25 g (1 oz)	220	R
Cabbage	125 g (4 oz) boiled	8	G
Celery	2 large raw sticks	10	G
	hearts, canned 125 g (4 oz)	4	G
Cheese			
Camembert	25 g (1 oz) portion	88	G
Cheddar	25 g (1 oz) portion	120	G
Cream	25 g (1 oz) portion	232	R
Edam	25 g (1 oz) portion	88	G
Gorgonzola	25 g (1 oz) portion	112	G
Spreads	25 g (1 oz) portion	82	G
Cottage cheese	25 g (4 oz) carton	132	G
Chicken	125 g (4 oz) portion, roast, weighed with bone	116	G
	125 g (4 oz) portion, roast	216	P
	75 g livers (3 oz portion)	120	G
Chocolate	Dairy Milk 125 g (4 oz)	653	R
	Wholenut, 125 g (4 oz)	665	R
	plain, 125 g (4 oz)	640	R
Chutney	20 ml (1 heaped tbsp)	122	R
Cod	steamed, 125 g (4 oz)	92	G
	grilled, 125 g (4 oz)	180	G
Coffee	average cup, black	4	G
	average cup, with 15 ml (1 tbsp) milk	10	G
Corn	whole kernel, ½ cup	75	G
Cornflakes	average for 50 g (2 oz) serving	210	R
Crab	125 g (4 oz) boiled, meat only	144	G
Cranberry sauce	15 ml (1 tbsp)	56	R
Cream	single 30 ml (2 tbsp)	62	R
	double 30 ml (2 tbsp)	131	R
Cress	125 g (4 oz) raw	16	G
Cucumber	125 g (4 oz)	20	G
Damsons	125 g (4 oz)	45	G
Dates	125g (4 oz)		

Courtesy of Slimcea Slimming Service, 21 New Row, London WC2

Food	Quantity	Calories	Group
	(weighed with stones)	244	R
Dill pickles	1 large	8	G
Dried milk	25 g (1 oz)	150	R
Duck	125 g (4 oz) roast meat, no bones	356	R
Eggs, hen	boiled	80	G
	scrambled (two)	270	P
	omelette, two egg, plain	212	P
Fats	25 g (1 oz) dripping	262	R
	25 g (1 oz) margarine	226	R
	25 ml (1 oz) olive oil	264	R
Figs	125 g (4 oz) green	48	G
	125 g (4 oz) dried, raw	244	R
Fish fingers	three	162	R
Flour (wheat)	25 g (1 oz)	100	R
Frankfurters	2 large	310	R
French dressing (oil and vinegar)	15 ml (1 tbsp)	86	R
Gooseberries	125 g (4 oz) raw	20	G
	125 g (4 oz) stewed without sugar	16	G
Grapefruit	half (no sugar)	18	G
Grapes	125 g (4 oz) black	56	G
	125 g (4 oz) white	68	G
Haddock	125 g (4 oz) steamed with bones	84	G
	125 g (4 oz) smoked, poached	72	G
Ham	125 g (4 oz) baked, lean	448	R
	125 g (4 oz) boiled, lean and fat	492	R
Herring	125 g (4 oz) grilled	190	P
Honey	15 ml (1 tbsp)	60	R
Ice-cream	average per 100 ml (3½ oz) portion	193	R
Jams	average 10 ml (2 tsp)	74	R
Juice (fresh)	small breakfast glass orange	38	G
	grapefruit	39	G
Kidneys	125 g (4 oz) grilled	120	G
Lamb	chop, lean grilled 125 g (4 oz)	310	P
	125 g (4 oz) leg, roast	332	P
	125 g (4 oz) stewing, neck end	368	P
Lard	25 g (1 oz)	262	R
Leeks	125 g (4 oz) boiled	28	G
Lemon	150 g (5 oz) average size	20	G
Lettuce	average head of round lettuce	24	G
Lime juice cordial	1 average glass diluted	65	P
Liver	125 g (4 oz) grilled	180	G
Liver sausage	125 g (4 oz)	385	R
Luncheon meat (canned)	125 g (4 oz) average	380	R
Macaroni	125 g (4 oz) boiled	128	R
	with cheese, small portion	475	R
Marmalade	10 ml (2 tsp)	74	R
Marmite	10 ml (2 tsp)	18	G
Marrow	125 g (4 oz) boiled	8	G
Mayonnaise	15 ml (1 tbsp)	110	R
Melons, yellow	125 g (4 oz) portion	16	G
Milk	300 ml (½ pt) whole	160	P
	300 ml (½ pt) skimmed	100	P
Mushrooms	125 g (4 oz) grilled	36	G
Mustard & cress	125 g (4 oz)	12	G
Nuts, mixed	125 g (4 oz)	376	R
	125 g (4 oz) slightly salted	20	G
Onions	125 g (4 oz) boiled	15	G
	spring — 4	10	G
Oranges	1 fresh	40	G
	juice — small glass	38	G
Parsnips	2 medium boiled	64	G
Pastry	125 g (4 oz)	592	R
Peaches	1 whole, fresh	36	G
	canned, 2 halves with syrup	79	R
Peanut butter	25 g (1 oz)	180	R
Peanuts	125 g (4 oz)	684	R
Pears	1 medium	36	G
	125 g (4 oz) canned with syrup	88	R
Peas	125 g (4 oz)	70	P
	tinned, 125 g (4 oz)	95	P
Pineapple	fresh average slice	26	G
	canned with syrup 50 g (2 oz)	44	R
Plums	2 large, approx.	36	G
Pork	leg, roast, 125 g (4 oz)	360	P
	loin, roast, lean and fat, 125 g (4 oz)	513	R
	125 g (4 oz) chop, grilled, lean	152	P
	125 g (4 oz) chop, grilled, lean	152	P
	125 g (4 oz) chop, lean and fat	400	R
Potato crisps	average 25 g (1 oz) packet	161	R
Potatoes	125 g (4 oz) portion, old, boiled	92	R
	1 medium, baked in jacket	96	R
	2 small roast	140	R
	125 g (4 oz) new potatoes, boiled	84	R
	instant, 30 ml (2 tbsp)	200	R
Prunes	125 g (4 oz) dried, stewed, no sugar	76	G
Rabbit	125 g (4 oz) stewed with bones	104	G
Radishes	6 small	8	G
Raisins	25 g (1 oz)	70	P
Raspberries	125 g (4 oz)	28	G
Rhubarb	125 g (4 oz) stewed, without sugar	4	G
Rice	50 g (2 oz) boiled	70	R
Salmon	125 g (4 oz) portion, fresh, steamed	228	P
	125 g (4 oz) smoked	178	P
	125 g (4 oz) canned	156	P
Sardines	canned, 4 drained	180	P
Shrimps	125 g (4 oz) shelled	128	G
Sole	125 g (4 oz) grilled	90	G
Soup:	canned — 300 ml (½ pt)		
Consommé		39	G

Cream of chicken		137	R
Cream of tomato		195	R
Vegetable (thick)		126	R
Spaghetti	1 cup cooked, 125 g (approx 4 oz)	155	R
Spinach	125 g (4 oz) boiled	28	P
Strawberries	125 g (4 oz) fresh	28	G
Sugar	13 g (½ oz)	56	R
Syrup — golden	15 ml (1 tbsp)	42	R
Tea	1 cup, no milk or sugar	under 1	G
	1 cup with 15 ml (1 tbsp) milk	10	G
Tomato	1 raw medium size	8	G
	sauce, 15 ml (1 tbsp)	20	P
	juice, small glass	25	G
Trout	125 g (4 oz) steamed	100	G
	125 g (4 oz) smoked	133	G
Turbot	125 g (4 oz) steamed	76	G
Turkey	125 g (4 oz) roast	224	P
Turnips	125 g (4 oz) boiled	12	G
Veal	125 g (4 oz) leg, roast	280	P
	125 g (4 oz) stewing	280	P
Vinegar	any amount	nil	G
Watermelon		nil	G
Whitebait	125 g (4 oz) fried	608	R
Yogurt (1 carton)	natural	75	G
	flavoured	115	P
	real fruit	160	R
Yorkshire pudding	75 g (3 oz)	189	R
Alcoholic drinks:			
Beer	Draught bitter 300 ml (½ pt)	88	R
	Lager — 300 ml (½ pt)	120	R
	Pale Ale — bottled, draught, 300 ml	155	R
	Stout — 300 ml (½pt)	210	R
Bloody Mary	average glass	140	R
Brandy	liqueur glass	75	P
Campari	average measure	110	R
Champagne	small wine glass	90	R
Cider	dry — 300 ml (½pt)	100	R
	sweet — 300 ml (½ pt)	120	R
Gin	single measure	55	P
Sherry	dry — small sherry glass	65	P
	sweet — small sherry glass	75	P
Scotch whisky	single measure	58	P
Wines	red — small glass	65—75	P
	white, dry — small glass	60—70	P
	white, sweet — small glass	90	R
Port	small glass	165	R
Non-alcoholic drinks:			
Cola	standard bottle	80	R
Cordial			

(diluted)	orange — 1 glass	35	R
	lemon — 1 glass	35	R
	grapefruit — 1 glass	35	R
Low calorie	tonic water	Nil–1	G
	bitter lemon	Nil–1	G
	ginger ale	Nil–1	G
	soda water	Nil	G
Sparkling	tonic water — 1 bottle	52	R
	bitter lemon — 1 bottle	78	R
	ginger ale — 1 bottle	35	P
Tomato juice	125 g (4 oz) bottle	25	G

The greedy girl's calorie chart

If ever your will-power weakens and the craving for fish and chips or a chocolate bar overwhelms you, run your eye down this forbidding calorie chart of super-fattening foods. The shock is guaranteed to kill your appetite!

Toasted cheese sandwich	345
Mars Bar	265
Shepherd's pie	210
Fried egg and bacon	230
Bœuf bourguignon	425
Baked beans on toast	150
Doughnut	220
Twenty peanuts	100
Six Brazil nuts	380
Carton fruit yogurt	150
Apple pie and custard	360
Spaghetti Bolognese	370
Yorkshire pudding	130
Scotch egg	220
Four fish fingers	240
Fish and chips	688
Asparagus with butter	190
55 g (2 oz) cream cheese	460
Walnut whip	169
Barbecued spare ribs	300
Curried lamb	430
Veal goulash	355
Shish kebab	330
Vichyssoise	200
Boiled sweet potatoes	92
Frozen cod in shrimp flavour sauce	155
Tinned ravioli with tomato sauce	188
Baked Alaska	300
Jam sponge and custard	668
113 g (¼ lb) coconut ice	444
Hot dog with onions	301
Kentucky Fried Chicken and chips	525
Portion of popcorn	278
Stick of rock	250
Slice fried bread	182

Packet potato crisps	160
Fried sausage	157
Bag Maltesers	194
Coq au vin	600
Steak and kidney pie	335
Birds Eye beefburger	160
Chicken and vegetable pasty	482
Penguin milk chocolate biscuit	140
113 g (¼ lb) fried scampi in butter	240
One pickled onion	12
Duck in orange sauce	846
113 g (¼ lb) pâté	320
Wimpy	292
Milkshake	266
170 g (6 oz) veal and ham pie	570
Fried rice	357
Boiled rice	140
One shortbread finger biscuit	73
Paella	715
Chocolate-covered ice-cream bar	130
Crème caramel	140
Mini Boursin cheese	65
Coquilles Saint-Jacques	140
Gazpacho	221
One slice toast, butter, marmalade	201
Scrambled egg on buttered toast	426
Chicken biriani	713
Chapati	120
Porridge, sugar and milk	305
Moules marinière	147
Trifle	250
Taramasalata	310
Mug of cocoa, with sugar	267
Chocolate marshmallow	74

Note Amounts are based on an average portion for an adult

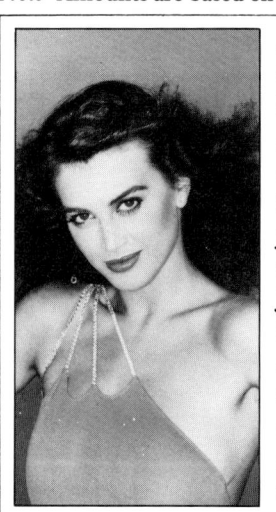

AMANDA PAYS, model: *"I usually remain at a steady weight by eating a normal balanced diet. For breakfast I have tea with honey, fresh fruit and muesli with milk. Lunch is always light — just cheese and an apple. Dinner is my main meal and I love Japanese or Chinese food or any white meat with vegetables. I put on weight if I eat too many sweet things in which case I just cut down on food for a few days. I don't fast — I love food too much!"*

150-calorie meals

If you are an obsessive calorie counter — or on the classic 1000-a-day calorie diet — you will find the following suggestions for 150-calorie meals helpful:

1 egg boiled or poached with a crispbread or followed by an apple or pear

1-egg omelette filled with boiled mushrooms or two tomatoes or three anchovy fillets, plus green salad

75 g (3 oz) cottage cheese or 35 g (1½ oz) Edam or Gouda with celery and green salad

100 g (4 oz) cod or haddock fillet with runner beans and grilled tomato

75 g (3 oz) tinned salmon with salad

100 g (4 oz) grilled haddock or plaice with 50 g (2 oz) frozen peas

100 g (4 oz) crabmeat with green salad and cucumber

1 medium rasher of bacon with tomato and mushrooms, all grilled

2 thin slices of ham or 3 of liver sausage or 4 of salami with lettuce, cucumber and watercress salad

50 g (2 oz) braised liver with runner beans and 1 small braised onion

2 thin slices of lamb or beef or 75 g (3 oz) chicken with cabbage, green beans and a little gravy

Half grapefruit sweetened with sugar substitute and a sandwich made with one slice bread, tomato, cucumber and watercress

1 carton plain yogurt plus one apple or celery and carrot sticks

1 large banana and 1 starch-reduced roll

1 tin of slimmers' soup

2 crispbreads spread with Marmite or meat or fish paste

1 glass of milk plus an apple, orange, pear or peach

2 frankfurters with 30 ml (2 tbsp) sauerkraut

50 g (2 oz) peeled prawns with salad plus one slice brown bread

Bowl of fresh or frozen, not tinned, strawberries with single cream from top of milk

The seven-day sweet tooth diet

This diet, based on energy-giving clear honey, will satisfy your sweet tooth yet keep you within 1,000 calories a day.

Daily allowance of liquids: 300 ml (½ pint) fresh milk; as much coffee or tea (include milk from allowance); artificial sweetener; 150 ml (¼ pint) orange or grapefruit juice, or 300 ml (½ pint) tomato juice; drink eight glasses of water a day.

DAY ONE: *Breakfast:* ½ grapefruit topped with 5 ml (1 tsp) honey; 1 thin slice bread, scrape butter; honey and egg flip — warm 150 ml (¼ pint) milk with 6 drops vanilla essence. Blend 1 egg, 10 ml (2 tsp) Gale's honey, 10 ml (2 tsp) each bran and wheatgerm. Pour in milk, stir. *Lunch:* 2 small hard-boiled eggs; green salad with dressing — 10 ml (2 tsp) lemon chopped and mixed with 15 ml (1 tbsp) mayonnaise and 5 ml (1 tsp) honey. *Dinner:* 100 g (4 oz) sole brushed with melted butter and grilled; lemon wedge; 1 grilled tomato; 100 g (4 oz) runner beans; baked apple —make slit around medium cooking apple, re- move core, stuff with 13 g (½ oz) dates (chopped) and 10 ml (2 tsp)

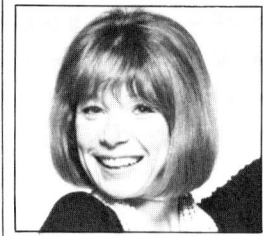

SHIRLEY MACLAINE, superstar: *"To keep thin, I jog and do exercises. I eat mostly protein, seven very small meals a day. And I drink a lot of water and skimmed milk. Then I go to bed and dream about chocolate cake."*

honey, pour 15 ml (1 tbsp) water over top. Bake in fairly hot oven for about an hour.

DAY TWO: *Breakfast:* Grapefruit as Day One; 1 slice of toast with 50 g (2 oz) mushrooms, brushed with melted butter and grilled, *or* honey and egg flip. *Lunch:* 1 slice of bread, scrape butter, spread with mix of 50 g (2 oz) cottage cheese, 10 ml (2 tsp) honey, ½ red pepper (chopped). *Dinner:* Glazed chicken — place chicken leg in foil and pour over top 15 ml (1 tbsp) honey with 3 ml (½ tsp) ground ginger. Seal foil and bake in fairly hot oven for 30 minutes, open foil and bake a further 15 minutes; 50 g (2 oz) cabbage; 75 g (3 oz) cauliflower; baked pear — peel and halve pear, roll halves in lemon juice. Fill with 13 g (½ oz) dried fruit and 10 ml (2 tsp) honey. Put halves together, place in ovenproof dish. Pour water over top and bake in fairly hot oven for 50 minutes.

DAY THREE: *Breakfast:* Grapefruit as Day One; 25 g (1 oz) Edam cheese grilled on 1 slice toast, or honey and egg flip. *Lunch:* 100 g (4 oz) fresh or frozen prawns; large plate of cabbage, celery, carrot salad with dressing as Day One. *Dinner:* Spanish omelette — use 2 eggs, 1 onion (chopped), 1 tomato (sliced), ½ green pepper (chopped) and mixed herbs; 125 ml (5 fl oz) yogurt mixed with 38 g (1½ oz) dried apricots (chopped), 10 ml (2 tsp) honey, 5 ml (1 tsp) each bran and wheatgerm.

DAY FOUR: *Breakfast:* Grapefruit as Day One; boiled egg; 1 slice bread, scrape butter, or honey and egg flip. *Lunch:* 1 slice bread, scrape butter, topped with 50 g (2 oz) cottage cheese, lettuce, 1 egg (sliced). *Dinner:* Kidney kebabs — grill 8 halved lamb's kidneys, 2 tomatoes (halved), 50 g (2 oz) mushrooms; 100 g (4 oz) braised celery; rhubarb — stew 175 g (6 oz) rhubarb with 15 ml (1 tbsp) honey.

DAY FIVE: *Breakfast:* Grapefruit as Day One; 75 g (3 oz) poached haddock; ½ slice bread, scrape butter, or honey and egg flip. *Lunch:* 38 g (1½ oz) Edam, cubed and mixed with chopped celery, 38 g (1½ oz) grapes (halved), 1 small apple (chopped) and dressing as Day One. *Dinner:* 150g (5 oz) lean lamb cutlet; 100 g (4 oz) spinach; 1 grilled tomato; 3 slices fresh or tinned pineapple.

DAY SIX: *Breakfast:* Grapefruit as Day One; 25 g (1 oz) lean gammon, grilled; 1 slice bread, scrape butter, or honey and egg flip. *Lunch:* 100 g (4 oz) tinned salmon, oil drained off; lemon wedge; green salad; ½ slice bread, scrape butter. *Dinner:* 75 g (3 oz) lean roast beef; 75 g (3 oz) cauliflower; 50 g (2 oz) runner beans; stewed rhubarb as Day Four.

DAY SEVEN: *Breakfast:* Grapefruit as Day One; poached egg; 1 slice bread, scrape butter, or honey and egg flip. *Lunch:* 1 slice bread, scrape butter, spread with 50 g (2 oz) cottage cheese, 25 g (1 oz) sultanas mixed with 10 ml (2 tsp) honey. *Dinner:* 100 g (4 oz) lamb's liver, brushed with butter mixed with 5 ml (1 tsp) mustard, and grilled; grilled tomato, 75 g (3 oz) carrots; banana snow — whisked egg white mixed with mashed banana, 5 ml (1 tsp) lemon and 15 ml (1 tbsp) honey.

The crash-off-ten-pounds-in-one-week-diet

This diet dates from 1938, when beauty expert Helena Rubinstein devised a speedy, simple and safe way to shed pounds, fast. It is important that you keep to the diet without cheating in order for it to be fully effective; please note that the diet was designed by Madame Rubinstein for one week, and no longer!

FIRST DAY

Breakfast
½ grapefruit
1 cup black coffee (no sugar)

Lunch
½ grapefruit
1 egg
1 slice Melba toast

Dinner
2 eggs
1 tomato
½ head lettuce
½ grapefruit
Tea (no sugar or milk)

SECOND DAY

Breakfast
½ grapefruit
1 cup black coffee (no sugar)

Lunch
1 orange
1 egg
½ slice Melba toast

Dinner
Grilled steak
½ head lettuce
1 tomato
½ grapefruit

THIRD DAY

Breakfast
½ grapefruit
1 cup black coffee (no sugar)

Lunch
½ grapefruit
1 egg
½ head lettuce
Tea

Dinner
½ grapefruit
Grilled steak
½ head lettuce
Tea or black coffee

FOURTH DAY

Breakfast
½ grapefruit

1 cup black coffee (no sugar)
Lunch
½ grapefruit
Small carton cottage cheese
1 tomato
1 slice Melba toast
Tea
Dinner
½ grapefruit
Grilled steak
Watercress or lettuce
FIFTH DAY
Breakfast
½ grapefruit
1 cup black coffee (no sugar)
Lunch
1 orange
1 lamb chop, grilled
½ head lettuce
Tea
Dinner
½ grapefruit
2 eggs
Lettuce and tomato
Tea
SIXTH DAY
Breakfast
½ grapefruit
1 cup black coffee (no sugar)
Lunch
1 orange
1 lamb chop
Tea
Dinner
1 poached egg
1 slice Melba toast
1 orange
Tea
SEVENTH DAY
Breakfast
½ grapefruit
1 cup black coffee (no sugar)
Lunch
½ grapefruit
2 eggs
Lettuce and tomato
Tea
Dinner
2 lamb chops
Lettuce and tomato
Tea or coffee

Avoid all sweets, starches, sugar and cream. Use vinegar and oil dressing on salads only.

Breakfast: The slimmer's ally

If you are one of the four million women in this country who start the day on an empty stomach, you are more likely to be overweight than the girl who sits down to a hearty breakfast. As the morning progresses, the non-breakfast-eater grows increasingly hungry, blood sugar levels sink and the temptation to drink more than one cup of milky coffee and eat a mid-morning bun is often too strong to resist. By lunchtime, you are ready to down a large calorie-rich meal — and probably do.

Researchers have proved conclusively that you will lose more weight by having several small meals in the day than by confining mealtimes to lunch and dinner. Not only are you less likely to cheat on your diet, but there is evidence that the meal pattern of the day affects the metabolic rate of the body, so that with the same food intake, a couple of larger meals can be more fattening than several smaller ones.

Ability-measuring tests developed by psychologists have shown that the person who skips breakfast works slower and with less concentration than his colleagues; there is a marked increase in efficiency after lunch. Check through the following breakfast suggestions — all suitable for slimmers —to find one suited to *you*.

Five 300-calorie breakfast ideas

● Glass orange or grapefruit juice
Ready-to-eat cereal with 1 tsp sugar and half a banana or fresh berries
Coffee or tea with skimmed milk
● Orange or grapefruit sections
Small carton cottage cheese
Lightly buttered slice wholemeal toast
Coffee or tea with skimmed milk
● Glass orange or grapefruit juice
Soft or hard-boiled egg
Lightly buttered slice wholemeal toast
Coffee or tea with skimmed milk
● Glass tomato juice
Two slices grilled bacon on wholemeal toast
Coffee or tea with skimmed milk
● Glass orange or grapefruit juice
Cooked cereal with 1 tsp sugar
Coffee or tea with skimmed milk

Liquid breakfast

This low-calorie breakfast drink is speedy to make and is ideal if you are too rushed to prepare breakfast — or cannot face eating first thing.
1 small carton natural low-fat yogurt
25 g (1 oz) dried apricots, soaked in water overnight, or any soft fruits: pear, peach or handful of berries

30 ml (2 tbsp) water
1 egg
7 ml (½ tbsp) clear honey, or to taste
Blend all ingredients together. Pour into tall glass.

Breakfast in a bowl

Muesli, soaked in low-fat yogurt or orange juice, makes a highly nutritional breakfast for the slimmer. Buy it ready made, or make it yourself from a mix of wheat flakes, rye flakes, barley kernels and millet flakes. A smaller proportion of wheatgerm and bran can be added; raisins and hazelnuts taste delicious in muesli, but add in moderation as they are fairly high in calories. Store muesli-base in a screw-top jar. Try chopping apple or orange segments into your breakfast muesli.

Gayelord Hauser's no-calorie counting, high-energy diet

Follow the recommendations of one of the world's leading nutritionists, Gayelord Hauser, who advocates a diet that gives you freedom from calorie-counting, offers the finest body-building foods and allows you to lose weight, too. The celebrated Hauser regime is high-protein, medium-fat and low-carbohydrate; it consists of fresh unprocessed fruits and vegetables, "wonder" foods such as wheatgerm and yogurt, plus a daily vitamin and mineral supplement. Hauser's advice: "Have delicious fresh food. Eat slowly. Chew well. Don't reach for snack after snack out of boredom or frustration." Your New Energy Diet starts here. . .

PROTEIN – HIGH The New Energy Diet stresses complete protein foods containing the eight amino acids the body cannot make itself. The main sources are meat – including glandular and organ meats, poultry; fish; eggs; milk; cheese and yogurt; fresh wheatgerm and soybeans (most other beans provide incomplete protein).

Gayelord Hauser believes you should have a good serving of protein at every meal. But, as many protein foods are very expensive, he says: fortify ordinary fare with the "wonder foods" – brewer's yeast, yogurt, wheatgerm, avocado. They are chock-full of protein, vitamins, and minerals. They store easily. And they are good mixers with other foods. In short, they are energisers to beat all energisers.

FATS – MEDIUM Fats have twice as many calories as protein or carbohydrates – nine calories per gramme instead of four. But even a reducing diet should contain an adequate amount of fat, as it is absorbed more slowly and staves off hunger longer.

What you must try to cut down on are the saturated fats – the heart hazards. Vegetable oils are what you want. But two cautions: avoid hydrogenated (hardened) products. And try to steer clear of over-processed liquid oils. As it is all but impos-

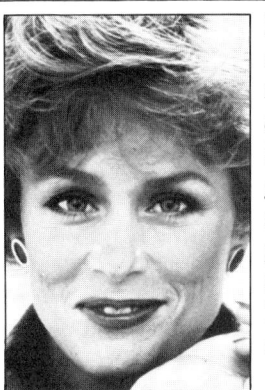

LAUREN HUTTON, model and actress: *"Breakfast is the* most *important meal. I usually eat just breakfast and dinner. For breakfast I have orange juice with ginseng in it, two eggs, sausage, toast and jam. You can eat all the good stuff like vegetables and salads and fruit,* never *eat sweets. The idea in losing weight is to shrink your stomach, so you eat smaller portions."*

sible to get pure crude vegetable oil, Gayelord Hauser suggests the cold-pressed oils you find in any good health-food store – they are the next best thing.

When you make your salad dressing, experiment – vary the oil you use from batch to batch. Corn oil is excellent and it is inexpensive. Half sunflower oil and half olive oil is a good combination. Safflower oil, alone, is a great favourite. So is sesame oil. And, whatever else you do, sprinkle in a few drops of wheatgerm oil – together with a pinch or two of vegetable salt.

One of the most important ingredients for good health and good looks in vegetable oils is linoleic acid. Safflower oil has the highest percentage. Then comes sunflower oil. And after that sesame seed, poppy seed, corn and soybean. If you like the taste of fresh sweet butter, you can enjoy Sunbutter – half-and-half mixture of fresh sweet butter and sunflower oil.

CARBOHYDRATES – LOW Carbohydrates provide fuel for the body and help assimilate other foods. That is their main job. Some carbohydrate is indispensable. But if you eat a lot of sweets, pastries and starchy foods, you are doing your health no good and you have blown your diet.

Refined sugar is one thing you can really do without – it is empty of everything except calories. The best carbohydrates, the ones which give you vitamins and minerals as well as calories, are whole grain flours, cereals, breads, fresh vegetables and fruits.

THE WONDER FOODS *Brewer's yeast* contains 17 different vitamins (notably all of the B family); 16 amino acids, including the vital eight; and 14 minerals. More than a third of what you get is protein (a much higher proportion than steak). And one teaspoonful has only seven calories. Try a teaspoon or two frothed in a blender with tomato juice, fruit juice or buttermilk – and add a little wheatgerm. This makes a great drink for your mid-morning or mid-afternoon energy break. Or sprinkle some

Excerpted from Gayelord Hauser's New Treasury of Secrets © 1975. *Published by Faber & Faber*

over your salad. If you don't like the taste – and it is very likely you won't at first – get the celery-flavoured kind that is sold at most health-food stores. Do not *ever* eat fresh yeast – that is meant only for baking. And one other point: when you start taking brewer's yeast, start slowly. If you are new to it, you may have a bit of trouble digesting large amounts until your system is used to it. Begin with half a spoonful and gradually work up to two or three teaspoons a day.

Nonfat dried milk gives you complete protein with rich quantities of riboflavin (B$_2$). You can make an excellent New Energy Milk Drink by mixing half a cup of dried milk with a quart of fresh skim milk in a blender – and adding a spoonful of brewer's yeast, if you like. Or simply make skim milk with double the usual amount of powder. This gives you a good boost of energy whenever you need it – in fact, a quart would actually provide you with more than a whole day's supply of complete protein.

Yogurt is another wonder food – an excellent source of protein, calcium and riboflavin. And it is a marvellous between-meal or bedtime snack. Yogurt is something you can take to quickly and become fonder and fonder of as time goes on. There are excellent yogurts on the market but if you culture your own from nonfat dried milk it is much cheaper and better for your diet. Eat it plain or with fresh fruit or as yogurt cheese in a romaine and watercress salad for lunch – together with sliced cucumbers, parsley and herbs. Or blend a cup of yogurt with a spoonful or two of unsweetened frozen fruit juice concentrate and drink it well chilled; it makes a very nutritious and pleasing energy break.

Wheatgerm, the world's best cereal, is protein-rich and full of vitamins – specially B. Add it to meat loaves or chopped meat. Mix it with tomatoes, chives and parsley for a tabbouli salad. Or sprinkle a little on yogurt: two wonders in one. If possible, get the fresh wheatgerm. It costs only half as much as the toasted kind, and will stay fresh for at least a month in the refrigerator. The best wheatgerm is milled in France by the Moulin de Paris – but there are plenty of fine brands to be found in this country as long as you avoid the sugared variety.

Six-course dinner growing on one tree. That is the *avocado*. This fruit – and it is a fruit – combines the protein of meat, the smooth texture of butter (but it is an unsaturated fat), the vitamins and minerals of vegetables and the flavour of nuts. A very ripe, soft avocado mashed with a few drops of lemon juice and spiked with herbs makes a delicious change from a vinegar-and-oil salad dressing – try it once in a while.

Your new energy diet plan

Breakfast is something people are either very pro or very anti. Gayelord Hauser is one of the pros. A breakfast with good protein, he says, keeps the blood sugar at an energetic level through the morning and beyond – it is your "energy determinator" for the whole day. Your plan for breakfast goes like this:

○ A glass of fruit juice – frozen or canned if you must, but by all means unsweetened.

○ Two-thirds cup of cottage cheese or 1 egg.

○ A slice of gluten, whole wheat or rye bread – toasted if you like and lightly sunbuttered.

○ A large cup of Swiss coffee – half freshly-brewed coffee and half foaming-hot skim milk.

○ Your vitamin-and-mineral supplement. Breakfast is the best time to take it – you benefit all day.

Mid-morning energy break – this is the moment to dip into wonder-food drinks made with brewer's yeast or non-fat dried milk or yogurt. Or try his New Energy Broth, for which the recipe is given further on. If you must have a coffee break, drink a big cup of Swiss coffee; that way you get energy, too. Make the coffee just as you did for breakfast – and to make it really foam, add the milk and the coffee together, holding one pot in the left hand and one in the right as you pour.

Lunch should be everything in one bowl – in other words, a salad. It is so simple and easy, especially when you are eating alone. Be sure you include a good portion of your favourite protein food – cold chicken, lean ham, lean beef, shrimp, tuna, salmon, hard-boiled eggs, yogurt, cheese, or soybeans – mixed with crisp greens. And then toss in some tomato, cucumber, green pepper and radishes, too, if you like.

For lunch at your desk, a pint of yogurt or two hard-boiled eggs and an apple or orange can be a nutritious and satisfying meal.

Mid-afternoon energy break – time for another wonder-food drink. Try a different one from the one you had mid-morning. A glass of chilled yogurt and frozen orange juice concentrate can give you plenty of first-class protein and quite an energy boost.

Dinner time is a relaxing time – whether you are with friends or at home alone. Enjoy a tall, cool glass of vegetable juice half an hour or so before sitting down to your meal. It can do wonderful things to unwind taut nerves and it helps erase fatigue after a busy day. What's more, it raises the blood sugar level enough

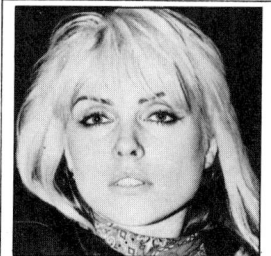

DEBBIE HARRY, singer: *"I look after myself by eating health foods and I don't have a particularly sweet tooth. Performing whilst on tour most nights keeps me very fit and in shape. I often find I've lost three or four pounds after one show!"*

so you have no urge to overeat. Try different juices together, such as celery, cucumber and green pepper with a tomato tossed in, too, just as you would do for a mixed-greens salad. And celery juice, alone, can be very refreshing – with just a few drops of lemon juice and a dash of vegetable salt.

Dinner should always be lean, light, and nutritious. The plan goes like this:

○ A good portion of lean meat – liver is excellent – or chicken without the skin, or fish. (See Gayelord Hauser's recipe for New Energy Burgers, Wonder Chicken, Sesame Halibut Steak and Liver Strips further on.) A large green salad with a tablespoon of vegetable oil and herb vinegar dressing. Or, occasionally, a platter of crudités served with spices, herbs and sea salt as a first course.

○ A short-cooked vegetable – such as courgettes, spinach, or green beans – that is steamed for just a few seconds and served with sunbutter. Or, from time to time, kasha or brown rice or baked potato. Gayelord Hauser has a wonderful, easy recipe for what he calls Lighthearted-Baked Potatoes – baked, scooped out, mixed with yogurt and chives and stuffed back in the shell – when you are having guests for dinner. And he has one recipe he calls Potato à la Garbo – split, scooped out within a half inch of the shell and then baked – for when you want to be alone.

○ Dessert can be fresh fruit – Gayelord Hauser's Compote with Honey or French Sherbet, for which recipes follow, or simply berries topped with yogurt or a bowl of freshly cut-up fruit. If the fruits are not sweet enough, add a few drops of kirsch or mirabelle. But never white sugar.

○ Coffee – either espresso or Sanka.

Always remember the pleasure principle. There are all sorts of ways to make dieting delicious and easy, whether you are at home or going out.

○ For instance, Gayelord Hauser's Sukiyaki, for which we give you the recipe, is a wonderful Saturday night dish when there are four or more – dieting you, and your non-dieting guests.

○ Talking of guests, be sure to make a little ceremony of coffee or Sanka with liqueurs (which *you* can skip) after dinner. Simply take a tray with all the makings into the living-room. Have a pot of Sanka piping hot and very strong as well as a *machinetta* of the real espresso thing. You will find that your friends who drink Sanka will be quite taken with the idea of having a little liqueur in it. You might also offer them a cup that is half espresso and half Sanka.

○ And suppose you are being taken out to dinner on Friday night. Striped bass for two is a perfect choice – perhaps with a watercress and endive salad. To begin, you might order oysters or consommé. And for dessert, strawberries *nature*. (The bass recipe is included so you can cook it at home.)

New Energy Broth
(Hauser broth)
1 cup finely shredded celery, leaves and all
1 cup carrots, chopped finely
1 cup onions, chopped finely
2 or 3 tomatoes cut in small chunks
½ cup spinach leaves, finely shredded
2 or 3 clumps of parsley
1.1 litre (2 pts) boiling water
A pinch of vegetable salt
Garnish of chopped parsley and chives

Put all shredded vegetables into the pot of boiling water. Cover and simmer for 30 minutes. Then add vegetable salt. Strain and serve with a garnish of parsley. Keep what is left over in a covered jar and store in the refrigerator – there is enough for several days. To vary the broth, add different herbs. Or a dash of celery-flavoured brewer's yeast if you could use some super-energy.

This broth is based on the ancient recipe worked out by the father of medicine, Hippocrates, about 400 BC. Gayelord Hauser's updated version has been bubbling on stoves all over the world since 1922.

New Energy Burger
(Inexpensive beefburger)
125 g (4 oz) lean chopped beef
5 ml (1 tsp) wheatgerm
5 ml (1 tsp) nonfat dried milk
5 ml (1 tsp) onion, chopped
5 ml (1 tsp) celery, chopped
5 ml (1 tsp) parsley, chopped

Mix all ingredients and make into a flat patty. Put into a heavy skillet with a little vegetable oil – or place on a lightly greased rack under a preheated grill – and cook very quickly, browning on both sides.

Wonder Chicken
1 chicken breast
30 ml (2 tbsp) wheatgerm
15 ml (1 tbsp) vegetable oil
1 sliver of garlic, crushed
A pinch of vegetable salt
A dash of paprika

Mix salt, oil, paprika and garlic. Apply to the chicken breast with a pastry brush. Roll the chicken in wheatgerm and lay it, skin side down, in a small baking dish coated with the remaining mixture. Bake for about an hour at 150°C (300°F, gas Mark 2). After about 45 minutes, turn skin side up.

Sesame Halibut Steak
1 halibut steak, 2.5 cm (1-inch) thick
5 ml (1 tsp) toasted sesame seeds
½ cup toasted gluten breadcrumbs
A pinch of thyme
A pinch of vegetable salt
A little vegetable oil

Place the steak in a small oiled baking pan. Sprinkle with salt and pour a few drops of vegetable oil over it. Combine breadcrumbs, thyme, sesame seeds, salt and a little more oil and spread on top of the steak. Place in a preheated 175°C (350°F, gas Mark 4) oven and bake uncovered for about 30 minutes – or until fish flakes easily.

Liver Strips

Take a piece of fresh tender liver. Cut it in noodle-like strips. If it is at all tough, sprinkle it with natural tenderiser and let it stand for 10 to 20 minutes. Then put 1 spoonful of vegetable oil in a heavy skillet. Sauté a sliced onion until golden brown. Add the strips of liver and sauté for just three minutes. Sprinkle with a bit of vegetable oil and serve at once. This is Gayelord Hauser's favourite recipe for liver – on evenings when he is having dinner alone.

Striped Bass for two

50 ml (2 fl oz) olive oil
1 small onion, chopped fine
2 cloves garlic, chopped fine
1 whole striped bass – about 900 g (2 lb)
150 ml (5 fl oz) dry white wine
Herbs:
Chives, 1 bunch, chopped
A pinch of thyme
A pinch of oregano
A pinch of rosemary, crushed
Salt and pepper to taste

Sauté onion and garlic in olive oil. When golden add fish and white wine. Simmer until the white wine is half evaporated. Add herbs. Cover and let simmer for 15–20 minutes – but do not turn the fish. Serve immediately. A salad of watercress and endive goes very well with this. And, for dessert, simply a bowl of chilled fresh fruit.

Sukiyaki

Heat a heavy iron skillet or wok. When the pan is hot, add 30–45 ml (2–3 tbsp) soy oil. Then add meat and chopped vegetables, in equal proportions, to give a good-size serving for each of your guests. The meat should be thinly sliced lean raw beef or chicken. The vegetables should be onions, celery and spinach. Slice onions thin; cut the celery into small sections and then sliver them the long way into strips. Place all ingredients in the pan at the same time. The steam begins to rise immediately and in a few minutes you can see the meat change colour and the vegetables begin to soften. At this time, you add a small amount of broth and 30 ml (2 tbsp) soy sauce and continue cooking for about 10 minutes. Covering the pan during the cooking will speed up cooking time, preserve the colour of the vegetables and prevent loss of vitamin C. The Japanese usually add little squares of soybean curd cheese (*tofu*) which resembles a thick salty custard; although it is a good source of protein it is not essential when the sukiyaki contains meat.

Crêpes Ratatouille

12 to 14 cooked crêpes, about 150 mm (6 in) in diameter (see below)
Ratatouille mixture (see below)
Parmesan cheese, freshly grated
Parsley, minced

Have crêpes ready. Spoon 2–3 tbsp of ratatouille into the centre of each crêpe. Fold up and place in a buttered baking dish. Bake in a pre-heated 190°C (375°F, gas Mark 5) oven for 10–15 minutes. Garnish with cheese and parsley. Serve at once.

Basic Crêpe Recipe

1 cup flour
Dash of salt
3 eggs
1½ cups milk
½ cup vegetable oil

Put milk, eggs, salt and flour into the blender and blend at top speed for 30 seconds. Scrape down lumps with a spatula. Blend at top speed another 15 seconds. The batter should have the consistency of smooth heavy cream. If any lumps remain, strain the mixture. Cover. Set aside in the refrigerator. The batter will thicken as it stands – let it chill for a couple of hours if possible. If you find it gets too heavy, beat in a few teaspoonfuls of water until the right consistency is reached.

Before preparing each crêpe, brush the crêpe pan with oil to cover the entire bottom. Heat pan over brisk heat until hot but not smoking. Remove from heat and pour in about 30 ml (2 tablespoons) of batter. Tilt to coat bottom. Set pan over medium heat and cook about 1 minute until the top of the crêpe is dry and the bottom is slightly browned. Turn and cook on the other side about 20 seconds. Flip out onto a plate. Repeat.

Ratatouille

¾ cup sliced onions
1 large clove garlic, mashed
1 sliced green pepper
1 cup plum tomatoes cut up
125 g (4 oz) aubergines, diced
125 g (4 oz) courgettes, diced
30 ml (2 tbsp) olive oil
Salt and pepper to taste

Heat oil in frying pan. Sauté the onions and garlic until golden. Add the pepper. Continue cooking until they are barely soft. Then add the tomatoes, aubergines and courgettes. Bring to a boil. Reduce heat to a simmer and cook, covered, until all the vegetables are done – about 10 minutes. Season to taste with salt and pepper.

French Sherbet

1 cup thick yogurt
½ cup fresh or frozen fruit juice
¼ cup honey
15 ml (1 tbsp) lemon juice
Vegetable salt
2 fresh egg whites, stiffly beaten

Mix yogurt with fruit juice. Add honey, fresh lemon juice and a pinch of vegetable salt and mix thoroughly. Place mixture in freezer until quite firm. Then remove to a bowl and stir until smooth. Now fold in the egg whites. Return to the freezing tray.

This is an excellent dessert to have when you are making dinner just for yourself. It is easy to do, and you can make enough to have on hand for a couple of evenings during the week.

The good food lover's diet

You love to cook – but have a weight problem? This five-day diet allows you to prepare and eat tasty meals, and lose a few pounds, too!

FIRST DAY

Breakfast

Eggs-a-Caper

1 egg
25 g (1 oz) Edam cheese, grated
Seasoning
Few capers
1 tomato
1 slice of wholemeal bread, toasted

Scramble seasoned egg with grated cheese, diluted with a little water, in a non-stick frying pan. Stir in the capers and serve on toasted bread. Garnish with tomato.

Lunch

Summer Sandwiches

4 finely-cut slices of wholemeal bread
12.5 g (½ oz) butter
75 g (3 oz) tinned salmon
125 g (4 oz) cucumber, finely sliced

Make two sandwiches from the 4 slices of bread, each very lightly spread with butter and filled with the salmon and cucumber slices

Dinner

Spicey Steak

5 ml (1 tsp) tomato purée flavoured with a little fresh garlic
5 ml (1 tsp) red wine vinegar
Seasoning
175 g (6 oz) fillet or rump steak
25 g (1 oz) slice lean smoked ham
12.5 g (½ oz) butter
25 ml (1 fl oz) dry red wine
Squeeze lemon juice

Coat steak with mix of tomato purée, vinegar and seasoning; leave for half an hour. Dot surface of steak with butter and grill to medium rare. Set aside on a warm dish. Pour juices from grilled steak into frying pan and use to lightly fry ham; place on top of steak. Make a sauce by adding wine and lemon juice to juices in pan; heat thoroughly. Pour over steak. Serve with 75 g (3 oz) boiled new potatoes and a tomato and onion salad dressed with vinegar.

SECOND DAY

Breakfast

Full o' Goodness Bowl

25 g (1 oz) wholegrain breakfast cereal
1 eating apple, sliced
Few sultanas
150 ml (¼ pt) milk
Dot honey

Stir fruit into cereal; pour milk over and sweeten with honey.

Lunch

Cheesey Asparagus Rolls

3 fine slices wholemeal bread, flattened with a rolling pin
3 fine slices Edam cheese, same size as bread
6 asparagus spears, tinned

Place a slice of cheese and 2 asparagus spears on each of the pieces of bread; roll them up tightly.

Dinner

Bacon Beanfeast

Seasoning
1 onion, peeled and sliced into rings
2 apples, peeled, cored, and sliced into rings
12.5 g (½ oz) butter
Seasoning
10 ml (1 dsp) chopped chives
4 rashers bacon

Lightly fry seasoned apple and onion rings in butter, and allow to cook under cover for short while until soft. While apple and onion rings are cooking, grill bacon rashers. Toss bacon with apple and onion rings; garnish with chopped chives, and season. Serve with salad made from bean sprouts, grated carrot and 15 ml (1 level tbsp) chopped nuts.

THIRD DAY

Breakfast

Citrus Pickup

1 grapefruit, peeled and segmented
1 orange, peeled and segmented
25 g (1 oz) stem ginger, sliced

Mix all together and leave overnight, covered in 'fridge, for juices to combine.

Lunch

Mint and Mushroom Salad

125 g (4 oz) Edam cheese, cubed
25 g (1 oz) sultanas
50 g (2 oz) button mushrooms, cleaned and quartered
Several lettuce leaves
(1 dsp) freshly chopped mint
10 ml (1 dsp) white wine vinegar

Toss cheese, sultanas and mushrooms together; spoon on to lettuce leaves; drizzle on dressing made from the mint and vinegar. Eat with two slices crispbread. Follow with an apple.

Dinner

Fish Niçoise

125 g (4 oz) cod steaks
6 g (¼ oz) butter
1 small onion, peeled and sliced
Little fresh finely chopped garlic
½ green pepper, sliced
2 anchovies, chopped
Few black olives, chopped
Seasoning
1 tomato, sliced
15 ml (1 tbsp) tomato purée
115 ml (4 fl oz) red wine

Gently cook onion, garlic and pepper in the butter. Add anchovies and black olives. Sandwich the mixture between the cod steaks and place in ovenproof dish. Top with tomato slices, and pour over a sauce made from the wine and tomato purée. Bake in a hot oven for about ½ hour. Serve with 75 g (3 oz) boiled or steamed rice mixed with half a green pepper, well chopped, and a large green salad.

FOURTH DAY

Breakfast
Fruity Yogurt
Small carton low-fat natural yogurt
1 apple, peeled and chopped
25 g (1 oz) sultanas
Fold fruit into yogurt. Serve with 1 glass orange juice.

Lunch
Double Decker
3 slices Pumpernickel bread
125 g (4 oz) lean roast beef, sliced
Few lettuce leaves
1 tomato, sliced
Seasoning
Make a double decker sandwich with the bread. Fill two halves with the beef, lettuce and tomato, seasoning to taste.

Dinner
Stuffed Veal
2 × 125 g (4 oz) veal escalopes, beaten thin
50 g (2 oz) Edam cheese slices
15 ml (1 tbsp) chopped walnuts
15 ml (1 tbsp) sultanas
15 ml (1 tbsp) parsley, chopped
12.5 g (½ oz) butter
115 ml (4 fl oz) white wine
Place cheese slices on escalopes. Mix together walnuts, sultanas and parsley; place half of the mixture in centre of each escalope. Roll each one up; tie with string. Brown them in butter, then allow to simmer gently for about 20 minutes in the wine. Serve on a bed of 50 g (2 oz) boiled rice, removing strings first. Spoon over sauce from pan. Accompany with sweetcorn.

FIFTH DAY

Breakfast
Square Meal Starter
1 glass orange juice
1 poached egg
1 toasted slice of wholemeal bread, lightly spread with butter.

Lunch
Ploughman's Feast
75 g (3 oz) chunk French bread
75 g (3 oz) Edam cheese
Stick celery
1 tomato
A spoonful Branston pickle

Dinner
Oyster Cocktail
6 oysters, served with a drizzle of Tabasco sauce.

Steak Tartare
125 g (4 oz) fillet steak, well minced
Ground black pepper
15 ml (1 tbsp) oil
5 ml (1 tsp) red wine vinegar
Dash Tabasco sauce
1 shallot, chopped
1 gherkin, chopped
1 egg yolk
Mix all ingredients together. Serve in a mound on a dish surrounded with a few onion rings, the chopped hard boiled white of an egg, a few gherkin slices, and some capers. Accompany with a large green salad and a slice of wholemeal bread.

Souped-up slimming

Here are soups which are substantial enough to be satisfying meals in themselves. Based on the *cuisine minceur* (slimming) method of cooking, these soups leave plenty of calories to spare for breakfast and dinner – even with the addition of a wholemeal roll and salad. Ideal for the office dieter, some of the soups can be prepared the night before and taken to work in a vacuum flask.

Hot Gazpacho
Serves 4; approximately 120 calories per portion.
400 ml (¾ pt) tomato juice
300 ml (½ pt) stock
2 onions, sliced
225 g (8 oz) tomatoes, chopped
1 green pepper, chopped
1 red pepper, chopped
30 ml (2 tbsp) chopped parsley
2 garlic cloves, crushed
Seasoning
100 g (4 oz) lean ham, chopped
Put all the ingredients, apart from the ham, into a saucepan. Simmer for 20 minutes. Blend the soup in a blender and put into a clean pan. Add the ham and heat through gently.

Soupe Florentine
Serves 4; approximately 160 calories per portion.
450 g (1 lb) fresh spinach
Grated rind of ½ lemon
400 ml (¾ pt) skimmed milk
300 ml (½ pt) stock
Pinch grated nutmeg
Seasoning
2 egg yolks
4 eggs
Put washed spinach into a pan with the lemon rind, skimmed milk, stock, nutmeg and seasoning. Simmer for 15–20 minutes. Blend soup with the egg yolks and heat through gently. Pour into 4 pre-heated ovenproof soup dishes and carefully crack an egg into each. Heat in a moderate oven until the eggs are set.

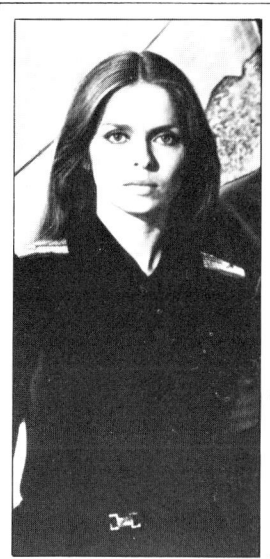

BARBARA BACH, film star:
"I have two diets that work for me. One is the boiled chicken diet. You boil a chicken, remove the skin and eat boiled chicken for every meal, as much as you like — but nothing else. You can lose five pounds easily in three days, but I don't think it's healthy for any longer than that. The other diet works a little slower: live on yogurt exclusively. I lose five pounds in a week on that. When I diet, I make sure I'm kept very busy, and fill in my days doing all sorts of things to keep me away from food."

Courgette Soup au Gratin
Serves 4; approximately 160 calories per portion.
450 g (1 lb) courgettes, sliced
1 onion, chopped
30 ml (2 tbsp) chopped parsley
Seasoning
400 ml (¾ pt) stock
300 ml (½ pt) skimmed milk
Pinch grated nutmeg
100 g (4 oz) Edam cheese, grated
Put courgettes into a pan with onion, parsley, seasoning, stock, skimmed milk and nutmeg. Simmer gently for 20 minutes. Blend soup and pour into 4 pre-heated ovenproof soup bowls. Sprinkle with grated cheese and heat in a moderate oven until cheese melts.

Hot Chowder
Serves 4; approximately 100 calories per portion.
1 small cauliflower
4 sticks of celery, chopped
1 onion, sliced
600 ml (1 pt) stock
300 ml (½ pt) skimmed milk
Seasoning
175 g (6 oz) smoked haddock, flaked
150 ml (¼ pt) fat-free yogurt
Slices of lemon
Trim outer leaves and stalk from cauliflower, then chop roughly and put into a pan with the celery, onion, skimmed milk and seasoning. Simmer until vegetables are tender. Blend the soup and put into a clean pan. Add the haddock and simmer for 5 minutes. Stir in the yogurt and heat gently. Garnish with the lemon.

Potage Paysan
Serves 4; approximately 132 calories per portion.
2 onions, chopped
225 g (8 oz) carrots, chopped
175 g (6 oz) sliced mushrooms
2 leeks, sliced
600 ml (1 pt) stock
150 ml (¼ pt) skimmed milk
45 ml (3 tbsp) tomato purée
Seasoning
225 g (8 oz) lean boned chicken, chopped
Put all the ingredients into a saucepan. Simmer for 20 minutes, and serve with crispbread.

The pasta diet

If you always put spaghetti at the top of your list of forbidden foods, take heart. Pasta *can* be part of a successful slimming regime. The point to remember is that it is the accompaniments to pasta which are fattening: if you substitute low-calorie toppings for rich, creamy sauces you will be able to eat pasta as a treat. A cereal bowl of cooked pasta will add only 200 calories to your daily allowance, and has the advantage of needing just a green salad and fresh fruit to supply a satisfying and healthy meal.

Pasta is made from hard durum wheat, ground into semolina; water is added to make a paste and eggs are added in the manufacture of noodles. Pasta is high in protein content, 24.5 g (1 oz) per average portion, equal to the protein found in three large eggs or 75 g (3 oz) hard cheese, plus traces of vitamins and minerals. The difference between wholemeal and "white" pasta is the same as the difference between brown and white bread; wholemeal pasta has a slightly nutty flavour, takes a little longer to cook than the conventional variety and can be used in any pasta recipe.

Tomato sauce, the classic accompaniment to spaghetti, makes an ideal slimmer's sauce: both tomato paste and tinned tomatoes are extremely low in calories and are good sources of vitamin C. Use a soft cheese such as Edam to garnish, and substitute a dollop of warmed low-fat yogurt for butter. Stir low-fat yogurt into sauces for a creamy consistency and add finely grated raw cauliflower, rather than flour, to thicken. Noodles tossed in warmed cottage cheese thinned with low-fat yogurt and sprinkled lightly with a Dutch cheese makes a delicious low calorie *Fettucine Alfredo*. All the following slimming pasta recipes are grand enough to be served at dinner parties.

Lasagne Florentine
Serves 6; approx 250 calories per portion.
225 g (8 oz) lasagne
15 ml (1 tbsp) oil
450 g (1 lb) fresh spinach

Salt and pepper
150 ml (¼ pt) chicken stock
1 onion, grated
30 ml (2 tbsp) cornflour
Juice ½ lemon
5 ml (1 tsp) salt
5 ml (1 tsp) mixed herbs
1 ml (¼ tsp) garlic powder
150 g (5 oz) carton low fat natural yogurt
225 g (8 oz) carton cottage cheese
1 egg
125 g (4 oz) chopped cooked button mushrooms
50 g (2 oz) grated Dutch cheese

Cook lasagne in boiling salted water with the oil until just tender – about 10 minutes. Drain well in separate sheets. Wash spinach and cook until tender in a little seasoned water. Drain well. Mix the stock with the onion, cornflour, lemon juice, salt, herbs and garlic powder. Stir in the yogurt and spinach. Mix the cottage cheese with the egg. Spoon a quarter of the cottage cheese mixture into the base of a greased ovenproof rectangular dish. Top with a third of the lasagne, a quarter of the cottage cheese mixture, and a third each of the spinach mixture and the mushrooms. Repeat layers until all ingredients have been used, finishing with spinach and mushrooms. Sprinkle with grated cheese and bake at 190°C (375°F, gas Mark 5) for 30 minutes.

Chicken Noodle Waldorf

Serves 6; approx 210 calories per portion.
175 g (6 oz) ribbon noodles
350 g (12 oz) cooked boned chicken, chopped
1 eating apple
Juice ½ lemon
4 stalks celery, chopped
1 egg
550 ml (1 pt) boiling water
2 chicken stock cubes
15 ml (1 tbsp) cornflour
5 ml (1 tsp) salt
2.5 ml (½ tsp) pepper
2.5 ml (½ tsp) powdered cinnamon
1 ml (¼ tsp) ground nutmeg
2.5 ml (½ tsp) mixed spice

Cook noodles in boiling salted water for 4 minutes. Drain well. Put half chicken in base of casserole. Core and chop apple and toss in lemon juice, mix with the celery, egg and cooked noodles. Spread noodle mixture over chicken and top with remaining chicken. Dissolve stock cubes in boiling water and mix with cornflour, seasonings and spices. Pour over noodles and chicken. Cover casserole and cook at 175°C (350°F, gas Mark 4) for 50 minutes.

Tuna Macaroni Salad

Serves 6; approx 175 calories per portion.
100 g (4 oz) shortcut macaroni
150 ml (¼ pt) low fat natural yogurt

1 small onion, grated
10 ml (2 tsp) honey
10 ml (2 tsp) mustard
Juice ½ lemon
5 ml (1 tsp) cider vinegar
Seasoning
200 g (7 oz) can tuna, drained and flaked
½ medium-size white or red cabbage, shredded
2 carrots, grated
2 green peppers, cut into thin strips

Cook macaroni in boiling salted water until just tender. Drain. Mix yogurt together with onion, honey, mustard, lemon juice, cider vinegar and seasoning. Stir this dressing into pasta while it is still warm. Stir in the flaked tuna, cabbage, carrot and pepper. Chill before serving.

Spaghetti Ducchini

Serves 4; approx 230 calories per portion
225 g (8 oz) wholemeal spaghetti
15 ml (1 tbsp) oil
400 g (14 oz) can tomatoes
Salt and pepper
Grated rind and juice of half a lemon
10 ml (2 tsp) honey
15 ml (1 tbsp) tomato purée
5 ml (1 tsp) basil
30 ml (2 tbsp) chopped parsley
175 g (6 oz) mushrooms, chopped
1 onion, finely chopped
1 crushed clove garlic
2 carrots, grated
1 green pepper, chopped
2 stalks celery, chopped
4 courgettes, chopped

Cook the wholemeal spaghetti in a large pan of boiling salted water with the oil, until just tender. Drain well. While spaghetti is cooking, prepare sauce. Put the tomatoes into a pan with the seasoning, lemon rind and juice, honey, tomato purée, basil and parsley. Bring to the boil and add the vegetables. Simmer for about 5 minutes. Stir the sauce into the spaghetti and serve. Each portion can be sprinkled with 25 g (1 oz) of grated Dutch cheese, which adds an extra 80 calories per serving.

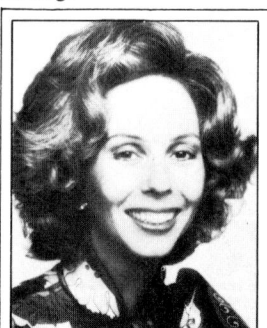

MARION MONTGOMERY, singer: *"I always go on the Scarsdale Diet when I need to lose weight. Occasionally I go to a health farm for a rest, and it puts me in the right frame of mind to adopt a healthy eating pattern. I also recommend a good massage with a good-looking man at least once a week!"*

Forbidden foods

For dieters who can't resist an occasional sinful snack here are some delicious diet treats that are easy to prepare, extra low in calories and just as tasty as the "real" things.

Granité de Mocha
Stir 2 tablespoons chocolate spread (120 calories) and 1 teaspoon instant coffee powder into crushed ice. Eat before it melts.

Chocolate Balls
From *Dr Atkins' Diet Revolution*, a quick recipe for a tasty snack: combine 1 cup of double cream and 1 tablespoon cocoa in the top of a double boiler. Heat until cocoa melts. Soften 1 tablespoon gelatine in 1 tablespoon cold water; add to mixture along with 2 tablespoons peanut butter. Heat until mixture begins to boil; remove from heat. Add 1 tablespoon crème de cacao, 2 tablespoons chocolate extract, 2 tablespoons low-calorie sugar. Blend well. Freeze briefly, then shape into small balls, roll in chopped walnuts or coconut until coated. Freeze again. Low in carbohydrates (about 1.7 g each) but not calories.

Avocado Starter
Mix 25 g (1 oz) tinned crabmeat, flaked (36 calories) with vinegar, drop or two artificial sweetner, salt and pepper to taste. Pile the mixture into a 175 g (6 oz) half of an avocado (150 calories).

Cheese and crackers
Spread wholewheat crackers (a mere 5–10 calories each) with a cheese produced from skimmed milk, like Jarlsberg or mozzarella (80–110 calories per ounce).

Add bezzazz to cottage cheese
Cottage cheese can contain as few as 123 calories per 125-g (4-oz) carton but does get boring. Quick remedy: cut up 2 shallots (8 calories), a celery stalk (6 calories), and ½ carrot (10 calories); stir into cottage cheese. Spice with salt, freshly ground black pepper, a dash of Tabasco sauce, and a pinch of dry dill.

Zealous Relish – a delectable sauce
Mince and mix together: 1 cocktail onion (trace of calories), ½ dill pickle (6 calories), small stuffed green olive (7 calories), hot chilli pepper to taste (trace of calories), and 3 anchovies (25 calories).

Wine Soda
For a refreshing low-calorie cocktail – dilute 50 g (2 oz) dry white or red wine (44 calories) with soda, lots of ice; add a sliver of lemon peel.

Melted cheese
Spread two slices wholewheat bread (130 calories) with mustard. Between them place 25 g (1 oz) sliced Cheddar cheese (110 calories), ¼ fresh tomato, sliced (6 calories) and 1 teaspoon bacon pieces (about 8 calories). Grill on each side till bread toasts.

Steamed spuds
Cut one medium, raw potato (90 calories) into bite-size cubes. Spread out on a vegetable-steaming rack placed over water in a saucepan. Sprinkle with 1 tablespoon parsley, freshly ground pepper, onion or garlic salt. Cover pan and cook until tender (at least 15 minutes).

Spiced pears
Diet dessert? Slice 1 medium, fresh pear (60 calories). Top with 2 tablespoons sour cream (60 calories), 1 teaspoon chopped walnuts (16 calories), and a shake of ground cinnamon and nutmeg.

The Scarsdale diet

Follow this new diet developed by American Dr Herman Tarnower and you will lose up to twenty pounds in fourteen days!

Diet Rules
1 No alcoholic beverages.
2 Do not stay on the diet more than fourteen days.
3 Abstain from everything not included here, and no substitutes.
4 No snacking between meals except raw celery and carrots.
5 Prepare salads without oil or mayonnaise. Use lemon and vinegar.
6 Serve all vegetables without butter.
7 Eat lean meat only.
8 Take coffee black, tea plain. You may use saccharine. Diet drinks are permitted.
9 You need not eat everything listed here, but don't make any substitutions or additions. The *balance* of foods on the diet is what maintains normal energy while you reduce. Indicated combinations must be strictly observed!

Menus
Breakfast (the same every day): Grapefruit, 1 slice of dry protein bread, toasted, coffee/tea

○ **Monday**
Lunch: Cold cuts of lean meat, tomato, coffee/tea
Dinner: Fish, combination salad (as many vegetables as you wish), 1 piece dry toast, grapefruit

○ **Tuesday**
Lunch: Fruit salad, as much as you want, any kind, coffee/tea
Dinner: Plenty of steak, tomatoes, lettuce, celery, olives, Brussels sprouts or cucumber, coffee/tea

○ **Wednesday**
Lunch: Tuna-fish or salmon with lemon-and-vinegar dressing, grapefruit, coffee/tea
Dinner: 2 lamb chops, celery, cucumber, tomatoes, coffee/tea

○ **Thursday**
Lunch: Cold chicken, spinach, coffee/tea
Dinner: 2 eggs, cottage cheese, cabbage, 1 piece dry toast, coffee/tea

○ **Friday**
Lunch: Assorted cheese slices, spinach, 1 piece dry toast, coffee/tea
Dinner: Fish, combination salad (as many fresh vegetables as you want), 1 piece dry toast, coffee/tea

○ **Saturday**
Lunch: Fruit salad, as much as you want, any kind, coffee/tea
Dinner: Cold chicken, tomatoes, grapefruit, coffee/tea

○ **Sunday**
Lunch: Chicken, tomatoes, carrots, cooked cabbage, or broccoli, or cauliflower, grapefruit, coffee/tea
Dinner: Plenty of steak, celery, cucumber or Brussels sprouts, tomatoes, coffee/tea

● If desired, you may have this substitute meal for any lunch: ½ cup low-fat cottage cheese, 5 ml (1 tsp) low-fat sour cream with sliced fruit, 6 walnuts or pecans, plus a diet drink.

Published by Bantam Books, 95p

The vegetable diet

This is the diet for you if you like to leave the dinner table feeling satisfied and not starving! Vegetables are low in calories – yet high in protein, vitamins and valuable minerals. Vegetables provide important roughage for your diet, too.
Drinks allowance: No alcohol, tea or coffe; instead, drink herbal tea or vegetable *bouillon*, available at health stores.

First Day
Breakfast
Small glass vegetable juice, fresh or canned
Large salad bowl of leafy greens, grated carrot and half sliced avocado. Season with salt and freshly ground black pepper; drizzle on a little lemon juice.
Lunch
Small glass vegetable juice
Baked green pepper stuffed with cooked brown rice.
Dinner
Small glass vegetable juice
Steamed vegetables: Layer in steamer three small new potatoes, one onion, three courgettes. Sprinkle with rosemary and steam for approx eight minutes. Serve with a large spoonful of low-fat natural yogurt.

Second Day
Breakfast
As First Day
Lunch
Small glass vegetable juice
One steamed or boiled artichoke. Serve with piquant sauce of natural low-fat yogurt spiced with chopped garlic and chives and seasoned with sea salt and freshly-ground black pepper.
Dinner
Small glass vegetable juice
Stir-fried chopped cabbage: fry a little mustard seed in vegetable oil and when grains turn black, add half a small cabbage, chopped, seasoning, and stir-fry for a couple of minutes. Serve with a bowl of brown rice and soya sauce.

Third Day
Breakfast
As First Day
Lunch
Small glass vegetable juice
Bean sprout salad: large bowl bean sprouts, one quartered tomato, 50 g (2 oz) crumbled Cheshire cheese.
Dinner
Small glass vegetable juice
Stir-fried mixed vegetables: three carrots, sliced lengthways, half an onion, chopped, two celery sticks, sliced lengthways and chopped in half. Stir-fry in vegetable oil; sprinkle dried coconut on top. Serve with a bowl of cooked brown rice and a spoonful low-fat natural yogurt.

Fruit and vegetable fast day

This purifying diet is not as stringent as most liquid fasts because it is vitamin-rich and loaded with energy-boosters.

Prepare all drinks in a blender, and if you are lucky enough to own a juice extractor, make your own fresh vegetable cocktail; if not, buy bottled carrot juice and check on the label that there are no additives. Between juices, you may drink as much bottled water or herbal tea as you wish. Sip all liquids slowly, and take time as you would over a meal.

Breakfast
Orange and Almond Froth
Juice of one fresh orange
1 egg
5 ml (1 tsp) honey
6 blanched almonds
1 cup milk made from low-fat skimmed milk powder
Blend thoroughly and serve in tall, chilled glass
Mid-morning
Carrot and Parsley Cocktail
Small glass carrot juice
Several sprigs fresh parsley
Blend ingredients well and serve in glass
Lunch
Tomato Cup
1 large ripe tomato, skinned and chopped
¼ large cucumber, chopped
1 small carton, 150 g (5 oz) low-fat yogurt
Pinch garlic, fresh or dried
Fresh chopped chives, if available
Blend all ingredients and pour into soup cup
Mid-afternoon
Carrot and Parsley Cocktail
Dinner
Blender Broth
170 g (6 oz) mixed raw chopped vegetables; eg, carrots, celery, leeks, spinach, cauliflower
600 ml (1 pt) water
Pinch salt
Simmer vegetables for twenty minutes in water. Blend. Serve hot.

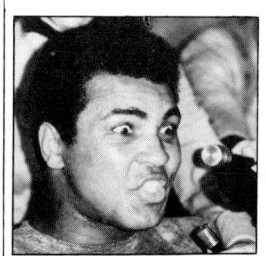

MOHAMMED ALI, heavyweight boxer: *"When I want to lose twenty pounds, I have a light breakfast. Then nothing until evening, when I have grilled meat or fish, and vegetables. I jog for twenty or thirty minutes every morning and have a workout. I do that for about six weeks."*

The milk and honey diet

You are allowed only 750 calories a day on this two-day diet, but unlike most semi-fasts you will benefit from the food and drink intake! Milk and honey combine to provide protein, calcium – and give you an energy boost, too.

In between meals you may drink as many non-alcoholic unsweetened drinks as you like and allow yourself an extra 150 ml (¼ pt) milk for coffee and tea.

Breakfast
Honey Flip
Beat one egg into a glass of milk; add two teaspoonfuls honey. If you prefer a sharper taste, add 1 tablespoon of lemon juice.

Lunch
Either not more than 75 g (3 oz) lean cold meat or not more than 250 g (8 oz) cottage cheese served with a selection from these salad vegetables: French or runner beans, beetroot, cabbage, carrot, cauliflower, celery, celeriac, cucumber, endive, lettuce, onion, radish, tomatoes, watercress.

Evening meal
As breakfast.
Note: After two days, return to your normal diet, but you could continue to replace your breakfast with the Honey Flip.

The lunchbox diet

Interesting and energy-giving – yet none of these lunchtime meals contains more than 350–400 calories. A polythene box, a thermos and a bit of trouble the night before are all that's required.

Pasta Niçoise, plus . . .
Cook 25 g (1 oz) whole wheat pasta rings; drain and cool. Skin and chop 2 tomatoes. Mix with half small onion, chopped, and a pinch mixed herbs. Add pasta. Top with 65 g (2½ oz) drained tuna fish and 25 g (1 oz) grated Edam cheese.
+ Carrot Juice (small bottle carrot juice, available from health stores)
+ Small banana
Potted Meat plus . . .
Mix 40 g (1½ oz) lean minced cooked beef or pork, 15 g (½ oz) low-fat spread, 5 ml (1 tsp) soy sauce and a good pinch raw brown sugar, salt and pepper. Pack in pot and cover with foil.
+ Apple and Prune Salad (to accompany pork)
Toss one diced apple, six chopped prunes and small bunch watercress in lemon juice.
+ Tomato Juce Cocktail
Pinch celery salt and a slice of lemon stirred into a small bottle or tin of tomato juice.
+ Citrus Fruit Salad
Toss segments from one orange and half a grapefruit in the juice of the other half of the grapefruit.
Chicken au Gratin, plus . . .

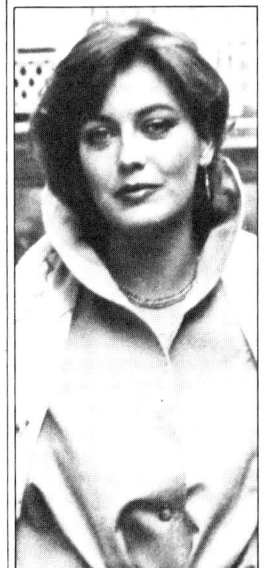

LESLEY - ANNE DOWN, actress: *"As an actress, one should be in tip-top condition most of the time, which can be difficult. I get on to the scales every morning — so that I can catch the problem before it goes too far. If my weight goes up more than three pounds I go on a diet for two days. I have been a non-meat eater for over a year now and think it is superb. I eat lots of fish, salads, fresh fruit, brown bread and brown rice and believe this is the best health and vitality diet going. Also, even on a diet, a few glasses of wine a day perks you up and I don't think it has any effect on weight at all."*

Remove skin from a 275 g (10 oz) chicken joint. Brush with Worcestershire Sauce and a little vegetable oil. Grill for 15–20 minutes, turning occasionally. Place 25 g (1 oz) of Edam cheese on chicken and grill until browned; allow to cool.
+ Ratatouille
Make from sliced aubergines, courgettes, tomatoes and onions, all cooked in a pan with a little water.
+ Sparkling Orange
Small bottle Perrier water with a slice of orange.
+ Grape Yogurt
Stir 50 g (2 oz) halved grapes into a small carton of natural yogurt.
Beef Carbonnade, plus . . .
Cook 125 g (4 oz) stewing beef with sliced onions, tomato purée, and a sauce made from 3 ml (½ tsp) flour and 75 ml (5 tbsp) ale and 75 ml (5 tbsp) stock.
+ Red Cabbage, Apple and Sultana Salad
Toss shredded red cabbage, half a diced apple and a few sultanas in 15 ml (1 tbsp) French dressing.
+ Sparkling Lemon
Small bottle Perrier water with a slice of lemon.
+ Raspberries in Orange Juice
Sprinkle 100 g (4 oz) raspberries with 30 ml (2 tbsp) orange juice.
Cheese and vegetable salad, plus . . .
Tear lettuce; cube 50 g (2 oz) Edam cheese and same amount of cucumber. Mix with 50 g (2 oz) cooked broad beans. Season and toss with 15 ml (1 tbsp) French Dressing.
+ Herb Tea
Sachets are practical for the office – drink as much as you like.
+ Cheese and Biscuits
Two low-calorie crackers with 25 g (1 oz) Dutch Edam cheese.

The three-day watercress and honey diet

This diet is delicious *and* nutritious: honey keeps your energy level from dipping and fulfils your craving for sweet things; watercress is renowned for its blood purifying properties, and should improve skin and digestion.

Note: Daily drinks allowance is unrestricted, although you should not exceed your daily milk allowance of 150 ml (¼ pt) milk. Alcohol is forbidden. When measuring honey for recipes, first dip your spoon in hot water and you will find the honey slips easily off the spoon.

Day 1

Breakfast
115 ml (4 fl oz) tomato juice
1 slice wholemeal bread
3 g (⅛ oz) butter
10 ml (2 tsp) Gale's clear honey

Lunch
Watercress Salad★ with honey salad dressing★
Iced yogurt drink★ (see p 9 of the Nutrition chapter)

Dinner
125 g (4 oz) canned salmon
50 g (2 oz) sliced avocado with a few slices of cucumber
Honey salad dressing★
50 g (2 oz) raspberries, 1 plum,
50 g (2 oz) grapes sweetened with 5 ml (1 tsp) clear honey
Daily milk allowance – 150 ml (¼ pt)
Approximate number of calories consumed: 830

Day 2

Breakfast
½ grapefruit sweetened with 5 ml (1 tsp) clear honey
1 slice wholemeal toast with 2 grilled tomatoes

Lunch
Watercress Salad★ with honey salad dressing★
Iced yogurt drink★

Dinner
Marinated lamb cutlets★
Hot watercress
50 g (2 oz) slice fresh pineapple with a sprig of mint
Daily milk allowance – 150 ml (¼ pt)
Approximate number of calories consumed: 740

Day 3

Breakfast
Slice of melon
1 slice wholemeal toast
4 large grilled mushrooms brushed with 8 g (¼ oz) butter

Lunch
Watercress Salad★ with honey salad dressing★
Iced yogurt drink★

Dinner
75 g (3 oz) lamb's liver grilled
3 g (⅛ oz) butter

1 grilled tomato
125 g (4 oz) boiled cauliflower
75 g (3 oz) boiled spinach
Half a banana sliced with 25 g (1 oz) grapes sprinkled with lemon juice and 5 ml (1 tsp) clear honey plus 2 chopped almonds
Daily milk allowance – 150 ml (¼ pt)
Approximate number of calories consumed: 785

★Recipes

Watercress Salad
½ bunch watercress
½ bunch parsley
25 mm (1 inch) cucumber, diced
½ chicory heart or lettuce heart
50 g (2 oz) chopped boiled lean ham or roast chicken or roast beef
Wash and trim salad ingredients and pick into small pieces. Turn into a bowl and mix with the meat. Add the salad dressing just before serving. Toss and serve immediately.

Honey Salad Dressing
15 ml (3 tsp) vinegar
2.5 ml (½ tsp) mustard
5 ml (1 tsp) clear honey
Salt, ground black pepper
A little garlic (optional)
Mix all ingredients together.

Marinated Lamb Cutlets with Hot Watercress (Serves 3)
3 lamb cutlets, weighing about 30 g–145 g (4½–5 oz) each, well seasoned on both sides with salt and pepper

Marinade: *Hot Watercress:*
Salt and pepper   *Allow 1½ bunches per head*
15 ml (1 tbsp) olive oil   Wash and trim cress
15 ml (1 tbsp) clear honey   then prepare as per instructions
30 ml (2 tbsp) lemon juice (fresh)   below.
2.5 ml (½ tsp) grated lemon peel
10 ml (2 tsp) finely chopped mint
A little chopped garlic

Put the seasoned cutlets into a bowl just large enough to take them in a single layer; blend together the marinade ingredients and pour over the cutlets. Leave to marinate for at least 4 hours (overnight if possible). To cook: remove cutlets from marinade and grill in the normal way, basting frequently with the marinade.

Watercress: Blanch the cress by dipping it rapidly into boiling salted water. Drain well and dry by blotting with a clean tea towel. Place in saucepan with a knob of butter and simmer gently until cooked. When serving pour some of the marinade juices over the cress.

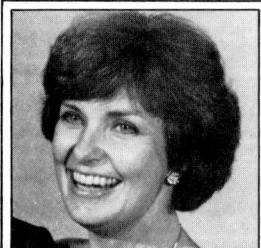

JOANNE WOODWARD, actress: *"The best way to lose weight is: don't eat! I eat breakfast, I rarely eat lunch and very little dinner. I do ballet every day and I run to class and back again. I eat health foods, and I'm a semi-vegetarian."*

The three-day Dutch cheese lover's diet

If you want a quick weight loss in a short space of time, try this no-starvation, tasty diet based on Dutch cheese. Calorie count per day is 1000. You are allowed to drink as much herbal tea as you like; try and limit coffee intake.

First Day

Breakfast
½ grapefruit
Small carton low-fat natural yogurt

Lunch
1 slice Pumpernickel bread topped with 40 g (1½ oz) sliced Edam cheese and 2 sliced radishes
1 orange

Dinner
Chicken and Cheese Supreme:
Cook 25 g (1 oz) rice, and add to it 75 g (3 oz) cooked chopped chicken, a few capers and 1 raw green pepper, thinly sliced. Make a cheese sauce from 20 ml (1½ level tbsp) cornflour, 45 ml (3 tbsp) milk, 45 ml (3 tbsp) water, 62.5 g (2½ oz) grated Edam cheese and seasoning. Add sauce to chicken mixture. Serve with steamed green beans or carrots.

Second Day

Breakfast
Chilled Coffee Shake:
Whisk together 1 egg, 25 ml (1 fl oz) milk, 5 ml (1 tsp) coffee powder, few drops liquid artificial sweetener; pour into tall glass.

Lunch
Mix together 50 g (2 oz) cooked ham, cut into cubes; 50 g (2 oz) Edam cheese, chopped; 2 rings of tinned pineapple, drained of syrup and chopped; 2 cups finely shredded raw green cabbage; 25 g (1 oz) unsalted nuts of your choice. Toss in dressing of small carton low-fat natural yogurt mixed with 5 ml (1 tsp) ready-to-serve mint sauce.

Dinner
Cheesey Bacon Grill:
Grill crisply 2 rashers back bacon and chop into small pieces. Mix with 37.5 g (1½ oz) grated Edam cheese, and season with ground black pepper. Spoon onto centre of heatproof plate and grill until cheese begins to bubble and brown. Serve with a large portion of spinach.

Third Day

Breakfast
25 g (1 oz) any wholegrain breakfast cereal with 25 ml (1 fl oz) milk.

Lunch
Mix together 50 g (2 oz) grated Edam, 2 carrots, grated. Season.
1 apple
1 small carton low-fat natural yogurt

Dinner
Dutch Omelette:
Mix 2 eggs with 15 ml (1 level tbsp) tomato paste and make omelette, using knob butter in frying pan. Make filling from 30 ml (2 tbsp) cooked peas, 1 sliced stewed onion, 50 g (2 oz) grated Edam, seasoning. Serve with 2 tomatoes, sliced, and 25 g (1 oz) wholemeal bread.

The five-meal-a-day diet

Eat throughout the day – you'll never have time to be hungry. The daily calorie count? Just 1200.

To follow the plan, choose one menu from each of the five groups in the columns below. Any combination will provide the variety of foods you need, including two servings each of protein-rich foods and milk, and four each from the bread and cereal, fruit and vegetable groups. To plan your own menus, choose foods that follow the same general plan. Don't forget to check calories and serving sizes so you won't overdo the calories.

Breakfast: a serving of bread or its equivalent in cereals, crackers, etc, and one of skimmed milk, buttermilk or yogurt. Total: 200 calories.

Midmorning: a moderate serving of fruit – ones high in vitamin C, like citrus fruits, are best – plus a serving of skimmed milk or alternatives like cottage cheese, yogurt or hard cheese, and extras (eg, crackers). Total: 200 calories.

Lunch: a 50 g (2 oz) serving of protein-rich foods like meat, fish, poultry, eggs or cheese, plus a serving of bread or an equivalent (see breakfast list) and a vegetable. Total: 200 calories.

Dinner: a 75 g (3 oz) serving of protein-rich foods, two of breads and one each of fruits, vegetables. Total: 400 calories.

Midevening: anything to add the remaining 200 calories.

Breakfast
(about 200 calories)
1 cup ready-to-eat or ¾ cup hot cereal
250 ml (8 fl oz) skimmed milk

225 g (8 oz) plain yogurt
1 slice rye or white toast

25 g (1 oz) Swiss cheese on 1 slice wholemeal toast

½ cup cottage cheese
1 slice rye or white toast

Midmorning
(about 200 calories)
125 ml (4 fl oz) orange juice
½ cup cottage cheese
2 rye crispbreads

Large bunch grapes
25 g (1 oz) hard cheese

2 tangerines or 1 pear
250 ml (8 fl oz) buttermilk or skimmed milk

½ cup fresh fruit
25 g (1 oz) Cheddar cheese on 2 crackers

1 large apple
250 g (8 oz) plain yogurt

1 cup cherries, other berries
250 ml (8 fl oz) skimmed milk

Lunch
(about 200 calories)
50 g (2 oz) lean ham as open sandwich on bread or toast
Carrot sticks

2 hard or soft-boiled eggs
1 crispbread

Celery stalks
37.5 g (1½ oz) Swiss or Cheddar cheese melted on 1 slice toast
Cucumber wedges

50 g (2 oz) sliced chicken on 4 crispbreads
Sliced tomato

½ cup cottage cheese
4 Melba toasts
Shredded lettuce

25 g (2 oz) turkey on small roll
Chopped lettuce

2 poached eggs on 1 slice toast
Green-pepper strips

Dinner
(about 400 calories)
Grilled chicken breast with twist lemon
1 cup parslied rice
½ cup spinach
1 small apple

75 g (3 oz) hamburger on bun
Peach half on lettuce

75 g (3 oz) ham or lamb
Large baked potato with bouillon
½ cup chopped broccoli
½ cup pineapple in own juice

125 g (4 oz) grilled turbot seasoned with salt, pepper, oregano
1 cup noodles
½ cup green beans
1 tangerine

Tuna salad with low calorie dressing in toasted sandwich
Cucumber salad
½ small banana in orange juice

125 g (4 oz) steak, grilled
Chopped onion
Ketchup
Large boiled potato
Unsweetened blackberries

125 g (4 oz) pork chop, grilled with orange slices
¾ cup sliced sweet potatoes
½ cup asparagus or cabbage
1 small bunch grapes

Midevening
(about 200 calories)
½ cup chocolate pudding
Coffee or tea

2 cups lightly-buttered popcorn
Bottle diet soda

Small bottle beer

3 chocolate chip cookies
1 cup espresso coffee

¼ cup shelled pecans

Iced tea with lemon

1 cup unshelled sunflower seeds
Bottle diet soda

Are you a carbo addict?

Emma Powell shows you how you can lose weight – yet still enjoy your favourite fattening foods!

How hooked on carbohydrates are you? Imagine . . . the smell of new bread, the sight of that thick bar of chocolate as you tear away the foil wrap, the crunch of a crisp sweet biscuit, the taste of a chewy toffee or a large, soft pile of mashed potato.

If your saliva glands are tingling and your hands are almost reaching out for the nearest bite of sweet or stodge you *are* probably hooked. And with you, at a conservative estimate, is over half the population of this country. But, if you are trying to lose weight, your reaction won't be just one of pleasure. For these, by a long process of brain-washing, are the "forbidden foods", the ones that make you fat. And the would-be slimmer who cannot cut them out completely, experiences a quite genuine sense of guilt.

Stop feeling guilty, weak-willed or just a hopeless addict. You can slim and include sweet and stodgy foods in your diet – in fact, if you have a particularly sweet tooth, you will almost certainly achieve better results with a diet that allows carbos in controlled amounts.

Recent research by *Slimming Magazine* in conjunction with Mars Ltd proves just this point. Two panels of slimmers, starting from the same weight levels, in the same age groups and physical conditions, but all carbo addicts, were tested with separate diets. One panel followed a traditional low-carbo diet, the other, a diet of 1,500 calories a day – comparable with the calorie intake on a low-carbo method – but with menus which allowed limited amounts of crisps, peanuts, ice cream and biscuits, plus the delightful indulgence of one whole Mars Bar every day.

At the end of the eight weeks trial, the panel on the low-carbo diet had lost, on average, 4 kg (9.1 lb) per head; those on the Mars Bar diet, a much more significant 5.5 kg (12.1 lb). The dropout percentage, perhaps the most important factor was interesting, too. Fifty-eight percent of the women on the low-carbo diet just couldn't "stand the course". On the diet that did allow sweet and stodgy foods, only thirty-one percent failed to make it to the final weight-check. (The Mars Bar diet is available from The Mars Health Education Dept, Stanhope House, Stanhope Place, London W2. Please enclose a stamped addressed envelope.)

Of course it is wise to be sensible about carbohydrates. Because they tend to be the foods most readily available, easily eaten, because, psychologically, they are often associated with safe, loving childhood moments, it is very, very easy to go overboard. And, on top of all that, too much sugar will ruin your teeth and play havoc with your skin.

Control is sensible, but if you are the slimming failure whose carbo cravings stopped your diet efforts getting off the ground, here is the diet for you. . .

The basic diet menus allow for three normal meals a day. The treats are your extras. If you are a nibbler you may choose up to ten items from the Small Treats selection; if you prefer something more substantial to satisfy that craving, choose two from the Big Treats selection. Your overall calorie intake will be equivalent to that of a low carbohydrate diet. But we have been generous with the goodies to get you started on your slimming campaign and to prevent you feeling underprivileged.

Think of this, not just as a slimming diet, but as a way to learn to live with your carbo craving. Aim to end your dieting with, if possible, only five items from the first list or one from the second. That way, you won't just be slimming – you'll be learning to keep yourself well treated for life, safely, and nutritiously!

Diet
You are allowed each day: 300 ml (½ pt) standard Silver Top milk; 12.5 g (½ oz) butter or margarine for cooking or spreading; and normal portions of any of the following vegetables – green salads, cucumber, radishes, tomatoes, green pepper, spring greens or cabbage, runner beans, sprouts, broccoli, cauliflower, leeks, onion, spinach, celery, swedes, turnips, carrots, mushrooms (not fried).

Breakfast
Large egg, boiled or poached, or 1 medium egg scrambled with a little milk, no butter, or two well-grilled rashers streaky bacon or 1 well-grilled rasher back bacon or 1 well-grilled chipolata sausage plus tomatoes, or 150 g (5 oz) smoked haddock, boiled or steamed, or 75 g (3 oz) grilled kidney and tomatoes, plus 1 thin slice bread (or toast) from large loaf and 5 ml (1 tsp) marmalade.

Lunch and dinner
Choose two from this selection a day. Use Small Treat items to augment the basic meal suggestions.

Small pork chop or medium lamb chop, well-grilled; 2 medium slices any roast meat, trimmed of fat; 150 g (5 oz) raw weight steak, grilled; generous helping smoked salmon; generous helping buttered shrimps; 175 g (6 oz) gammon steak, grilled and trimmed of fat; generous veal escalope, grilled; 1 baked chicken drumstick or small chicken joint; one 2-egg omelette filled with prawns or mushrooms or tomatoes; 2 fried fishcakes; one 175 g (6 oz) portion fish, shallow-fried in breadcrumbs; 250 g (8 oz) white fish – sole, plaice, haddock, cod or hake – grilled with a brushing of fat, or up to 175 g (6 oz) dressed crab; 175 g (6 oz) braised or grilled kidneys or liver (any variety); 1 bowl thick soup, any flavour, plus thick slice of bread from large loaf or 2 good slices salt beef plus 15 ml (1 tbsp) pickle; 75 g (3 oz) minced beef stewed with onion, tomato or carrots (gravy, not thickened) – serve with rice or spaghetti from Small Treats; 125 g (4 oz) salmon cutlet grilled or boiled, or ¾ of a 200 g (7½ oz) tin canned salmon, well-drained or 125 g (4 oz) slice roast chicken or turkey; one 175–200 g (6–7 oz) smoked trout; 4 fish fingers grilled; one 125 g (4 oz) cheeseburger; 4 frankfurters or hot sausages.

Small Treats
You may have up to ten a day. 10 ml (2 tsp) sugar (for fruit or drinks); 1 small banana; 125 g (4 oz) beetroot, weighed boiled; 6 dates; 2 dried figs; 1 small roast potato; one 15 ml (1 tbsp) gravy; 1 medium slice melon; 1 apple, orange or pear; 125 g (4 oz) grapes; ½ large grapefruit plus 5 ml (1 tsp) sugar; 1 medium slice fresh pineapple; 2 small chocolate finger biscuits; 1 small shortcake biscuit or Swiss cream; 1 large digestive, ginger or bourbon biscuit; 2 sponge fingers or marie biscuits; 1 thin slice bread or 2 Primula crispbreads; 15 ml (1 tbsp) currants or sultanas; one ice lolly; 50 g (2 oz) potato – boiled or plain mashed; 37.5 g (1½ oz) rice, weighed boiled; ½ tube fruit gums; 5 ml (1 tsp) drinking chocolate, or Ovaltine with milk from allowance; 150 ml (¼ pt) glass grapefruit juice, or 300 ml (½ pt) tomato juice; 1 glass fruit squash using not more than 30 ml (2 tbsp) concentrate; 2 barley sugar lumps, or 3 Murray-mints; 1 whole packet chewing gum; 1 liquorice stick; 3 fruit-flavoured boiled sweets, 3 Ritz crackers; 9 Twiglets, or 12 Cheeselets.

Big Treats
You may have two a day instead of the ten Small Treats, or one from this list and five from the other.

Average bowl of cornflakes or rice crispies with 1 small 5 ml (1 tsp) sugar and a little milk; 1½ dinner rolls, or 1 thick slice of bread from large loaf, buttered normally; 1 small slice chocolate gateau; 2 Scotch pancakes, thinly buttered with a 5 ml (1 tsp) jam; 37.5 g (1½ oz) milk or plain chocolate; 1 small pancake with lemon juice and 5 ml (1 tsp) sugar; large bowl chocolate blancmange, or bigger one of sorbet; 2 small creme caramels; ½ family vanilla block of ice cream; big bowl of soufflé; 1 tube Smarties; 26 lumps of sugar; 30 ml (2 tbsp) portion apple crumble; 1 doughnut; thin slice of fruit cake; 5 cheese sandwich biscuits; 2½ orange sandwich biscuits; 4 shortbread rounds; 4 milk chocolate mallows; 4 plain chocolate wholemeal biscuits *or* rich short-bread; 1 medium slice chocolate sponge cake, ginger or florida sponge, *or* 2 chocolate ripple rolls, jam tarts, *or* jam ripple rolls; 1 chocolate eclair plus 1 Small Treat item; 1 small packet crisps; 1½ real fruit yogurts; 2½ slices bread from large loaf, cut thin; 1 large potato baked in jacket, or 3 pieces roast potato, or 125 g (4 oz) portion chips; 175 g (6 oz) rice, weighed boiled; 1 small Cadbury's Fruit and Nut bar or Mars; Bounty Bar or 1½ Rowntree's Walnut Whips.

This diet is based on about 1,500 calories a day and if you stick to it without cheating you should lose weight steadily. As it is not a crash diet, it is suitable for long-term slimming, but if after a few weeks you find you are no longer losing weight, you should cut down on the Treats until you reach your target.

Less weighty problems

You may think that, if you manage to lose weight, all your troubles will be over but that is not always true. Many people find it difficult to adjust to the new person they have become and, in the most severe cases, make it an excuse to pile the weight back on.

This is the end of the rainbow; where is the crock of gold?

Fat girls tend to think that thin girls have a wonderful life and only fatness comes between themselves and their heart's desire. But life can be tough for slim girls, too. Yes, it is more fun to be slim and that is your reward for all your hard work and self-denial, but you are going to have to work even harder if you are to become the sparkling conversationalist, brilliant dancer or wonderful lover you wanted to be.

Here is the rainbow's end, here is the gold, but I'm scared

The very successful dieter who has lost a lot of weight some-times has an even more unexpected problem. If you used to hide behind acres of flesh, you learned to cope with your problems in certain ways: you could be "one of the boys" because none of the boys were likely to lust after you. With the

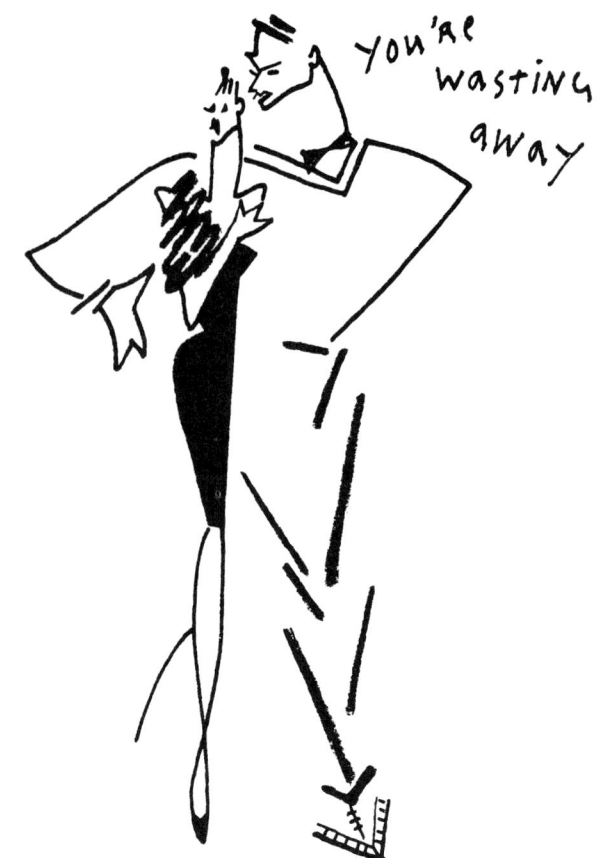

you're wasting away

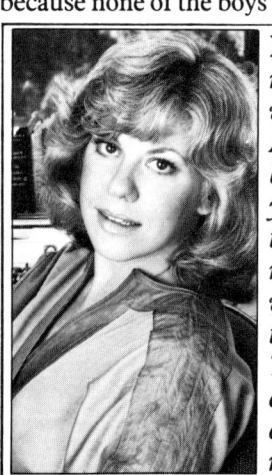

ERICA JONG, writer: *"I had never been able to control my weight until I started doing yoga. And it helps control my metabolism. I lost fifteen pounds last year, and I've been able to maintain it because of yoga. I'm not model-thin, but I don't feel overweight. I eat three meals a day; that way, it's easier not to binge. The secret is to do anything you can really live with, even if you cheat once and eat chocolate mousse."*

weight gone, lust begins to raise its disconcerting head — perhaps for the first time. Suddenly you are getting admiring glances from men in the street, wolf-whistles instead of cat-calls. Suddenly, at the age of twenty, thirty, or more, you have become thirteen again and have to learn to deal with men.

Even if you had a steady relationship before you began your diet, the new you is going to notice some changes. Now there is an added element of choice in your relationships, and your man will notice it, too. Do not be surprised if *he* starts acting strangely, he needs to be reassured that you will not flit off with someone else.

If you are prepared for these problems, you have a good chance of solving them. Certainly, you should not let them spoil an ideal opportunity for a new, and better, future.

This may sound exaggerated, but if you have been fat virtually all your life, you may have paid the penalty by not having had a full relationship with the opposite sex. Don't get swept off your feet by the first to come along!

EXERCISE

Slot any kind of workout into your daily regime and it's not only your body that will benefit: your energy level will rise, your health will improve — and your skin will glow! Scared to get into training when you're out of condition? If you're not in shape to start a sport, let the pros show you how: from the right breathing technique and ways to save your back from strain, to the correct clothes to wear. Follow simple diagrams for spot exercises that reshape your body, warm-ups that tone and firm flab, plus limb-stretching yoga and ballet movements. And if you can't decide which sport's for you, these pages provide the low-down on all the options — from jogging to roller disco. There's no excuse now to sit in a heap because you'll discover that when you're tired is a great time to exercise and recharge your batteries. So get moving, exercise is *fun!*

Which sport is right for you?

You can't decide whether to take up jogging or swimming? Like to try yoga? All the benefits — and limitations — of today's most popular sports are outlined below. Follow our comprehensive guide and see which suit your body — and lifestyle — best!

The ideal exercise regime includes at least one aerobic exercise, ie a physical workout that increases the vigour and stamina of the cardiorespiratory system (heart, blood vessels, lungs). Heart and lungs, like other muscles, weaken and atrophy from disease; when these organs are properly conditioned, however, they become stronger and we become less vulnerable to heart attacks and strokes, which is why aerobics are considered to be life-prolonging and the lack of them considered to be life-threatening.

While all the exercises listed here offer some aerobic benefits, two of them (yoga and calisthenics) are important principally for the good effects they have on the musculoskeletal system. Well-worked muscles are also vital to sustaining good health, since the more flexible and stronger your body, the less likely it is to succumb to pain or injury.

Also, since tight, well-toned muscles are much more attractive than saggy ones, yoga and/or calisthenics will help you to look your sleekest as well.

JOGGING

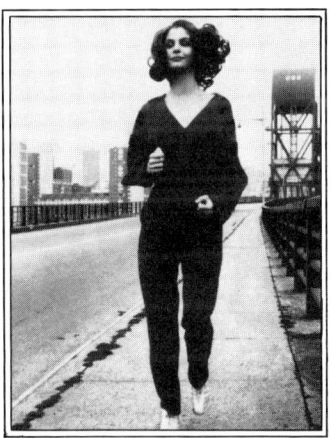

This is the most popular physical activity in America today. Fans on both sides of the Atlantic testify that the experience elevates the spirit as well as strengthening and toning the body. Experienced women joggers usually run from four to six miles, but even a one-to-two mile daily stint (easily accomplished in under half an hour) can work wonders for your complexion, circulatory system, and state of mind. Jogging is better for you than any of the "stop and start" exercises (eg tennis or gymnastics), since the action of heart and lungs is both intense and continuous. Only swimming and skipping with a rope provide comparable aerobic benefits. Jogging also helps keep your figure trim: besides toning and strengthening the legs, it has a firming effect on the muscles of the buttocks, generally a badly underworked area.

According to fitness experts, a modest two-mile jog every day will keep your cardiorespiratory system in peak condition. To begin, you need a pair of running shoes (Plimsolls or sneakers do not supply sufficient support), and a soft dirt or clay surface. (Jogging on cement can cause injury to the foot and leg.) Always begin with five minutes or so of warm-up exercises: shoulder and leg stretches combined with knee bends will do nicely. At first, simply jog until you tire (perhaps no more than one-eighth of a mile), walk until you feel vigorous again, then start again to run lightly. Build up your stamina before you start concentrating on speed, and never push beyond your physical capacity. If your heart is pounding and your legs cramp, stop and walk for a while.

Watchpoints You will be less likely to suffer "shin splints" (painful bruises to the calfbone) and/or sprained tendons if you build stamina *slowly* and are careful always to run on a soft surface. Besides doing warm-ups beforehand, you should always allow yourself a cooling-down period — five minutes of light physical activity, like walking, is ideal. If you just flop, the sudden withdrawal of air from fully oxygenated lungs can result in dizziness or even fainting.

SWIMMING

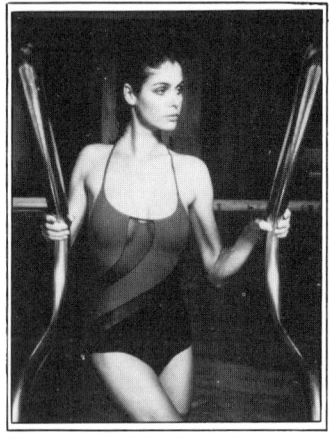

This guarantees one of the most enlivening cardiovascular workouts of all (only sprinting is significantly more strenuous), as well as possibly the most *psychologically* refreshing form of exercise: there is nothing like the sensation of weightlessness to drain away the day's tension! Indeed, swimming has been called the perfect exercise, in that it works the *whole* body without placing undue strain on any part. Jogging, on the other hand, although aerobically valuable, is very hard on the feet.

Some special benefits of swimming When the body is submerged in water, blood circulation automatically increases, and lung ventilation deepens. Then, as you begin to move (ie swim), both circulation and ventilation are further increased. The most vigorous stroke and the one providing the best cardiovascular workout, is the Australian crawl: on your belly, propelling yourself with an arm-over-arm motion, your head ducking rhythmically in and out of the water. The side, back and breast strokes, which allow for momentary rests between motions, are somewhat less efficient, but still good for heart and lungs. As long as you are moving in the water, your body will be benefiting.

In addition to providing an excellent aerobic workout, swimming is a tremendously good way to stretch and firm the muscles: almost any stroke uses all the muscle groups. It is so good for you that doctors will often recommend it as therapy for patients suffering from any of a wide range of disorders, including bad back, arthritis, and elevated blood pressure. The gentle action of the water provides an invigorating supply of blood to damaged or aching limbs, while the sport's relaxing properties soothe psychological distress.

Because swimming strengthens the entire musculoskeletal structure, particularly the spine, it is good *preventive* exercise as well. Most of our back problems derive from the fact that, as bipeds, we must remain in a stressful upright posture (other mammals distributing weight on four legs rarely suffer slipped discs). Swimming eases this strain in two ways — first, the sport is performed in a prone position, and second, it strengthens the abdominal muscles that support the spinal column.

Where to swim Public swimming pools are inexpensive and generally well-maintained and, if you live in a city, you can probably select from several health clubs with pools.

How much swimming to aim for A good workout involves thirty to forty continuous Olympic-sized laps, but, as with jogging, you must work up to this. Three or four laps, followed by five minutes of rest, followed by more laps until you tire, is a fine beginning for the novice swimmer. Stamina builds quickly in this sport, though, and you will be surprised at how easily your capacity increases.

WALKING

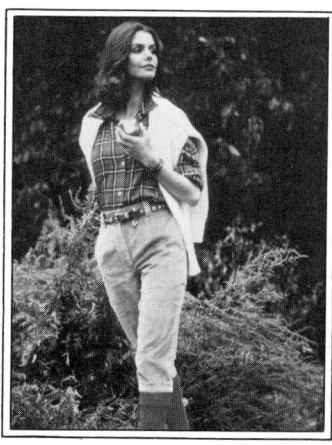

In its way, a long, long walk may be as good for you as an hour's swim in the pool. The walker's easy, continuous motion, which can be sustained for hours, even by those of us who are only in moderately good condition, affords a gentle but excellent cardiovascular workout. Long *brisk* walks bring greatest benefits (walking two and a half miles in thirty-five minutes is the aerobic equivalent of running one and a half miles in thirteen minutes or of swimming 550 m [600 yds] in fourteen minutes).

When you walk, more than half the body's muscles are used: all the foot, leg and hip muscles; the back, abdominal and rib muscles; even the arm, shoulder and neck muscles move as you swing along in stride.

Walking also benefits the parts of the body involved in digestion and elimination and serves as a natural tranquillizer.

The more you walk, and the more regularly, the better. If possible, walk to and from work — or at least to and from a bus stop farther than your usual one! Set aside a few hours at the weekend for a hike: walk briskly, and swing your arms from side to side, thus ensuring that your torso, and not just your lower body, becomes involved. It's important to get the whole of you moving. Research the best walks in your area by contacting local hiking clubs and park authorities, and check to see if your town offers walking tours of interesting or historically significant areas.

BICYCLING

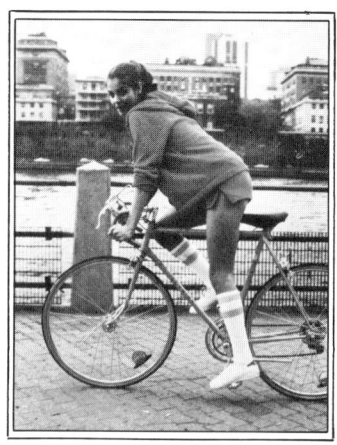

This offers a good cardio-vascular workout (cycling six miles in thirty minutes is the aerobic equivalent of jogging one and a half miles in twenty minutes), while it strengthens back and leg muscles. As with almost any exercise, more is better, but even a brief stint on your bicycle will help refresh heart, lungs and muscles. An experienced cyclist should be able to negotiate twenty-five miles in about an hour and a half, which means moving briskly along at just under fifteen miles per hour. You probably won't be biking so fast at first, and surely not for as long (a two or three mile ride provides a good enough workout for beginners), but, if feeling ambitious, you might set that as your goal.

What kind of bike to buy Bikes come in speeds, with one, three, five and ten speeds the most common. Heavy, unwieldy one-speed bikes have pedal brakes and are just like the one you learned to ride on as a child. Three-speed bikes, somewhat lighter and with hand brakes, are adequate if the terrain is flat but not nearly so acceptable when you're trying to climb up a steep hill.

Probably you will want either a five or ten-speed bike, both of which assure an easy uphill ride. The crossbar on the man's ten-speed model actually makes for a structurally sturdier bike, but may take some getting used to if, like most women, you learned to ride on a girl's bike.

Racing (or backwards-tilted) handlebars, which are also a common feature on ten-speed bikes, can be difficult to master as well.

Watchpoint Traffic can be very dangerous in the city, and dogs are almost equally menacing on country rides. If you're riding for pleasure, stick to designated bike paths — or ride your bike in the park.

THE SOCIAL EXERCISES

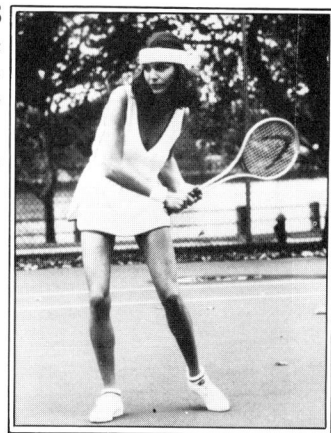

Most recreational sports are slightly less beneficial than solo workouts such as jogging or skipping with a rope. Naturally, though, the more vigorous the sport, the greater the stress on heart and lungs: squash is a better aerobic exercise than tennis, and playing singles works the cardiovascular system harder than doubles.

Though they are somewhat less valuable aerobically than other exercises described here, recreational sports can be much more fun than solitary laps in the park or pool. Hedonistic types who simply could not discipline themselves to do a quarter of an hour skipping with a rope before their morning coffee, have been known to make it to the tennis courts as early as seven in the morning.

What is important is to find the exercise that suits your temperament, and keep with it. Different sports work out different areas of your body: tennis strengthens the arms and tightens the buttocks. Horse riding is a terrific way to streamline hips and thighs. Golf strengthens and shapes shoulders.

And, though it's not strictly a sport, disco dancing works out very nearly all of your body. It differs from other recreational sports in that it does tax heart and lungs: dancing vigorously for fifteen minutes can be quite as strenuous as jogging two miles!

Watchpoint It's better and safer to pay for instruction than to attempt to struggle by on your own: an untutored backhand at tennis can damage the muscles of your arm — a fall from a horse can kill.

CALISTHENICS

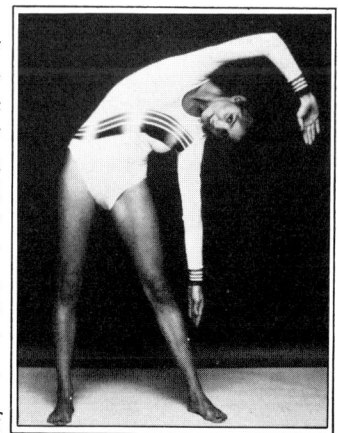

Calisthenics are principally muscle-stretching and strengthening exercises which are marvellous for your body shape though they do not ask much from your heart and lungs, unless done very vigorously and for an unusually long time. They do, however, lend a lithe suppleness to the body and a tautness to your muscles which can make you look skinnier and more shapely. The greatest advantage of calisthenics is that they may be done anywhere, at any time, and require no equipment. Jumping jacks will wake you up faster than your morning cup of coffee, and five minutes of workouts in the office at mid-afternoon will revive you a treat! Follow the shape-up routines in this section, or begin by taking a class, and put your expertise to work at home. If you join a gym to take calisthenic classes, you can then use the equipment provided, too. Start with supervision! Gymnastics turn calisthenics into a sport, and since some of the gym routines taught are extended and rather vigorous, you benefit aerobically while you strengthen and firm muscles. Performed regularly and over a long period of time, adult gymnastics will alter the contours of your body, slightly broadening the shoulders, lifting breasts, firming hip and stomach area.

YOGA

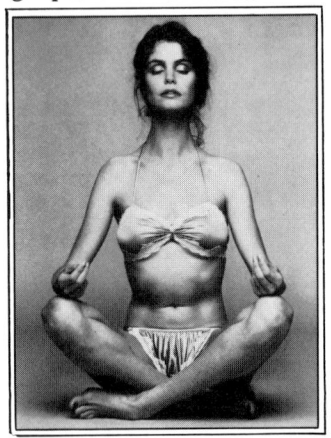

Imported to this country from India, yoga is a form of exercise which attempts systematically to renew each body part, beginning with the scalp and moving right down to the toes. Unlike most forms of exercise, yoga doesn't *build* muscles, but rather alternately compresses and stretches them. An obvious result of this is increased flexibility — a veteran yoga practitioner can assume poses that an acrobat might envy — but greater elasticity is only *one* effect of a discipline whose primary aim is to bring arterial (oxygen-carrying) blood to each part of the body, as it carries away veinous (waste-transporting) blood. Tension is drained away along with "bad blood", leaving the body more relaxed and vigorous.

The various postures of yoga are addressed to different parts of the body, though many of them involve the spine, which, in yogic thought, is the core of our strength and stamina. In the "cobra", for example (all positions are colourfully named), you lie prone, then raise the upper body until the spine is fully arched. As your torso curves upward, back muscles are compressed and supplied with arterial blood. This is a relatively simple yogic posture, but positions become more difficult and advanced as you progress in the discipline. In the "full lotus", for example, you sit with knees bent, placing the right foot high upon the left thigh and vice versa.

The full range of yogic postures is far too extensive and complex to be briefly described, since it includes positions that address themselves not just to spine and legs, but to the stomach, colon, intestines, liver, kidneys, gall bladder, and reproductive organs — even bones and joints. There are also special breathing exercises designed to refresh the lungs. In its most advanced form, yoga involves meditative techniques that clear the mind of accumulated toxins, but it would require a professional to explain how that works. Suffice to say that, physiologically, the benefits of yoga are vast and well-documented, as are its splendid effects on your figure. Yoga tones the muscles, and, while not precisely an aerobic discipline (there's no heavy work done by heart and lungs), its replenishment of arterial blood makes an important contribution to cardiovascular fitness.

No equipment is required and yoga can be done anywhere and at any time (while practitioners may *enjoy* maintaining a "locked lotus" for half an hour at a time, even a five minute yoga break can stimulate and refresh the body). And although advanced forms of this discipline can be quite complicated, the rudiments of yoga can easily be mastered, and instruction is usually inexpensive.

SKIPPING WITH A ROPE

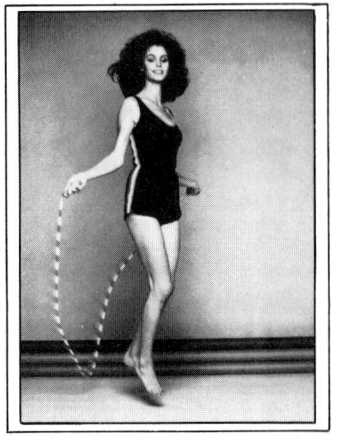

More popular in the States, though gaining popularity over here, skipping with a rope or "jumping rope" is a good, concentrated aerobic exercise. If you jump vigorously for five minutes, the benefits to heart and lungs are as great as one half-hour of jogging, and this form of exercise compares favourably with other sports: fifteen minutes of skipping is the aerobic equivalent of three sets of singles tennis or swimming 640 m (700 yds) in twenty minutes. Skipping also benefits the figure, toning arms, firming pectoral muscles, tightening buttocks, thighs, hips and developing the calf muscles. Skipping with a rope is convenient: you can do it anywhere, any time, with a minimum of equipment (running shoes and a rope are all you need). Go slowly at first, jumping a minute or so until your tire; rest, then begin again. Make fifteen minutes a day of continuous jumping your goal, but expect to build up to that gradually.

Jumping to music is fun and a good way to time yourself. If you skipped when a child, you probably remember how — but it's important to turn the rope with your wrists, not your arms, and to jump lightly on the balls of your feet. (If you can hear your feet as they strike the floor, then you are jumping too heavily.) Note that a simple running step is as beneficial as other fancier ones!

Questions you may ask about exercise

Is it necessary to limber up before exercising?
Yes, it's a good idea, particularly if you're jogging first thing in the morning. When you get out of bed your muscles are slack, and that's when it's easy to strain or pull them. The Health Education Council issue a free Health Pack which includes a useful chart of exercises (there's also a booklet on fitness, plus a Look After Yourself badge); write to them at London SE99. Meanwhile, do a few basic stretches, leg bends (knee to chest) and circle your arms and shoulders.

What about exercise during your period?
Although some women feel less energetic at this time, exercise won't do any harm. In fact, some women say it helps premenstrual tension and cramps.

Does it matter what time of day you choose to exercise?
The actual time you take exercise is immaterial so long as you're not doing it on a full stomach (leave at least an hour after each meal). The one time to avoid is immediately before going to bed, as exercise will mobilise the muscles, stimulate the brain and can stop you sleeping.

Why do my legs go red after I've been running for a few minutes — is it a danger sign?
No, it's simply a matter of circulation. As you get fitter this will probably improve and the redness will eventually disappear. Don't worry about it.

Is it safe to exercise during pregnancy?
Yes, except when it becomes uncomfortable in the last stages. In fact, women athletes seem to produce heavier and healthier babies and have far fewer miscarriages than other women.

Is it true that you can run or walk off a cold or flu?
No. Vigorous exercise if you are ill — particularly if you have a fever — can actually make you worse or lead to something more serious. Better to stay at home in the warm.

What to wear

Comfortable, strong shoes are essential for walking — it's misery otherwise. Not so important for cycling, but a rubber sole for grip is a good idea. For jogging or skipping it's important to have a decent pair of running shoes with a thick sole and some support for the instep.

Try to wear cotton clothing — at least next to your skin — it breathes as you sweat. Make sure nothing is too tight: a tracksuit is ideal, but otherwise not-too-tight jeans, a T-shirt and a jacket you can undo when hot are fine.

Women should always wear a bra that fits and supports them well. Bouncing bosoms can hurt (and they won't do your figure any good at all) and nipples can hurt, too, if they have been rubbing against a T-shirt.

Good habits to get into

- Leave the car at home on short shopping trips.
- Get off the tube one station earlier (or get on one station later) and walk the difference.
- Get out of the lift a few floors too soon, and take the stairs up to your flat or office.
- Walk or run up and down escalators.
- Don't wait for buses: start walking to the next stop. Run if the bus is beating you there.
- Park your car a short way from where you want to go.
- If you can, choose a pub or restaurant you can walk to.
- If you usually walk to the station or bus stop, try running.

How to start

Gently, especially if you're unfit, overweight or a smoker. It's easy to go mad on the first and second days and not be able to move on the third. Best plan is to start little by little, slowly and progressively. Do a few minutes more, or go a little faster each day until you reach a level that suits you. If you get pains in your chest or other symptoms, stop and see your doctor.
Note Anyone with a history of heart disease or problems with joints or muscles MUST SEE THEIR DOCTOR before starting on a fitness routine; likewise, anyone with a history of back trouble should ask their doctor's advice before embarking on any workout programme.

How to check your progress

The easiest way is by how you feel and how much you can do, but to make it more interesting and to check progress more accurately, you need to keep an eye on your heart rate. First establish what is the fastest it should beat after exertion: do this by subtracting your age from 200, then subtract a further forty (for unfitness), leaving you with the number of times your heart should safely beat per minute. When you start exercising, check your pulse every few minutes — do this by placing three fingers on the inside of your wrist under the thumb and counting the number of beats made in fifteen seconds, then multiply by four to get the rate per minute — if the count per minute is higher than your pulse rating, stop and wait for it to go down. Exercise in spurts of a few minutes, then rest. Gradually make the exercise periods longer until you can do ten minutes continuously, keeping the pulse rate at your level.

Excuses that won't wash

My legs ache from overdoing it yesterday.
If you're unfit, muscles are bound to ache but this will wear off if you keep going gently.

I'm sure the extra sleep will do me more good.
Not true, you'll feel far perkier after a run.
I haven't got time.
Make time, and you'll find that you'll need less time in order to do more.
Ouch, my head hurts.
Exercise and fresh air are marvellous for hangovers and will clear the cobwebs far quicker than cups of coffee.

Keeping company

It's obvious that you don't need a partner or to be a member of a team for any of the activities mentioned, but of all of them, jogging seems to be the most social activity. People just aren't so keen to jog around on their own. It's far more fun, they say, if you can encourage all or one member of your family, a friend or some office colleagues to get into gear with you. Offices, street communities, all sorts of clubs and local authorities organise jogs and runs, so ask around and you're more than likely to find dozens of healthy soul-mates.

Serious swimming is as much fun on your own as in company, but perhaps your enthusiasm will infect your friends. Walking and cycling will most probably become part of your personal transport system, but sunny weekends and thoughts of picnics in meadows may draw you to the country with a few friends in tow.

Set yourself a build-up programme

Start at the slowest rate and slowly build the speed and time spent until you are able to achieve the next level. Remember that you are not entering the Olympics, so do not push yourself to go faster than is comfortable.

	RATE	TIME SPENT	DAYS A WEEK
JOGGING			
1 mile	1 mile in 13 mins (walk)	13 mins	3–5
1 mile	1 mile in 12 mins	12 mins	5
1 mile	1 mile in 9½ mins	9½ mins	5
SWIMMING			
25 yds	25 yds in 35 secs	2½ mins	3–5
100 yds	100 yds in 2½ mins	2½ mins	5
300 yds	100 yds in 2½ mins	7½ mins	5
WALKING			
1 mile	1 mile in 15 mins	15 mins	5
3 miles	1 mile in 13 mins	39 mins	5
4 miles	1 mile in 13 mins	52 mins	4
5 miles	1 mile in 13 mins	65 mins	3
CYCLING			
1 mile	12 mph	5 mins	5
8 miles	20 mph	25 mins	3 or 4
SKIPPING			
½ min skip, 1 min rest, ½ min skip		2 mins	3–5
½ min skip, 1 min rest, ½ min skip, 1 min rest, ½ min skip		3½ mins	5
Build your skipping time with ½ min rest in between until you can do 6 mins without stopping		6 mins	3–4

Walk tall –
for health and beauty

Poor posture leads to unnecessary aches and strains — and an awkward gait. Exercising is more difficult, and less fun. Clothes do not fit as well. Good posture will give you good balance and easier movement, even easier sleeping. Is that enough to convince you of the importance of correct posture? Learn the feeling of good body balance by doing the following exercise three times a day before breakfast, lunch and dinner:
1 Place back against a wall with heels 7.50 cm (3 in) away, knees bent.
2 Push feet on the floor and tighten thigh and pelvic muscles. This forces waist to the wall and flattens the back.
3 Pull the shoulder blades down, not back, 2.50 cm (1 in); lift and expand the lower ribs.
4 Straighten legs; move slowly away from wall. Hold position, but relax muscles of arms and neck.

Check your posture as you move, then follow up by practising until the flow of movement comes naturally. Stand about 6 m (20 ft) from a full-length mirror. Bend arms to touch top of hips; press palms together. Walk slowly toward mirror, keeping eyes on hands reflected in it. Move so you keep hands moving steadily and directly forward. Do whatever comes naturally to keep hands from wavering from side to side or up and down. Every part of the body must be upright, and legs and torso moving smoothly to keep hands still. Do exercise daily until hands move smoothly.

Posture and balance are the basis of the regular activity and exercise everyone needs for vitality.

HOW DO YOU STAND?

To check your posture, stand sideways in front of a long mirror. Don't try to look your best; just stand naturally. Now use the table below to check what you see:

BAD POSTURE	GOOD POSTURE
Head forward, neck curved	Neck straight from hairline to shoulders
Protruding shoulder blades	Shoulder blades flat
Chest caved in	Bosom high
Deep curve in lower back at waistline	Shallow curve in back at waistline
Abdomen bulging	Abdomen flat, buttocks tucked in
Feet turning out	Feet straight ahead

FOLLOW THESE TIPS TO PREVENT BACK PROBLEMS — AND IMPROVE POSTURE!

● Save high heels for special occasions; they tilt your weight on to the ball of the foot causing you to stoop, which eventually leads to strained back muscles. If you must wear them, make sure you change to flat shoes or go barefoot at some time during the day.
● Don't wear very tight trousers or belts because the squeezing causes unnecessary pressure on the vertebrae.
● Don't carry heavy shoulder bags — they strain back muscles and make you stoop.
● If your job is sedentary, make sure your chair supports your back: you should not tower above your desk. Make a conscious effort to sit up straight, pulling neck and back muscles up.

How to strengthen your back

If your back isn't healthy you cannot exercise without danger of injury, but in any case the muscles in this part of the body are highly susceptible to strain. Follow the advice and exercise programme below which should help relieve back problems and build muscles up to be strong and supple.

Your back consists of the vertebral column (spine) and the soft structures relating to it. The spine provides the back with both stability and mobility. For stability it is dependent on the large muscles, ligaments, discs, normal curvatures, and bony joints. The inter-relationships of these structures, and their inter-dependency, form a complex entity.

The muscles of the back, for the most part, are very small, and span no more than two or three inches in length. These muscles, attached along the back of the vertebral column, help prevent too much flexion, or forward-bending of the spine. Conversely, the abdominal muscles, although not directly attached to the structures of the back, help prevent too much extension of the spine by providing a counterbalancing effect, and therefore play a vital role in back care. That is often why the unlucky woman with a protuberant pot belly and weakened abdominal muscles usually suffers from low back ache.

The discs between the vertebrae act as buffers, a necessity in walking or jumping. They help to reduce strain on the bony structures by absorbing shock. But it is important to note that these discs become avascular after the age of twenty-one. That is, they lose their blood supply, and it follows that there is a subsequent loss of water and "sponginess", which reduces the ability to absorb shock. Degenerative disc changes, then, are obviously not limited to the aged. An awareness of that fact is important for the safe performance of exercises.

If this anatomy sounds complicated and dull, just remember that when all these structures work well together, they help you to stand erect. Usually, they do that rather well.

Occasionally, however, one may get sudden and extremely severe back pain. It may occur after an unusual movement, or a movement of stress such as rotation, or bending down with knees straight. Sometimes the pain does not begin until a day or two later, but when it does, it can be severe enough to warrant a doctor's attention and, frequently, follow-up physiotherapy treatments.

Maybe you're one of the unfortunate thousands who suffer from a miserable aching in the low back area. It could be chronic back strain, due simply to poor posture, aging processes, or the residual effects of a previous injury. Even if you have no back complaint, it's easy to develop one if you neglect to take proper care. First of all, you should be aware that the small muscles and ligaments of the back are not meant for weight lifting — certainly not for lifting more than half your own body weight against the resistance of gravity. That is precisely what you ask them to do every time you bend down to touch your toes. They don't like you for that, and may go into spasms out of spite! That is what strained muscles usually do to protect themselves from further strain. Muscle spasm and pain work as defence mechanisms to protect the body and must not be ignored. Should you unknowingly or suddenly perform a movement beyond the elastic capabilities of your muscles or ligaments, they may actually tear, thus allowing for more serious injury to other soft structures of the back.

What does all this have to do with your exercise programme? Unless you have a written guarantee that your back is in good condition, don't stoop. That includes all exercises that involve bending down with straight knees and touching your toes. If you want to limber up, there are safer and more effective ways to do it. Most of us over twenty-one don't know if we have a weakness in our back until, unexpectedly, we put it out. Do yourself a favour — save it!

When muscles are strained, they usually react by going into spasm — that is, by shortening their length, which serves to increase or accentuate that normal curvature. The best way to relieve spasms is to stretch the muscles out. Bend one knee toward your chest and you automatically flatten out the low back curve. Needless to say, if one knee is good, two knees are even better.

You may have seen exercise men on television doing wonderful sit-ups. That's fine for them; they're paid to be in shape. But you may be asking for trouble if you make your over-indulged stomach muscles pull you up; if they are too weak to do the job without extra help, they call upon your little back muscles to tighten up and stabilise the area, and so your back begins to ache. How to avoid that? Bend your knees and come up that way. You have mechanically eliminated the possibility of muscle substitution; at the same time, you derive maximum benefit from the exercise, by using only those muscles for which the exercise was designed.

A very common error in exercise is to use momentum to get you where you couldn't get on muscle power alone, and that involves uncontrolled movement. Although you may want to stretch some muscles in the hope of becoming more limber, it's more likely you'll throw them into spasm in self-defence. Stretching a muscle does *not* improve tone, it only stretches it. You must contract the muscle — that is, make it work — to improve tone. So all your exercises must be controlled and within your capacity. So, before you begin your exercise programme, consider your normal everyday activities and how you can make them work for you.

Lifting Dropped a paper clip? Bend your knees and down you go with a straight back. Are you lifting a heavy carton? Let your legs lift it for you. You squat, you wrestle with it, then you use your powerful quadriceps — those big muscles in the front of your thighs — to get on your feet. If you still can't lift it, it's probably too heavy, so get some help.

Carrying If you have too much to carry properly, enlist another person or a trolly. Do use common sense. Or, divide your load so you carry half in each hand in shopping bags or even clutched in close. You thus lessen the strain on your back and heart. You carry the same load with much less effort.

Be concerned about what you wear on your feet around the house. Your feet are beautifully designed to give you excellent traction, and when you go barefoot you allow your muscles the freedom to do their work.

Standing If you have to stand all day, you may be subject to aching feet, cramped legs, sore back. Here is a technique to relieve the strain. Find a low stool and rest one foot on it. When you do that, you have mechanically straightened out the low back curve and brought relief to your low back muscles. Alternate your feet, and you find you tire less easily, as the strain is decreased. If a stool is inconvenient and you stand at a counter, use the bottom ledge of that counter for the same effect. Walking around helps, too, as the pumping action of your leg muscles assists venous return to the heart. And do sit down whenever you don't have to stand.

Sleeping If you find you are waking in the mornings with low back ache, there are a few techniques you can use while you sleep to help reduce the discomfort. If you like to sleep on your side, bend at least one knee. A pillow under the upper knee may also be of help.

A good bed is important, too. A firm box spring is probably enough, but a length of plywood under the mattress is helpful if you really need it. A soft mattress may feel comfortable when you lie down on it, but it requires too much muscle work for proper relaxation.

LOW BACK EXERCISES

If you are suffering from severe back pain, either constant or intermittent, check with a qualified doctor before beginning a programme of back exercises.

Choose a few of the following exercises and include them in your routine. Begin by doing them five times each day, holding the contraction for a count of five. If that begins to feel too easy, progress by increasing the number of times you do the exercise, until you reach twenty-five; then increase the length of holding time.

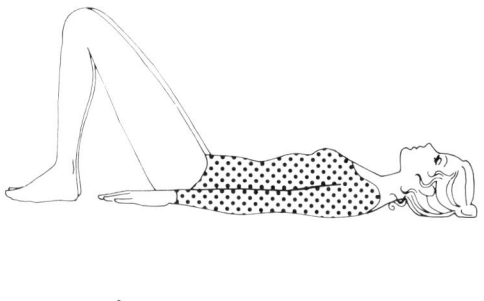

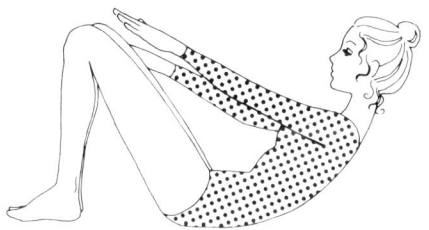

1 KNEE REACH Lie on your back with knees bent and feet flat on the floor. With both hands, reach out to touch your knees and try to sit up. Lift your head and shoulders, keeping your chin tucked in and tightening your abdominal muscles. Lower yourself slowly. Repeat.

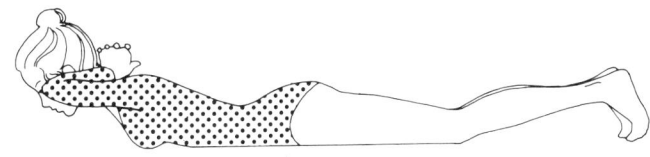

2 BACK STRETCHER (tough but worth the effort). Lie on your stomach, face down, and clasp your hands behind your head or neck. Raise your head and shoulders, keeping your chin tucked in. Hold. Lower and repeat.

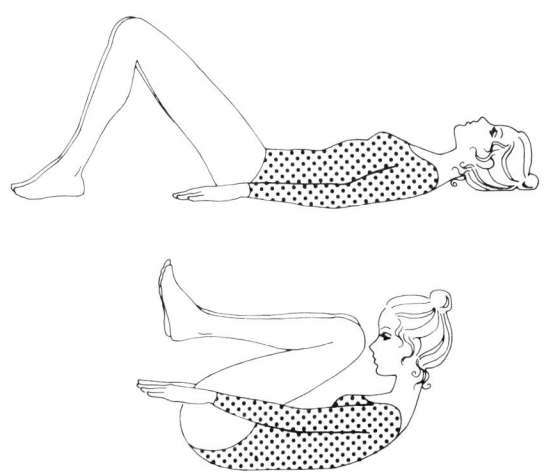

3 KNEES TO CHEST Lie on your back with knees bent and feet flat on the floor. Keep hands at sides, palms down, and use them only for support. Tighten abdominal muscles and slowly pull knees up to chest. Lower slowly to starting position. Repeat. You may progress by combining this exercise with the knee reach. Do them together, hold, and relax.

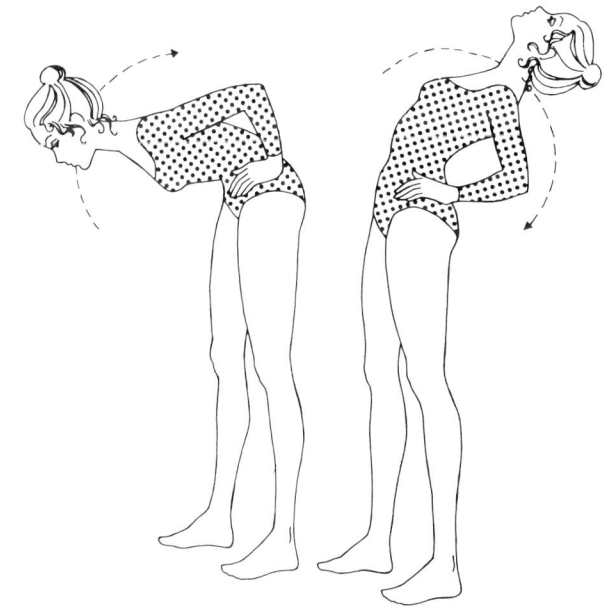

4 MERRY-GO-ROUND Stand up straight; space feet about 46 cm (18 in) apart. Place hands on hips and lean forward. Slowly rotate body from waist, moving clockwise. Feel a good stretch on those muscles. Go around five times and then repeat, going counter-clockwise.

Extract from EVERY OTHER DAY EXERCISE BOOK by Fran Lebo, Lester & Orpen Ltd, published in the UK by Penguin Books Ltd. © by Fran Lebo.

Dr Solomon's trouble spot exercises

The good news from this American fitness expert is that, with perseverance (that means regular *daily* exercising for at least a month) you can improve the lines and contours of your body by working on specific sets of underlying muscles. If you've ever felt your thighs could be less flabby, your buttocks a bit tauter and your hips slimmer, you'll want to start Dr Solomon's painless but rewarding body resculpting programme *now!*

THE GOAL: FIRM BEHIND

The problem Excessive weight and lack of exercise, together with the "sititis" common to modern living, aggravates the "droop" in the bottom. Sitting deactivates the buttock muscles by keeping them inactive and constricting the circulation in that area.

The programme You will find, first of all, exercises to uplift your behind by strengthening and firming the large buttock muscles. Then you will have some other exercises which firm and strengthen them, but also serve to increase the circulation in the area.

Technique tips As you do these exercises, whenever one leg is crossing over the torso, your head should be turning in the opposite direction.

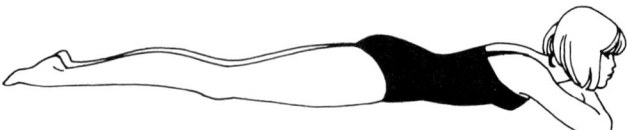

1a Lie on stomach. Legs straight and together, insteps pressed to floor. Hands on floor either under chin or under hips.

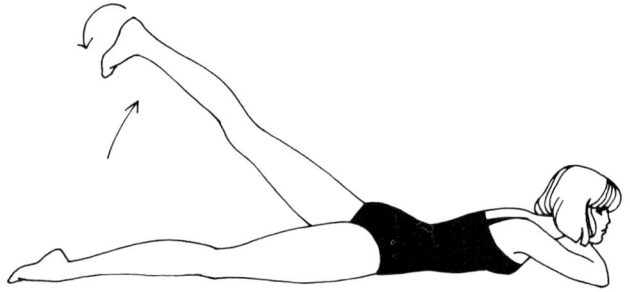

b Lift left leg high off floor, toes pointed. Hold. Lower leg to stem. Then the right leg. Repeat lift and add a flex and point to each foot when in mid-air. Alternate legs ten times; work up to twenty.

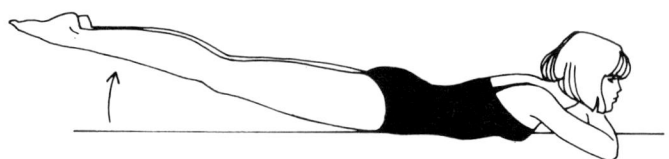

2 Lift both legs high off floor. Hold. Lower to stem. Keep knees straight and toes pointed. Tighten buttocks as legs lift, release buttocks as legs lower. Begin with five; increase to twelve.

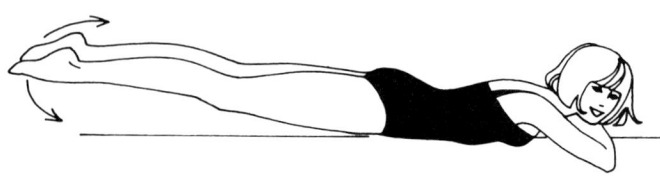

3 Lift both legs slightly off floor. Hold. Separate legs and scissor them wide to the side. Hold. Bring legs together. Hold. Repeat eight times. Lower legs to stem. Repeat sequence three times; increase to six.

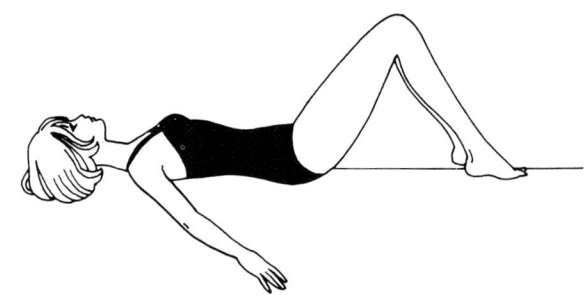

4a Lie on back. Knees bent. Feet flat on floor. Arms outstretched, shoulder level, palms to floor.

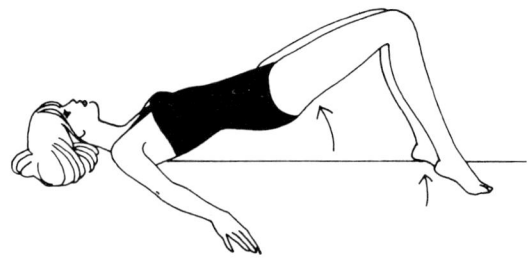

b Tense buttock muscles. Lift buttocks high off floor. Hold. While in high lift position, raise heels off floor, then lower heels to floor, eight times. Lower buttocks to stem. Repeat sequence four times; increase to ten.

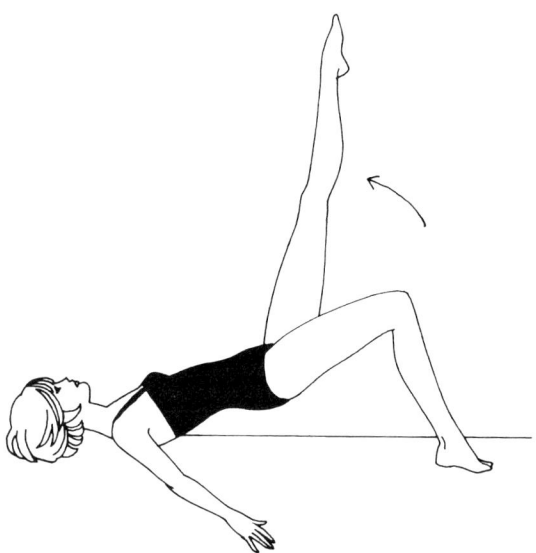

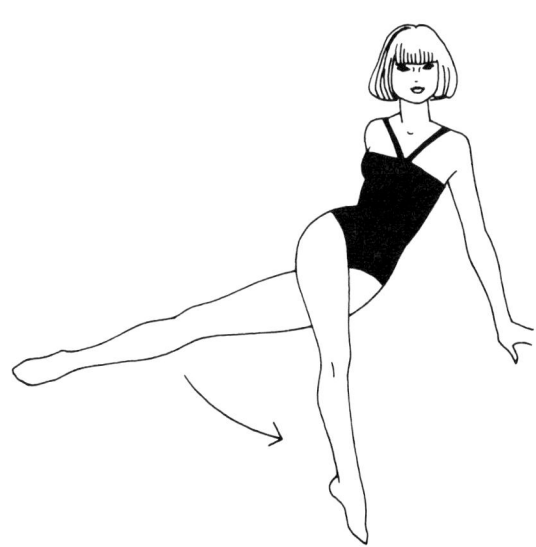

5 Lift buttocks off floor. Hold. Raise left leg toward ceiling. Hold. Bend knee. Lower buttocks to floor. Return to stem. Repeat to other side. Begin with four; increase to twelve.

b Lift right leg off floor. Cross right leg over left until foot touches floor. Hold. Lift right leg up and return to stem. Repeat with left leg to right side. Alternate sides. Begin with eight; increase to sixteen.

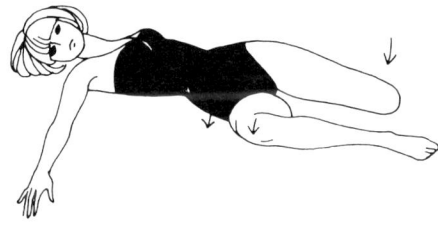

6 Separate legs, keep knees bent. Lift buttocks high off floor. Hold. Twist trunk to right side and lower hip to floor. Try to press both knees to right side on floor. Hold. Return to stem. Lift buttocks high off floor. Hold. Twist trunk to left side and lower left hip to floor. Try to press knees to left side on floor. Hold. Return to stem. Alternate sides. Repeat six times; increase to fourteen.

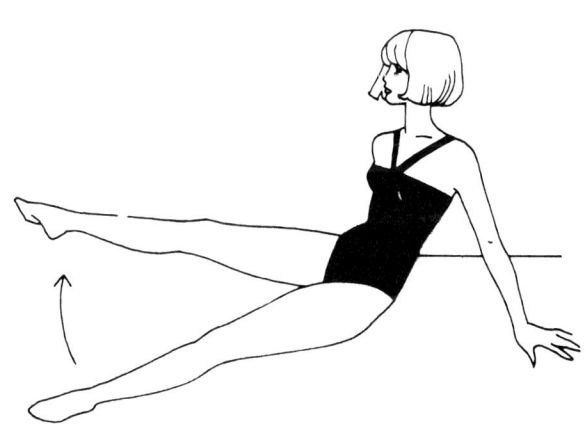

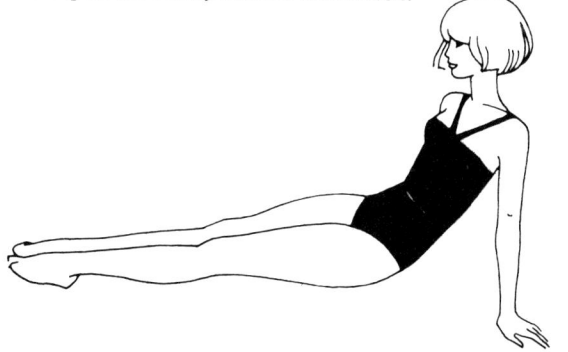

7a Sit on floor, legs straight and together. Lean back; rest on hands.

8 Lift right leg off floor. Cross right leg high over left until right foot touches floor. Hold. Swing right leg up again and far out to right side until foot touches floor. Hold. Slide leg back on floor to stem. Cross left leg over right until left foot touches floor. Hold. Swing left leg up again and far out to left side until foot touches floor. Hold. Slide leg back on floor to stem. Alternate sides. Begin with four; increase to twelve.

THE GOAL: SLIMMER HIPS

The problem Even if you have inherited a tendency toward heavy hips, you can help slim them down through "spot" exercising. The usual reasons for flabbiness and "spread" in the hip region are: weakened muscles resulting from inactivity, artificial support and/or incorrect diet.

The programme The programme for hips is designed to activate the large muscles in the hip and buttock area. This changes the contour of the hips, but you will derive a double benefit. You are involving your buttocks and thighs in inch-reducing as well. The exercises accelerate muscle activity, increase circulation and strengthen your muscles.

Technique tips Take time during these exercises to check your body position. In hip exercise especially, you must eliminate as much extraneous movement as possible: shifting your weight or changing your body position may cause muscle cramping and/or incorrect exercising.

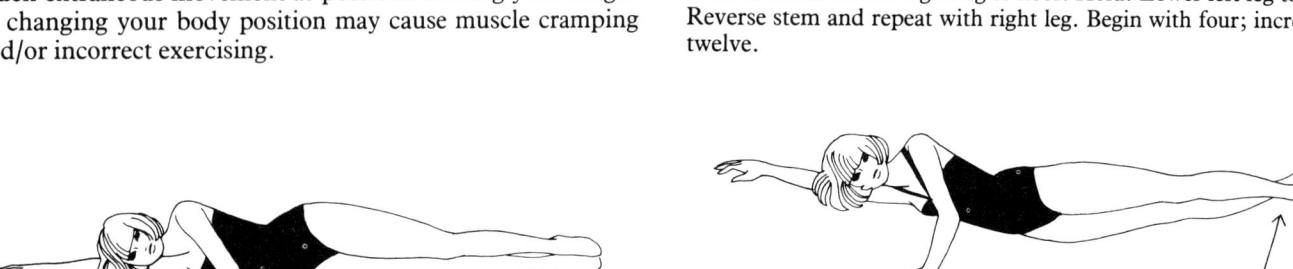

2 Lift left leg high off floor. Hold. Lift right leg up to meet left leg. Touch. Hold. Lower right leg to floor. Hold. Lower left leg to floor. Reverse stem and repeat with right leg. Begin with four; increase to twelve.

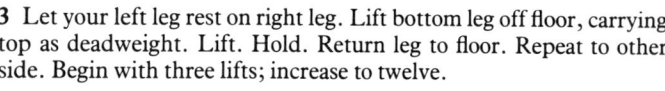

3 Let your left leg rest on right leg. Lift bottom leg off floor, carrying top as deadweight. Lift. Hold. Return leg to floor. Repeat to other side. Begin with three lifts; increase to twelve.

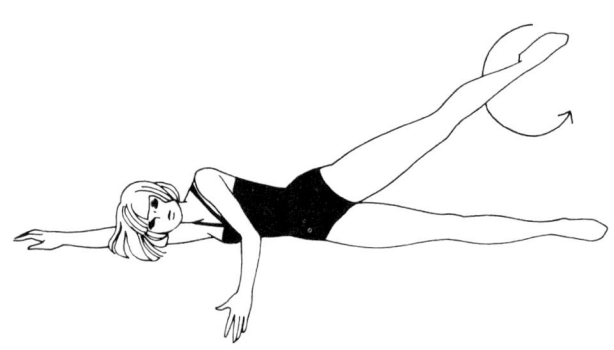

1a Lie on right side. Head resting on shoulder and outstretched arm. Left hand front, palm on floor for support, legs straight.

b Lift left leg and make a complete circle in the air. Move whole leg front-up-back-down. Try to make two circles before lowering leg. After two circles, reverse direction. Begin with four circles in each direction and work up to twelve. Reverse stem position and repeat with right leg.

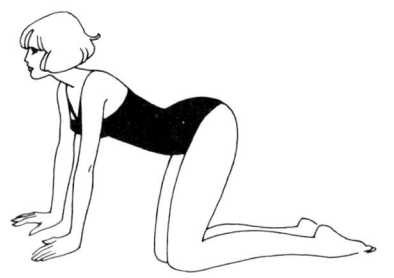

4 Kneel on hands and knees. Press insteps to floor. Head up. Straighten left leg back and lift it up as high as you can. Hold. Lower straight leg to floor until toes touch. Hold. Repeat five times on each leg; increase to fifteen.

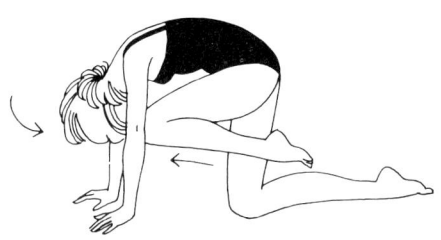

5 Bring left knee to nose as head lowers. Hold. Extend left leg back and up high, as head lifts. Hold. Repeat five times on each leg, increase to fifteen.

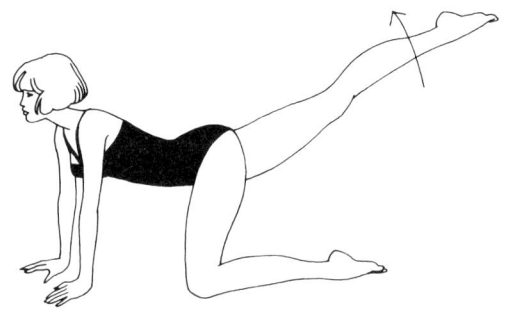

6 Extend right leg straight back, not higher than hips. Swing right leg way around to right side, then back, and around to left side. Keep leg off floor. Let your buttock and hip area follow the movement. Begin with six on each leg; increase to twelve.

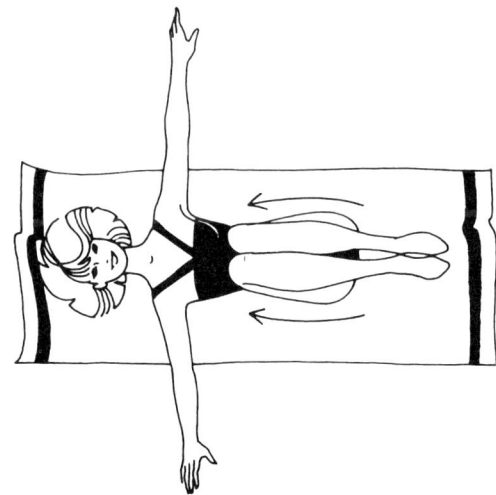

7a Lie on back. Knees bent to chest. Arms flat to floor, shoulder level. Palms down.

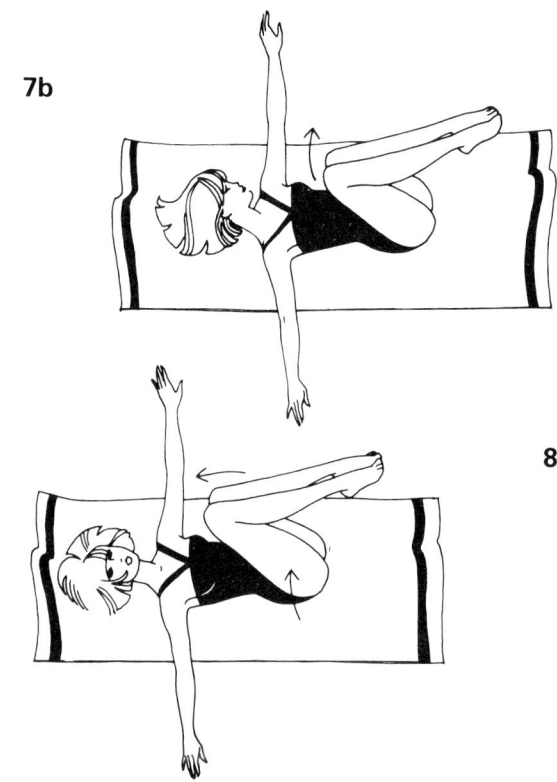

7b

8

b Slowly roll both knees to left side. Hold. Return to stem. Roll knees to right side. Hold. Return to stem. Keep knees together. Begin with eight; increase to twenty.

8 Keep knees pressed together. Lower hip to left side. Hold. Slide knees up to touch left elbow. Hold. Release knees to stem. Lower hip to right side. Release to stem. Begin with eight; increase to twenty on each side.

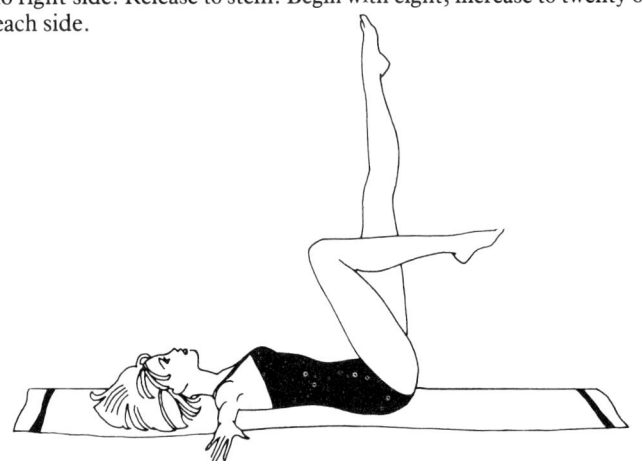

9 Extend left, then right, leg up toward ceiling. Start both legs moving as if cycling. Begin with ten; increase to thirty.

THE GOAL: TRIMMER WAIST

The problem The reason I include the midriff together with the waistline is that the rib cage provides such a convenient hanger for fat. It causes the midriff to expand and creep downward until there is a straight line from under the arms to the top of the hips. In fact, the problem is not one of the waistline, but one of no waistline at all.

The programme I will show you how to "awaken" the muscles in the midriff-waistline area. As you increase the activity and stimulate the circulation, you will notice a reduction in your waist measurement. This area responds beautifully.

Technique tips You will achieve a greater pull on your large areas during your stretches from either a floor or standing position by being careful of the way you hold your hands. Always have the raised hand palm upward. This produces a greater pull all the way down to your hips and buttocks.

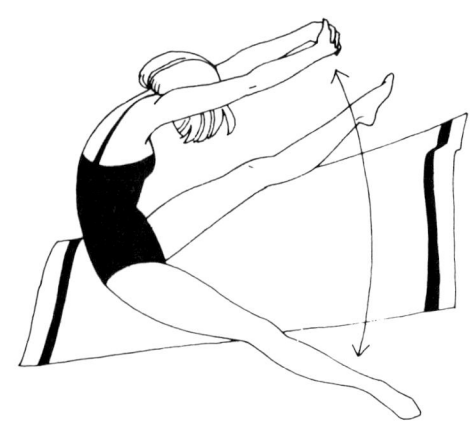

2 Clasp hands over head and turn upper trunk to left side. Slowly bounce over left leg four times. Try to touch hands to toes. Stop. Release to upright position. Turn trunk to right side and slowly bounce four times over right leg. Release to upright position. Begin with four; increase to twelve.

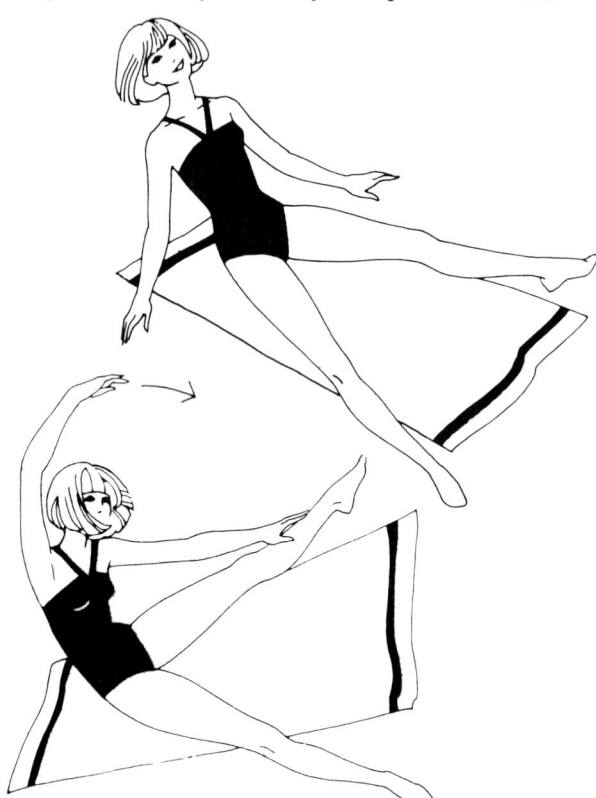

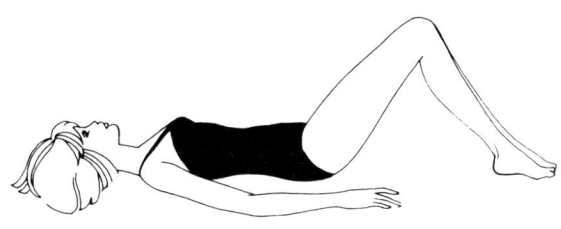

3a Lie on back. Knees bent and together. Feet flat on floor. Arms down at sides, palms down.

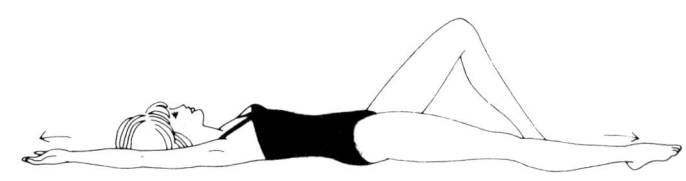

1a Sit erect on floor. Legs wide apart and toes pointed.
   b Grasp left ankle with left hand. Curve right arm over head, palm to the ceiling, and slowly bounce torso over left leg four times. Hold. Clasp hands over head and release trunk upright. Stretch up and pull waist off hips. Alternate sides. Begin with four; increase to twelve.

   b Simultaneously reach right arm back on floor as you stretch right leg forward, toes pointed. Stretch your leg and arm out as far as you can on the floor. Alternate sides. Begin with six; work up to twenty.

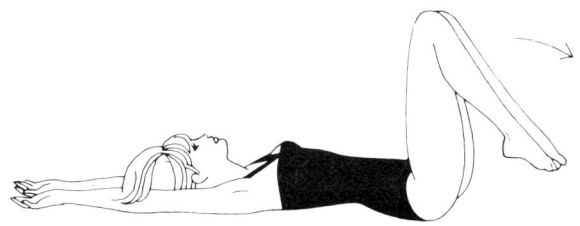

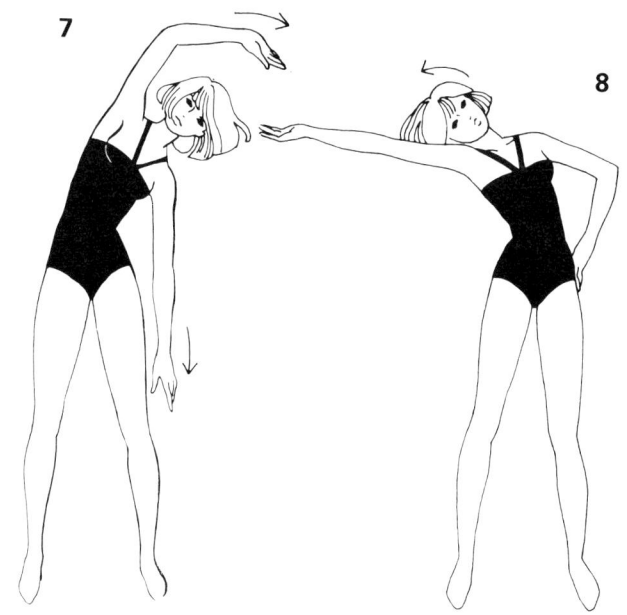

4 Lift both knees to chest. Hold. Keep knees bent and lower feet to floor, as arms stretch over head to floor. Hold. Lift both knees back to chest, as arms lower to floor. Hold. Repeat six times; work up to twelve.

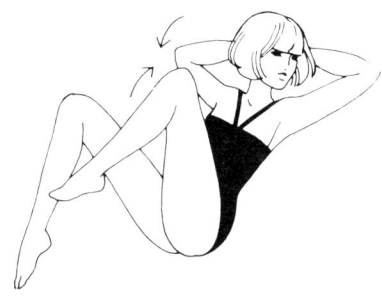

5 Lace fingers behind head at neck. Raise both knees off floor to chest as you lift head and shoulders up. Twist trunk and try to touch right elbow to left knee; then touch left elbow to right knee. Repeat four times. Begin with two sets of twisting and increase to twelve.

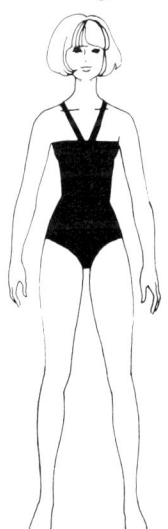

6 Stand erect. Legs wide apart. Knees over toes. Feet flat on floor. Arms down loosely at sides. Without moving hips or bending knees, move rib cage (chest) as far to the right side as you can. Hold. Release to the centre. Move rib cage over to the left side. Hold. Return to centre. Alternate sides. Begin with eight; work up to sixteen.

7 Curve right arm overhead, palm to ceiling. Bend deeply to the left side. Bounce over and try to slide left hand down leg toward ankle with each bounce. After four bounces release slowly to stem. Repeat four deep bounces to right side. Begin with two sets of four bounces to each side and increase to six sets.

8 Extend right arm out to side, shoulder level. Palm up. Tilt head and stretch out to right side, bending at waist. Stretch four times over right arm. Release to stem. Repeat side stretch four times to left side. Begin with four sets and increase to eight.

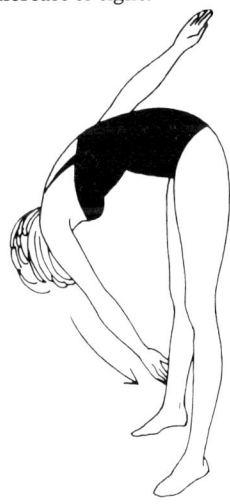

9 Bend and try to touch left hand to the outside of your right heel. Hold. Repeat twist and try to touch right hand to outside of left heel. Begin with six; increase to twelve.

THE GOAL: FIRM, SLIM THIGHS

The problem For every curve there is a muscle. And the curve is only as pretty as the muscle is firm and shapely. Thigh curves are four-dimensional because there are four regions to each thigh: front, back, inner and outer. Your thigh problem may exist in one region, two regions, three regions, or all of them put together. This very much depends on your diet, work, and life-style. Unfortunately, I discovered in working with my patients that the exercises for inner thighs did not generally firm the outer thighs. It became necessary to develop specific exercises for all four thigh areas and to encourage my exercisers to use the proper ones for their individual problems.

The programme The programme is broken down to deal with all four trouble areas in the thighs. You will find exercises that will tighten the inside and outside of the thighs, slim your legs, reduce fatty knees, and generally restore a firm, attractive outline and strength to the entire area.

Technique tips The most important tip is the one I have already mentioned. When you are lying on your back, always turn your head in the opposite direction from the working leg. NB Some of the exercises are labelled W. This W means that they are designed to be done with weights if you wish to increase demands in order to hasten results. A 450 kg (1 lb) weight on each ankle, or wearing skiing boots, will do.

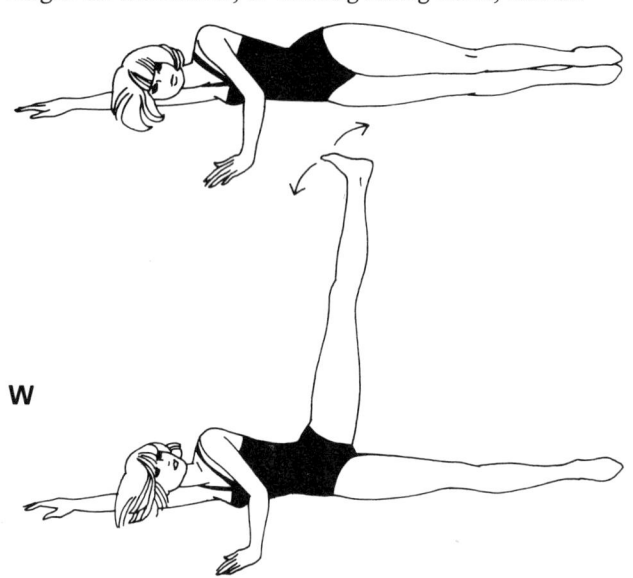

W

1a Lie on right side. Head resting on shoulder and outstretched arm. Left hand flat on floor by chest for support. Legs straight.

b Slowly raise left leg high off floor, toes pointed. Hold. Flex and point foot four times in mid-air. Slowly lower leg to stem. Begin with six high lifts; increase gradually to twelve. Repeat on other side.

W

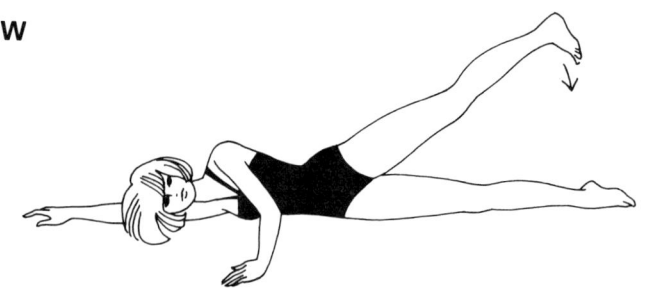

2 Turn right foot down with toes touching floor, heel turned up toward ceiling. Maintain this foot position. Lift and lower left leg six times; gradually increase to twelve. Repeat on other side.

W

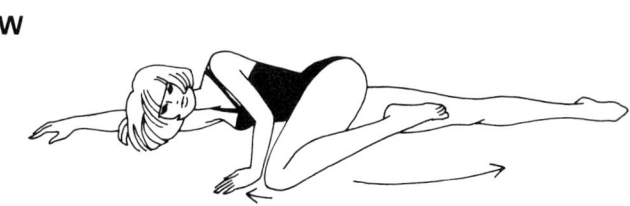

3 Bend left leg. Bring knee to left elbow. Hold. Extend leg straight out low, over right leg. Hold. Repeat. Continue bringing knee to elbow, then swiftly out straight. Begin with six; gradually increase to twenty. Repeat to other side.

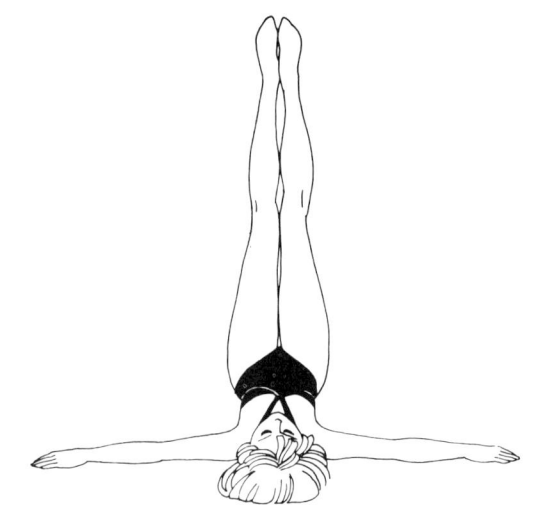

4a Lie on back, legs extended toward ceiling. Knees straight; arms flat to floor, shoulder level, palms down.

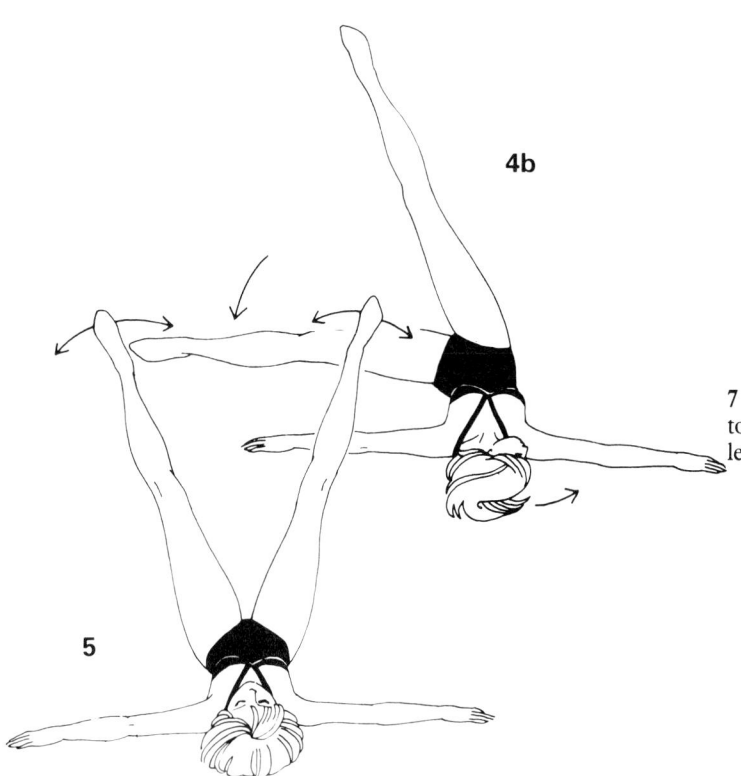

4b

5

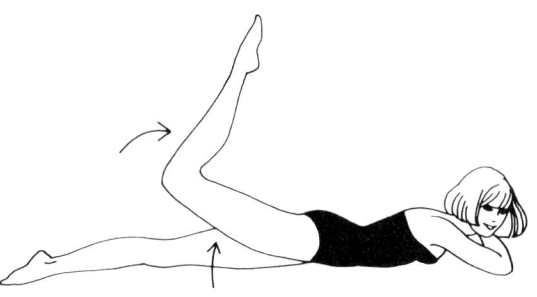

7 Lift right leg as high as you can. Hold. Bend knee, toes pointed toward your head. Hold. Straighten leg. Return to stem. Repeat with left leg. Begin with six; gradually increase to twenty.

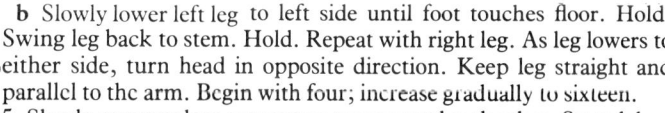

b Slowly lower left leg to left side until foot touches floor. Hold. Swing leg back to stem. Hold. Repeat with right leg. As leg lowers to either side, turn head in opposite direction. Keep leg straight and parallel to the arm. Begin with four; increase gradually to sixteen.

5 Slowly separate legs as you turn toes toward each other. Stretch legs apart as wide as possible, with toes turned inwards. Hold widest position. Now, turn feet until toes point out to sides. Slowly bring legs together until heels touch. Repeat. Stretch legs to widest position, then return to centre until heels touch. Begin with four; increase gradually to twelve.

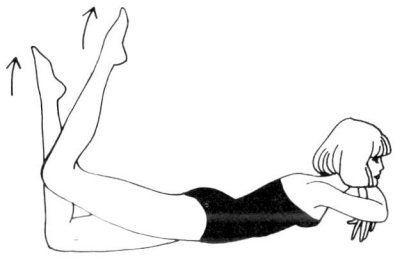

8 Bend both knees on floor. Hold. With a moderate pace, and alternating, lift and lower each leg with bent knee. Lift as high as possible. Begin with ten; increase gradually to thirty.

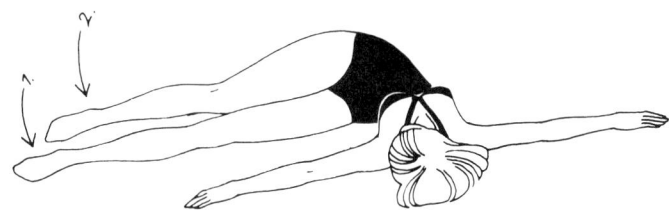

6 Slowly lower left leg to left side on floor. Hold. Lower right leg until resting on left leg. Hold. Release right leg to stem. Hold. Release left leg to stem. Hold. Repeat sequence to other side by lowering right leg to right side until foot touches floor. Alternate sides. Begin with four sets on each side; increase gradually to twelve.

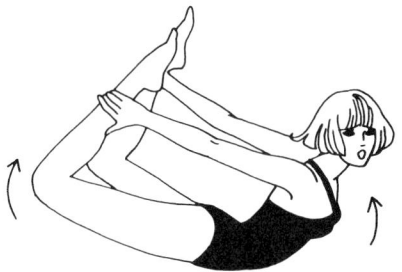

9 Bend both knees. Reach back and grasp ankles firmly. Hold. Raise head, shoulders, chest, thighs off floor. Hold for two counts. Lower on two counts. When chin touches floor, repeat. Begin with three; increase to twelve.

Exercises ballet dancers do

Did you ever see a ballet dancer on stage who wasn't enviably lithe and slim? Here, we show you how to do the warm-up exercises many top ballet dancers follow. They should whittle down flabby areas and make your body supple at the same time. Never exercise quickly when your body's cold; the secret is to start slowly so muscles won't pull.

NB To do all these exercises you'll need something to hold on to, like the back of a chair or a towel rail.

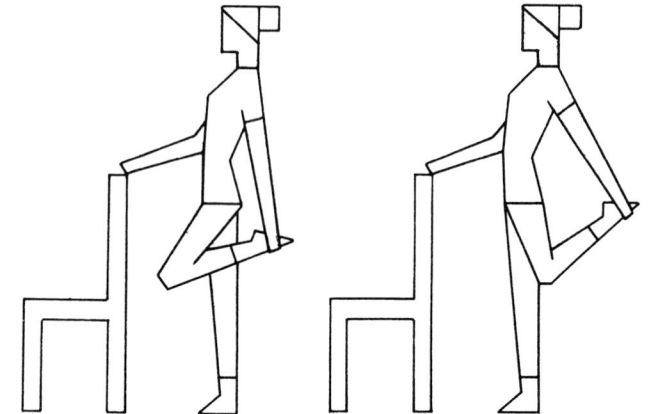

1 *A hip and thigh jerker.* Facing forward, hold on to the side with your right hand. With your other hand, grip left foot by the arch of the foot. Keeping right leg straight and still, try to pull left leg backwards. You must keep the line of your right foot, knee and thigh together and your body straight.

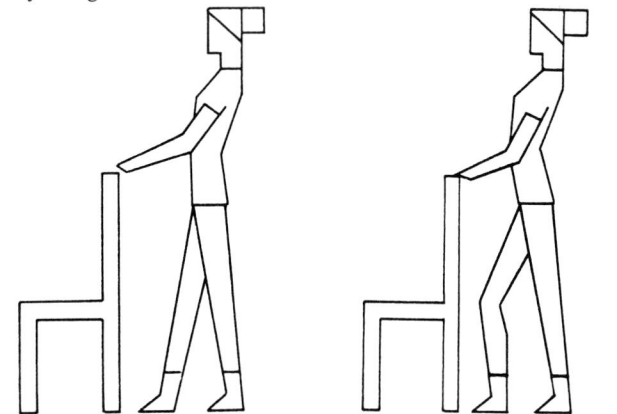

2 *Place left leg behind right leg.* Tighten muscles of your hips, tummy and thighs and bend the front leg forward at the knee so that you are leaning forward slightly. Take the weight on your hands — and feel the pull on the calf muscles of the left leg. Twice only, each leg, to start with.

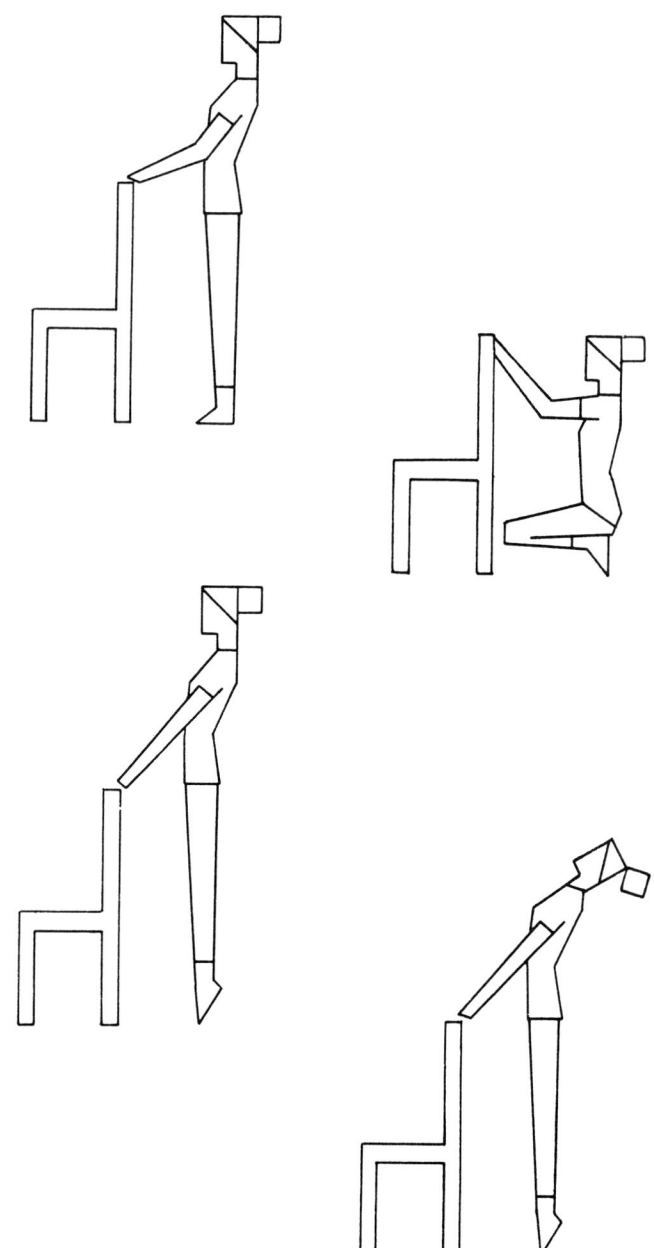

3 *An all-over toner.* Stand at arm's length away from a chair or table, holding it lightly with fingertips. Now crouch down on the balls of your feet, keeping ankles and knees together. Straighten that back! Rise slowly to a standing position, letting thigh muscles take most of the strain. Up on tiptoe, stretch upwards and backwards very slowly. Relax.

84

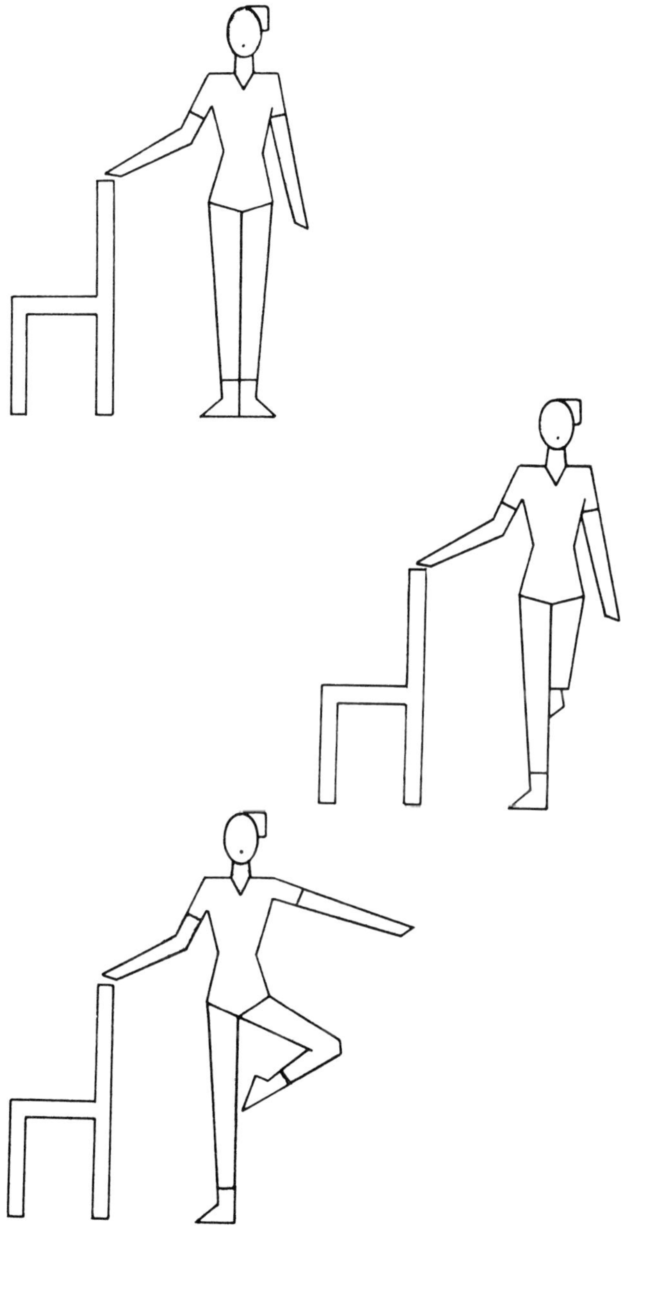

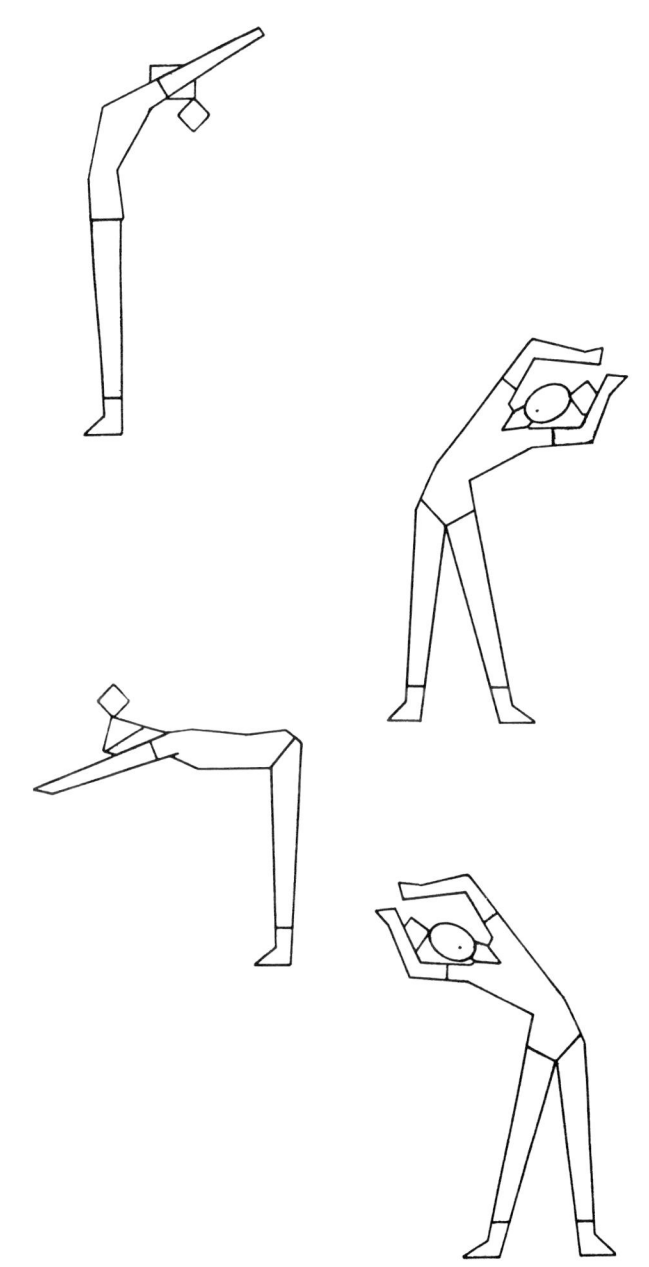

4 *This one's very hard if you're not a dancer.* But just attempting it will help flaccid thighs and bottom. Bend left leg until your toe is pointed at your right knee. Now swivel left leg outwards. Swing left arm up and outwards to keep balance. Return left leg to front.

5 *A waist trimmer.* Bend back as far as you can, then try to describe a complete circle with the upper part of your torso, using stretched-out arms to help swing you along. Legs must be kept straight, feet flat on the floor. Do this one gradually at first.

Special offer

It's funky, it's fun, and will keep you as lithe as a professional dancer. Switch on the Cosmopolitan Shape Tape the moment you wake up in the morning and launch into a ten to fifteen minute work-out that will make you feel fitter, slimmer and more energetic than ever before. The routine (adapted from the jazz dancing course at the world-famous Dance Centre by choreographer Arlene Phillips) will get you bending and stretching and toning up every muscle you have, plus quite a few you never knew existed. It's not easy, but the music will keep you moving and the warm, gravelly voice of commentator Tony Hertz will coerce you into extra effort.

The cassette, which can be played on a cassette recorder, comes to you with a beautifully designed wall chart which shows you exactly how you should look in action. It's the next best thing to having your own Dance Centre on the premises — and it's all yours for only £3.25.

Just send a crossed cheque or postal order (name and address in block letters on the back please) made payable to National Magazine Co Ltd, to: Shape Tape Offer, PO Box 4, Farnham, Surrey, GU9 8JB. The offer is available to readers in the UK and the Republic of Ireland but not overseas.

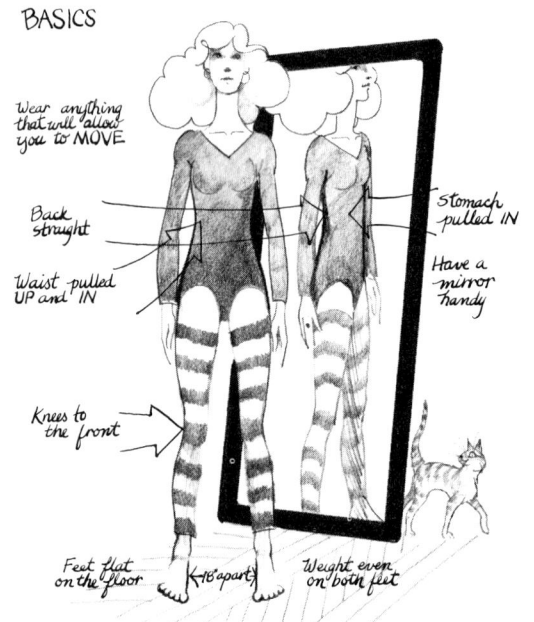

BASICS

Wear anything that will allow you to MOVE

Back straight

Waist pulled UP and IN

Stomach pulled IN

Have a mirror handy

Knees to the front

Feet flat on the floor

18 apart

Weight even on both feet

The first drawing in the chart shows how you should look *before* starting the action!

Body energisers

Follow this series of warm-ups daily to stretch and tone every inch of your body. Try them when you're tired and you'll find you feel energised, but not exhausted! Allow ten minutes to work through the routine to start with, but you can increase the number of times you do each movement as you grow more flexible. Follow them in the order shown.

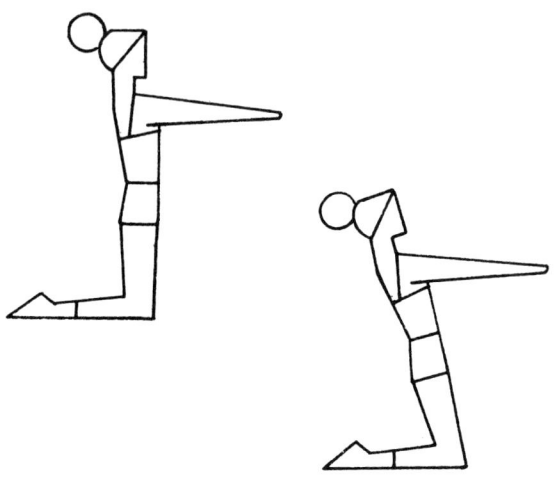

1 ANGLE POSE Kneel with arms extended and back at right angles to the floor. Now slowly bend back as far as possible, keeping back straight so your body forms a Z shape; hold. Return to first position. Repeat five times. Tones stomach and thighs.

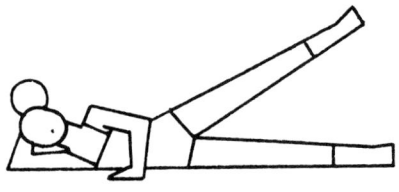

2 SCISSOR STRETCH Lie on your side, keeping body in alignment and top hip slightly tilted forward. Place corresponding arm on floor in front, so it supports body. Lift top leg as high as possible without swivelling hips; lower. Do this six times for each leg. Tones the waist and hips.

Exercises devised by Jan Boorer of the Gym 'N' Tonic Health Club, 4 Welbeck St, London W1; 01-580 4556.

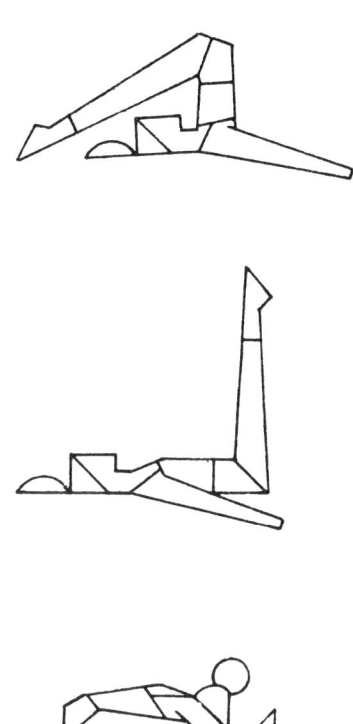

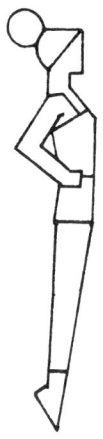

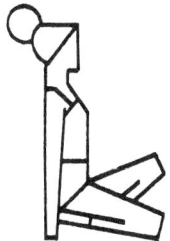

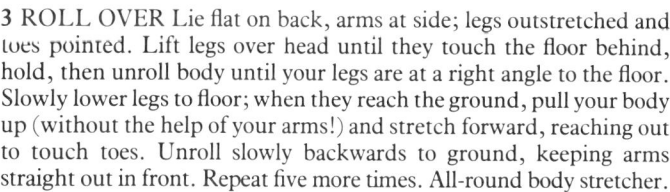

5 BODY BOUNCE With hands on waist, jump three times on your toes. Jump a fourth time, landing in a crouching position so that one knee is nearly touching floor, the other straight forward. Repeat exercise, alternating leg. Do six times for each leg. Good for circulation, giving greater energy output!

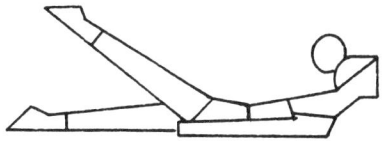

3 ROLL OVER Lie flat on back, arms at side; legs outstretched and toes pointed. Lift legs over head until they touch the floor behind, hold, then unroll body until your legs are at a right angle to the floor. Slowly lower legs to floor; when they reach the ground, pull your body up (without the help of your arms!) and stretch forward, reaching out to touch toes. Unroll slowly backwards to ground, keeping arms straight out in front. Repeat five more times. All-round body stretcher.

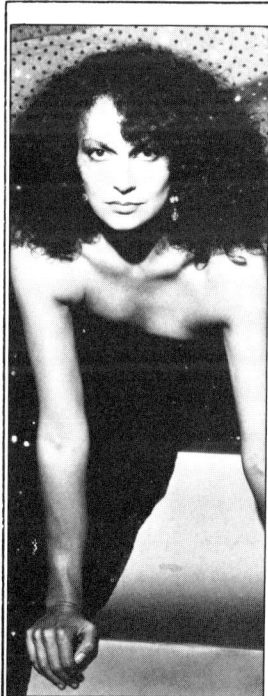

DIANE VON FÜRSTEN-BERG, *designer: "I think of exercise as a way to improve rather than repair the body — otherwise, it would seem so depressing. Once you begin to see yourself getting firmer and in better shape, though, working out becomes pleasurable and turns into a need. I have my own routine which I do five days a week in the morning. And I enjoy sports you can do alone, such as skiing, riding, walking and jogging. I don't smoke and don't drink much except for water, which cleans out the body. I try not to eat a lot of junk food although I'm a real chocolate addict. But that's why I exercise — because I don't really watch what I eat!"*

4 BACK LIFT Lie flat on your stomach, chin on floor and hands under hips. Raise right leg, at the same time raising head and chest so you feel one long pull on torso. Lower leg and body back to original position. Do six times for each leg. Stretches long muscles of the back, and calf muscles.

How to have a flat, firm stomach

Unless they are constantly exercised, stomach muscles easily slacken, resulting in a flabby, protruding stomach, even on the slimmest person. To make your stomach flat and taut, you have to work on all three sets of abdominal muscles: straight, oblique and transverse. Here, Nicholas Kounovsky, famous body builder, gives you one effective exercise for each set of muscles.

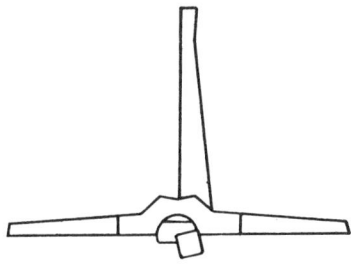

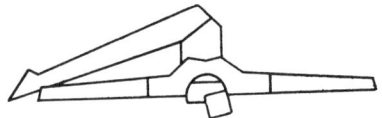

3 *This exercise is for the transverse muscles* Lie on floor. Start with arms outstretched, one leg pointing straight up. Keeping knee straight and arms flat on the floor, lower legs sideways and touch your toe to the floor. (The higher your "touch point", the better — aim at your hand.) Do two to six times; switch legs.

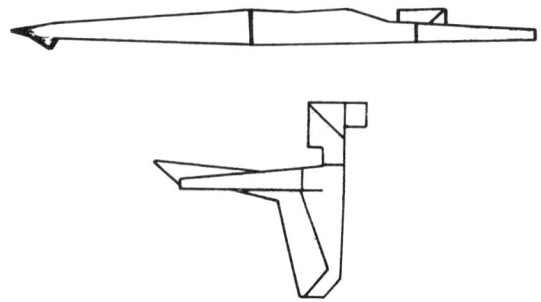

1 *For the straight abdominal muscles* Start from prone position. Sit up, swinging arms forward and jack-knifing knees to chest at the same time. (Keep toes pointed, elbows stiff.) You'll feel your tummy muscles tighten as they literally pull you off the floor! Start with two, and gradually work up to six.

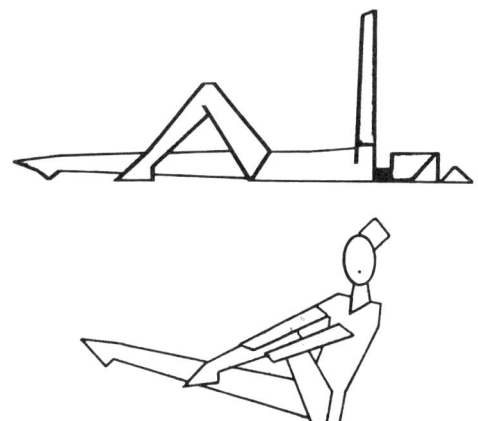

2 *For the oblique stomach muscles* Lie flat on back with one knee bent and arms pointing at ceiling. Sit up quickly, but keep the movement fluid. At the same time, lift legs a few inches off floor and swing arms to the same side as flexed knee. Alternate sides; work up to six on each side.

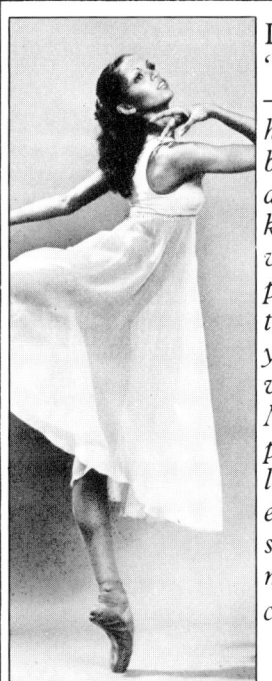

LYDIA ABARCA, *ballet dancer:* *"My exercise regime is strenuous — eight hours a day including rehearsal; I wear through a pair of ballet shoes after two performances. First thing, I work out the kinks and weaknesses in my body with a specialised limber-up programme, then in class the troupe practises simple exercises you can do to keep in shape whether you're a dancer or not. Most of the exercises are based on pulling, stretching movements. A lot of dancers have those stretchy exercise ropes with stirrups for strengthening leg muscles, and many of us go swimming when we can find the time."*

The ultimate flesh firmer

Though hips, stomach and thighs are the flab "danger zones", the upper part of the torso has trouble spots too: slack upper arms, bosom and throat, to name but three! Actress Lynda Carter, appropriate star of television's *Wonder Woman*, demonstrates in these simple hard-working exercises, how you can have a *décolleté* to be proud of!

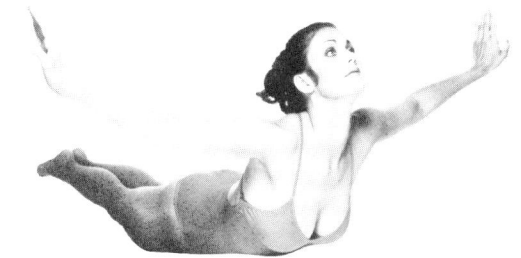

3 BACK BUILDER Swan-dive position strengthens muscles in back, keeps spine erect and supple. Raise and lower legs and upper torso slowly.

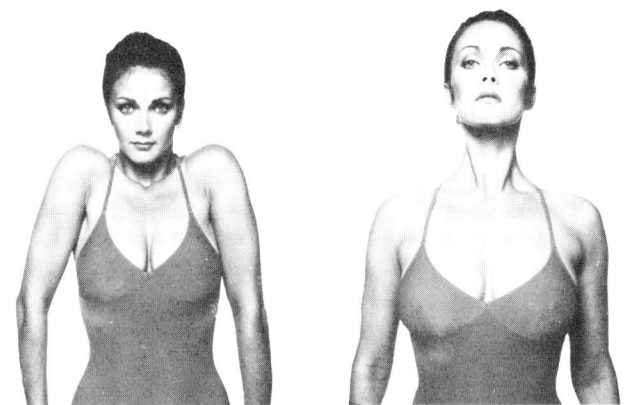

1 SHOULDER DE-TENSER Learn to carry shoulders down and back — not hunched with tension. Shrug shoulders as high as you can, then pull them right down and lift head as high as possible. Do slowly about ten times.

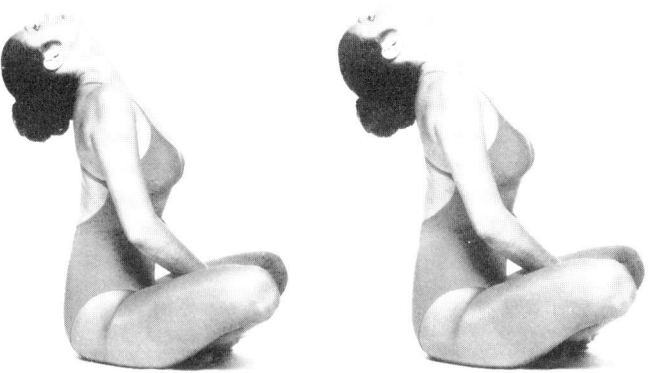

4 THROAT FIRMER Sit cross-legged, back straight. Pull head back as far as you can (you'll feel the pull in your throat muscles). Now open and close mouth slowly several times. Lower head, relax.

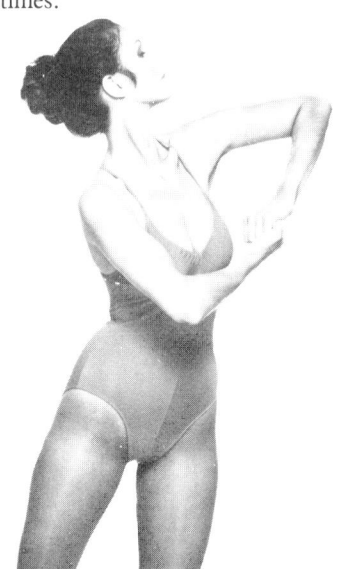

2 ARM DE-FLABBER Clasp hands, lift right elbow. Push down with right hand; resist with left. Switch sides.

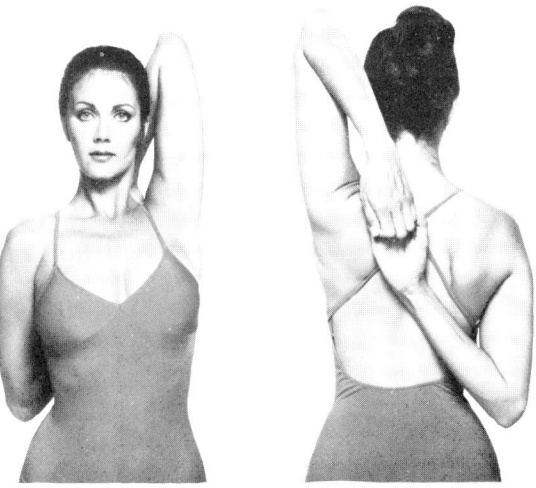

5 BACK FLATTENER Grip hands behind back as shown. Pull up with top hand, then down with the other. (Feel little back muscles working). Now switch hands and repeat. Do several times.

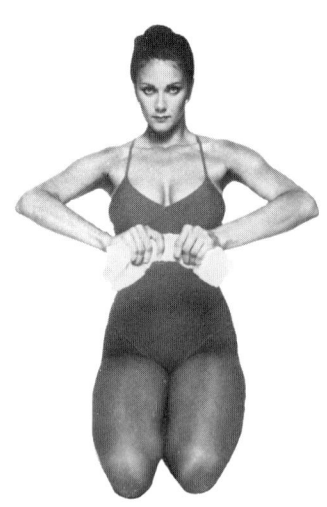

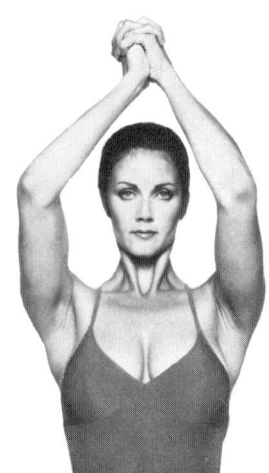

8 BOSOM SHAPER This one strengthens the pectoral muscles (they support the breasts). Grip hands above head; slowly bring elbows together.

6 FLAB FIGHTER This will keep upper arms firm and unflabby. Take a small towel, kneel and twist the towel in a wringing motion, first forward then back. Do this several times.

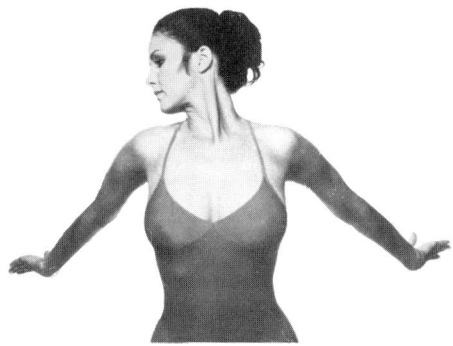

9 UNDERARM FIRMER Extend both arms out to the sides. Now, rotate arms forward from shoulder socket until palms face ceiling. Bounce arms backwards thirty times. You'll feel the pull in underarm muscles.

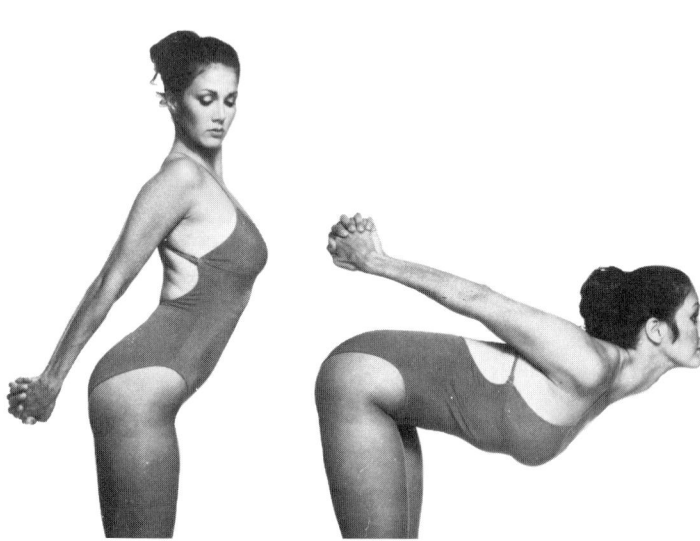

7 BREAST LIFTER This will raise and firm the bosom by tightening the small supporting muscles of the back. Grip hands behind you, arching back. Keep arms high, and bend over from hips. Hold, raise torso, relax.

Ski shape-ups

Begin these exercises in August and you'll be in form by the winter. The first one helps flexibility, the second one strengthens legs.

1 Stand up straight with feet close together. Using your best posture, raise arms all the way over your head, stretching upward and out. To a count of eight, raise and stretch both arms, reaching above your head and then to the right. Return arms to centre and then repeat the stretch to left. Do four of these stretches.

2 Lie on your back and roll legs up into the air until you're resting on your upper back. Support lower back with your hands and, keeping legs straight with pointed toes, slowly move legs back and forth in a scissor movement. Do this sixteen times; increase to twenty-four.

The benefits of basic yoga

Yoga exercises, claim devotees, are unsurpassed. They stretch and activate all the muscles in your body in a way no other exercises can. They seem to help relieve tension, take off inches and pounds, keep your skin glowing and wrinkle-free. They also help you to think more clearly, have lots more energy and improve your sex life! In fact, experts claim that yoga can be so revitalising that you go on looking forty-five for thirty years.

Tolin, one of New York's top yoga instructors, extols the rejuvenating effects of yoga but cautions against rushing into it and expecting miracles seven days on. "Work at it with daily discipline," he advises, "for your own needs. And go at your own speed." The postures here, supervised by Tolin, are a basic part of Hatha Yoga: the physical method as distinct from the meditative method. Hatha Yoga's goals are achieved through a combination of *asanas* (postures) and controlled breathing. Each posture is held for about ten seconds at first, working up to fifteen or twenty very gradually. Ten or fifteen seconds of complete relaxation are essential between postures.

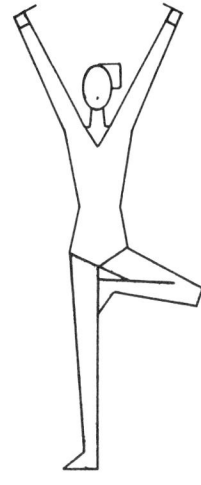

3 THE TREE This posture is excellent for improving one's balance. The left heel is lifted and tucked under the right thigh. The arms are raised above the head, palms facing forward, and are brought into prayer position. Considerable practice is required in order to do this posture well.

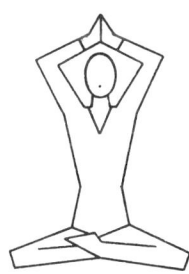

1 THE LOTUS This posture is named after the lotus plant, the national flower of India. It also symbolises everything about yoga. To assume the posture, the legs are crossed and intertwined, the eyes are closed, the arms are slowly raised over the head in a prayer position. The spine is kept very straight. The position is held as one concentrates on achieving complete relaxation.

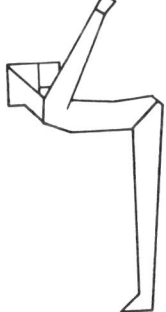

4 THE BACK CLASP Standing straight, knees locked, hands clasped behind the back, the body is bent forward at a 90-degree angle, as the arms are raised. This strengthens the chest muscles, and firms throat, bosom and upper arms.

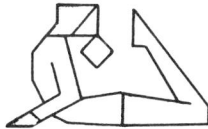

2 THE COBRA Head and legs are lifted while the body remains prone, hands pointing straight ahead. The aim is to be able to touch the head with the toes.

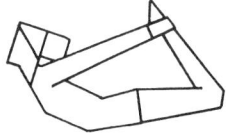

5 THE CRADLE This is for relaxing tension in the neck and back and toning bosom and buttocks. Head and legs are raised as far as possible off the floor and ankles are clasped; the body is kept prone.

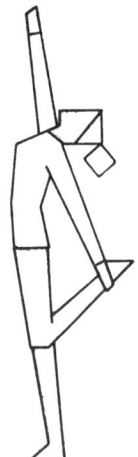

6 SALUTE TO THE SUN The left foot is raised and held in the left hand, the right arm is raised and the head lifted towards the ceiling — once the centre of balance is found. This posture is very good for relieving tension in the back and lower spine.

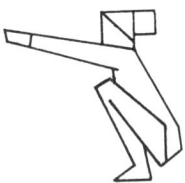

7 KNEELING ARCH Standing with arms outstretched, the body is lowered until the knees meet the chest, keeping the feet flat on the floor. This exercise is intended to firm buttocks and thighs.

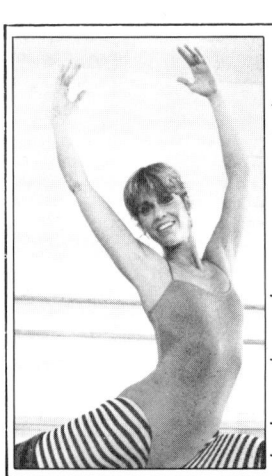

JANE FONDA, *actress: "When people ask where I get my energy, I say it's from hard workouts (I have to push myself), and watching what I put into my body. Exercise does a tremendous amount for emotional and mental stability. If you can get yourself to work out, no matter how tired or depressed you feel, the benefits go far beyond staying fat or thin — you also give yourself the energy to confront your problems."*

Put on your skates and dance!

Roller disco is *the* fun sport that keeps your muscles working as it keeps you moving. It also needs style, verve and a lot of practising to keep you upright. To help you cut a dash on the roller disco rink, follow these basic steps — then go on to invent a few of your own!

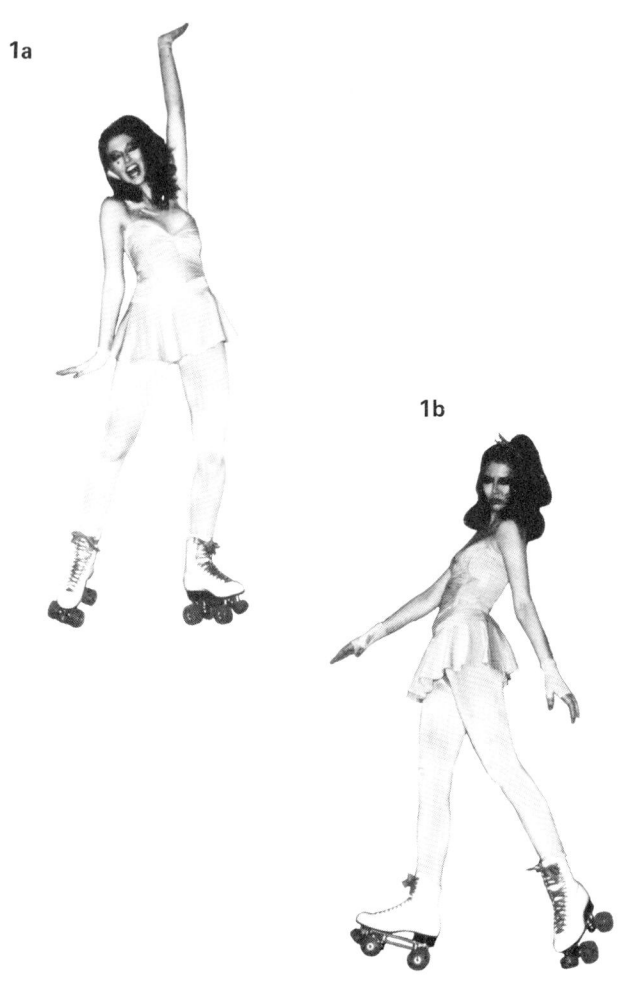

1a

1b

1a Start rolling with a forward push, the leading toe pointing out away from the body.
  b Lean into the motion, the body slightly forward. . .

Professional roller skates available from Beadle Roller Skates, 45 Finsbury Road, Wood Green, London N22; 01-888 3400. Ring or write to above for free catalogue and price list. Prices from £56.

2a

2b

2c

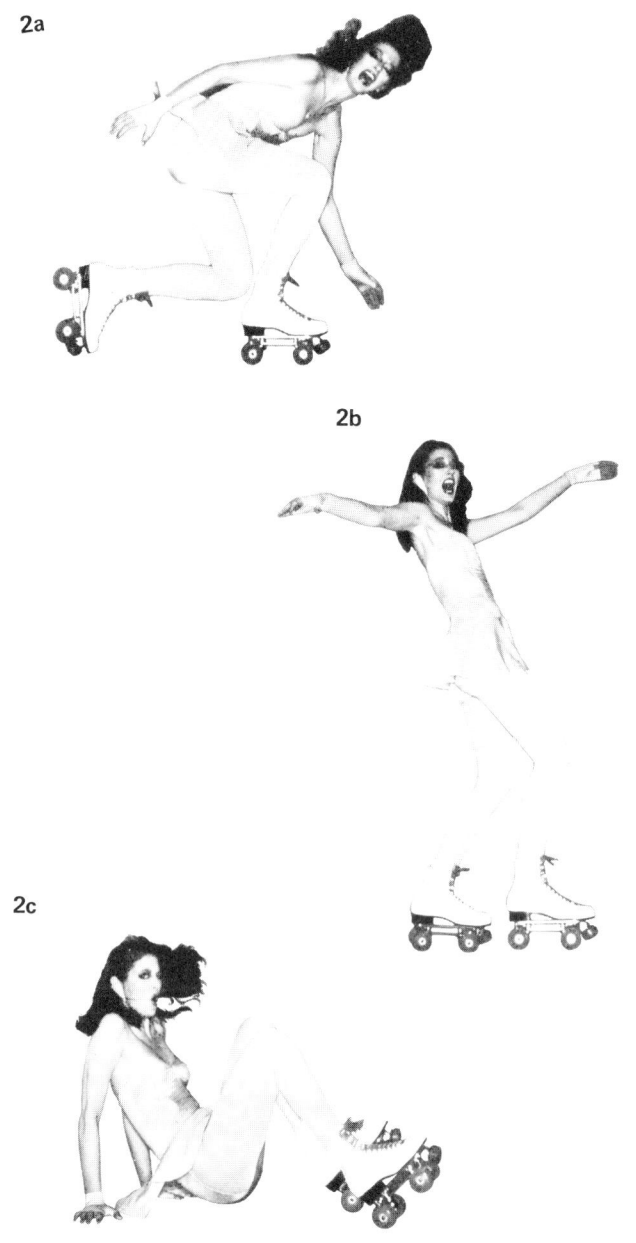

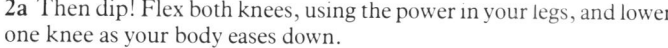

2a Then dip! Flex both knees, using the power in your legs, and lower one knee as your body eases down.

b Expect to fall — but do it right! Don't tense your body when you crash — wear gloves, elbow and knee pads for protection.

c If you begin to teeter, fall *forward* . . . not *backward* — otherwise you will hurt your spine.

3a

3b

4a

4b

4c

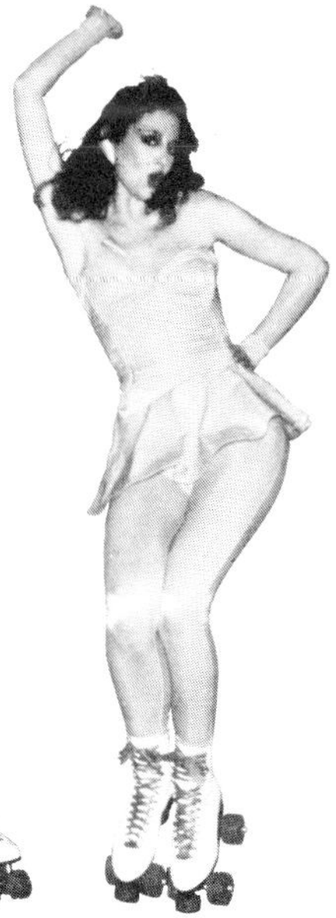

3a To whirl around curves, cross the right foot over the left. . .

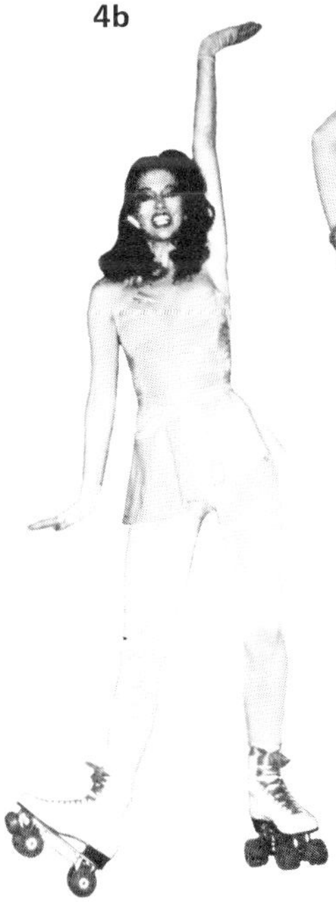

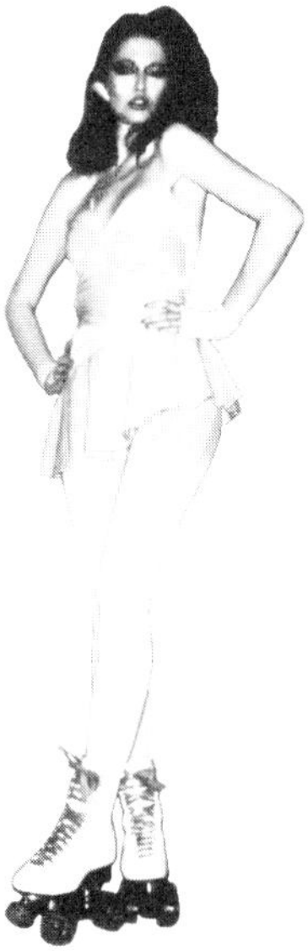

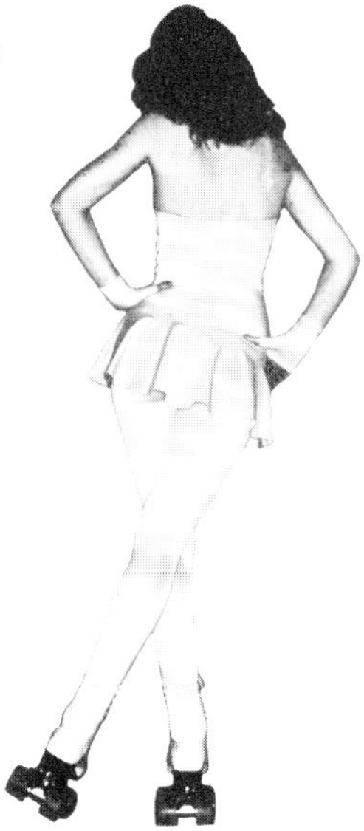

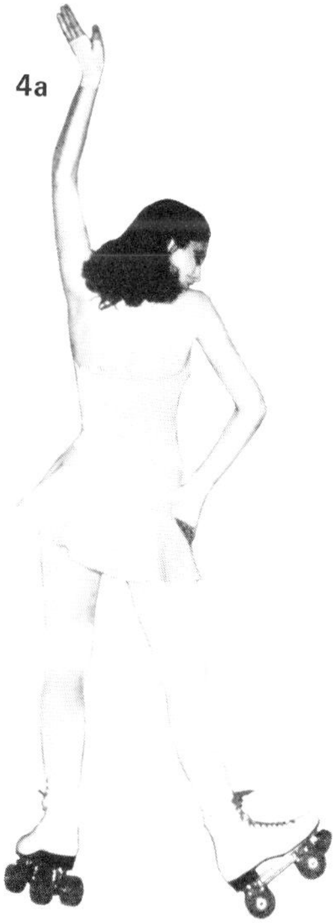

b Lift the left foot as it rolls behind the right.

4a To spin in place, balance firmly on one heel, locking the knee. . .

b Bend the other leg up and down, rolling along as you rotate on the stationary heel.

c Stop short by turning sharply, then flip up on to your toe-stops.

5a

5b

5c

5d

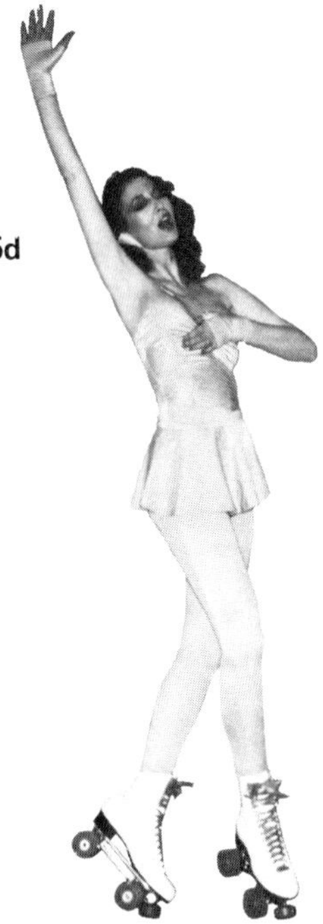

5a Use your toe-stops for more daring disco steps. Poise on one foot and kick up high!
b Leap forward. . .
c Raise your knee. . .
d And up on toe-steps!

6a

6b

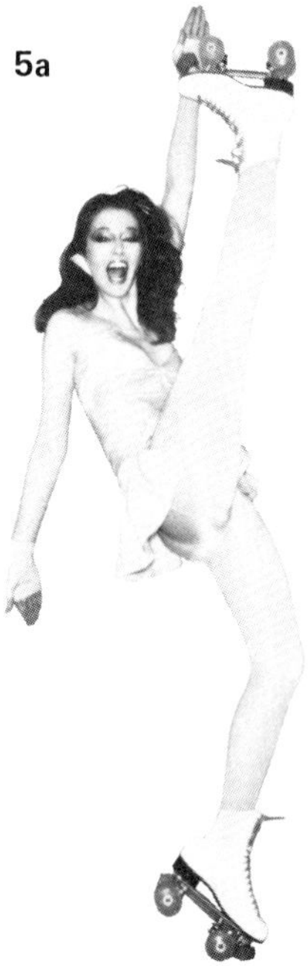

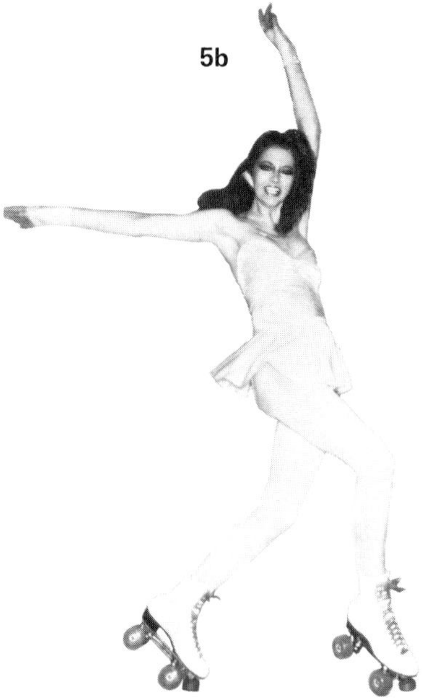

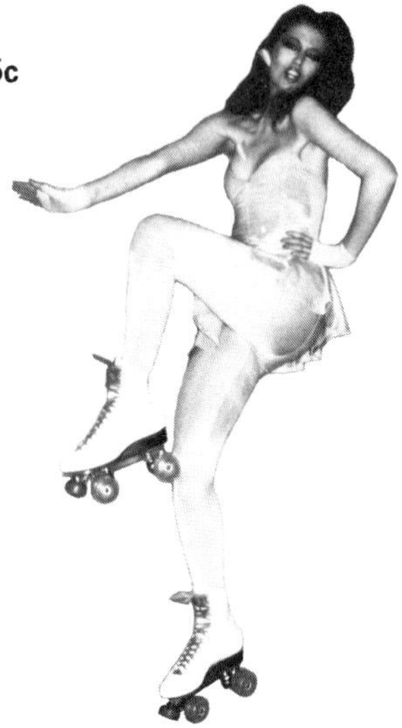

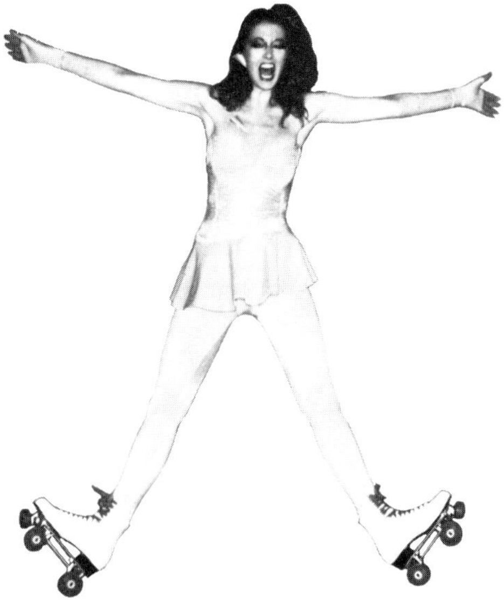

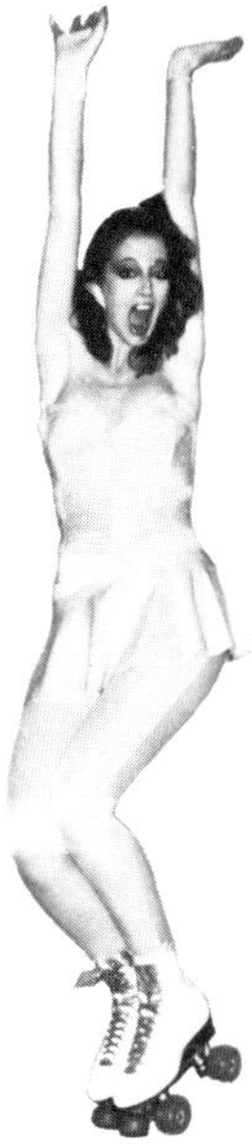

7a

6a Try a side-to-side jump!
b Flex your knees and balance on toe-stops as you flip your heels.
7a This one needs care — glide *slowly* into a spread eagle.

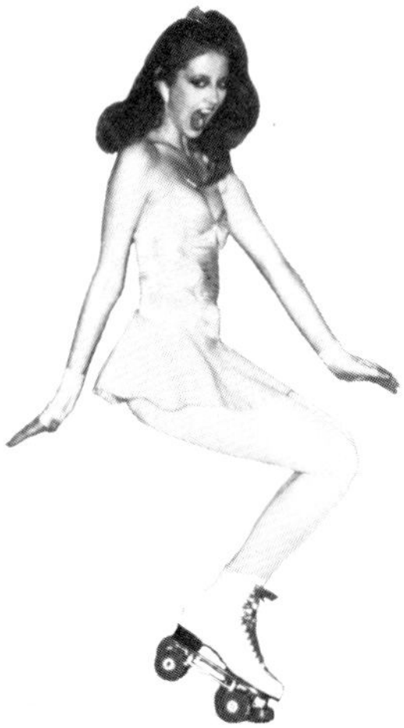

THE BODY

Learn how to pamper, treat and benefit your body from the tips of your toenails upwards . . . Discover how to turn your bathroom into a superspa, have your own health farm weekend (without the expense and within the privacy of your own home!) and how to give yourself sybaritic salon treatments that make you *feel* as well as look much better. All the equipment and know-how on body self-improvement starts here.

Make the most of your bathroom

Your beauty routine should centre around the bathroom. This is your private place where you can condition your skin, steam your face, relax in a herbal bath or paint your toenails! Look at the following checklist to select the right bathroom basics for *your* body beautiful.

LOOFAH Length of dry, rough-textured vegetable gourd. Buy it flat and it will swell in hot water. Chop it in two (before swelling) and you have two friction mitts—or keep it whole for sloughing skin on back, hips, etc.

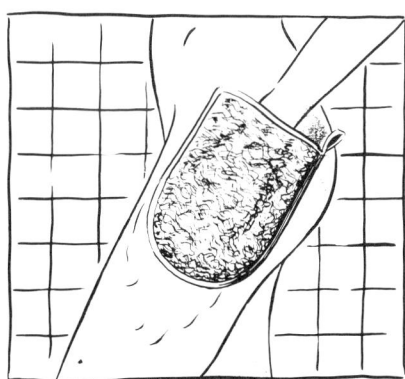

FRICTION STRAP/FRICTION MITT Buy the kind made from hemp and blended with horsehair. They are gentler than loofahs, but have the same basic function of smoothing rough skin. Friction straps have hand grips at either side so you can rub them across your back; slip your hands into friction mitts for easy, convenient use all over your body.

BACK BRUSH should have bristles of animal hair and be quite harsh to the touch; nylon bristles are too soft. The most useful kind of back brushes have a webbing loop over the brush, and the curved handle can slot free so you can use the brush separately as a friction rub.

BUF PUFS are small circles of polyester fibres which you rub on your skin to eliminate excess oil, stimulate circulation and smooth skin. Their effectiveness lies in the fact that *you* control the amount of pressure applied to the skin, and can vary this pressure according to the delicacy and sensitivity of your skin. You can buy a Buf Puf attached to a long handle to reach back and legs more easily, or a Buf Puf specially for the feet, but all have the same effect.

FLANNEL or washcloth, as the Americans call it, is generally only used on the body, not the face. This is a pity, as a flannel is useful to soak in hot water and apply to face or body to soften and loosen blackheads. A flannel should be made of cotton; soak in boiling water after every use as it collects bacteria easily.

NATURAL SEA SPONGE These are expensive but are lovely to use in the bath; they work up a good lather with soap and their mild exfoliating action keeps skin in good condition.

PUMICE STONE The oldest and one of the most effective methods of dealing with hard, dead skin, the pumice stone is simply a block of volcanic lava which you rub on hard skin spots such as heels, elbows, etc.

BATH PILLOW A luxury for bath fanatics, small plastic

or rubber pillows are placed at the back of your neck to ease muscle strain: for long lie-ins only! (Alternatively, you could use a rolled-up hand towel.)

SHOWER ATTACHMENT If you do not have a shower already, you can buy a rubber hair-wash shower very cheaply, and attach it to bath taps. It is useful for a home hydrotherapy treatment, see page 100, and for firming the bosom, see page 112.

Retexturising your skin

With the correct and daily use of friction mitts, scrubs, etc you will be able to literally plane away any roughness, lumps or bumps on the skin. "Chicken skin"—the name applied to clusters of small raised bumps often found on thighs and sides of hips—is not, as is often thought, cellulite, but is due to poor circulation, and can soon be broken down with the continual use of a sloughing agent. After this important retexturising step, when fresh new skin cells are exposed, your skin is at its most receptive for moisturising.

● The hardy Swedes and body-conscious Frenchwomen use friction mitts to increase circulation and keep skin smooth *before* entering the bath: this might be too harsh for your skin to begin with. Use friction mitts in the bath to work up a soapy lather and use them on problem areas in steady, circular motions; you will find that, with constant use, you will be able to increase pressure. Even on smooth, silky skin you can use friction to promote healthy circulation and prevent lumps and bumps from appearing.

● Spotty, greasy backs benefit greatly from a soapy scrub with a back brush every day. Use a rotary motion and do not be afraid to scrub quite hard. Always rinse the soap off your back very thoroughly afterwards with fresh water.

● Body scrubs are similar to facial scrubs. You can buy them in the form of dry granules or as grains suspended in a moisturising cream which you rub on skin to slough off dead cells. It is cheaper and as effective to look in the kitchen cupboard for some oatmeal or cornflour, and use that; keep a jar corked by the bath and reach for it whenever you see rough or dingy-looking patches of skin.

● Champneys Health Resort keep big buckets of sea salt by their showers; you can do the same. Keep a large bowlful by your bath and grab handfuls to rub into your skin. This treatment is particularly beneficial for greasy, large-pored skins, but may be a little too harsh for dry and sensitive skins.

● A similar treatment, with a moisturising plus, is to mix corn or vegetable oil with enough sea salt to form a paste. Rub well into the skin before entering the bath. It will wash off in the bath, and will leave your skin feeling beautifully soft and silky. You can, if you wish, follow with a loofah or friction mitt rub-down.

● Other good, abrasive pastes to try are: yogurt with almond meal; sugar with vegetable oil.

● Beauty expert Joan Price of the Face Place salons advocates the brush-on/peel-off masks for use on rough elbows, heels, knees, etc, as she says they roll off a lot of dead cuticle that tends to accumulate in these areas. Allow the mask to become tacky; rub off.

Skin conditioning treatments

Your most basic skin softening—and conditioning—treatment is the daily massage you give your body with your favourite nourishing cream. Always apply this after the bath, when skin is warm and slightly damp; this increases effectiveness of the cream, as it seals in moisture. Use strong massage movements on legs and arms, working in the direction of the heart. It is the rubbing movements, as much as the moisturising, that promote a healthy circulation.

Later on, you can read how to make your own nourishing creams and oils for the body; listed here are several special skin-softening treatments that are worth trying when a simple moisturiser does not seem adequate.

● A paraffin wax treatment is one of the luxuries a health farm offers, and something you can try yourself. The warm wax is brushed onto the skin, left to dry and peeled off to expose fresh, beautifully soft skin underneath. It can be used on hands (a friend will have to help!), feet, thighs—anywhere on the body. An added bonus of this treatment is that it has the ability to draw off excess body fluids and acts as a good muscle de-tenser; health farms often use it on the back for this purpose. You can buy large blocks of Low Melting Hard Paraffin Wax from larger Boots branches. Melt in a pan till wax is comfortably hot to the skin—test on the inside of your wrist—and apply with a large, soft brush to the area you wish to treat. Cover in baking foil and leave for approximately twenty minutes. Unwrap foil and you will find that the wax has hardened to a malleable consistency which will peel off easily.

● Marina Andrews, owner of the Town and Country beauty salons, suggests this bath-soak treatment for clients with rough or "chicken-skinned" problem areas: half fill the bath with hot water, then add a mix of one tablespoon olive oil and one of white vinegar; top up bath with water. Use friction mitt on rough skin in circular movements in the oil-and-vinegar bath. Afterwards, pat dry and massage in Vaseline, dabbing off excess with towel or tissues.

● Africans and Asians have less lined skins because they have a greater oil absorption through their diet, Marina points out, about a 50 percent increase on ours. Take a tablespoon of vegetable oil daily or—when they are in season—eat an avocado! Use the shell to rub on rough skin patches and leave the oils on for twenty minutes for greater penetration.

● One of the world's most exclusive health spas, The Golden Door in Escondido, California, offers this treatment to clients which you can try yourself. They recommend it for dry, rough knees—which are real age giveaways—but you could use it for elbows, feet or hands. Cocoa butter, available from many health food stores, is, on its own, a marvellous skin softener and is doubly effective when used in this programme:

Before bedtime, apply a mix of cocoa butter thinned out with olive oil, to the problem area, and rub in. Soak for five minutes in a hot bath to which you have added a handful of baking soda plus two handfuls of bran. Using a flannel, massage with the hot water, working in the oil and cocoa butter. Do not use soap. Dry lightly after bathing, reapply cocoa butter and oil mixture, and bandage lightly with cheesecloth for the night.

The next morning, apply body lotion or baby oil to the area. The second night, follow the same procedure, but massage knees in the hot bath with coarse salt and not the flannel. Finish treatment as before. The third night, repeat the same routine, but use a mixture of cornmeal and oatmeal as a scrub. By this time you should already have noticed an improvement!

You may discontinue this "blitz" programme after the third day, repeating one phase of it once or twice weekly as necessary. Keep up the cocoa butter and oil applications at night and use lotion by day. To keep the skin extra soft in between, rub with the cut side of a cucumber.

Soaps and bath additives

Soaps

There are countless soaps on the market, all with the same purpose: to cleanse the skin. You may be a little confused over the difference between them, what effect they have on your skin, and which is suitable for your skin type. Below is a breakdown of the eight most widely-used types of soap, to help you choose the right one for you.

GLYCERINE SOAPS Glycerine is a by-product of the fatty acid used in all soap-making. It is transparent, mildly scented and is good for sensitive, dry skins, as it disturbs the skin's natural pH balance only marginally. (The Skylab astronauts used it in Space to retain the ecological balance of their skin!)

SUPERFATTED SOAPS have added oils, fats and creams to moisturise dry skin. The additives leave a thin film on the skin to protect and lubricate. Those with greasy skins should avoid superfatted soaps.

MEDICATED SOAPS contain mild antiseptics and anti-bacterial agents in varying amounts. They are specially formulated for very greasy and acne-prone skins as they deep-

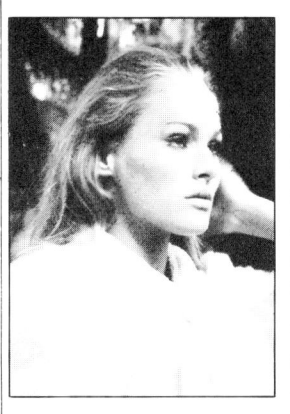

URSULA ANDRESS, *film actress: "I use only soap and water on my skin when I bathe but if my skin is feeling dry I'll add a few drops of bath oil. I always massage moisturiser into my body after the bath to keep it smooth and supple. I hardly wear any make-up these days because I think it is ageing. I attribute my glowing skin to soap and water — and playing masses of sports!"*

cleanse and dry the skin. If you use a medicated soap and find it becomes too drying, switch to a milder brand and use a small amount of moisturiser after washing.

UNSCENTED SOAPS are designed for sensitive skins as many people find the scent content in soaps causes allergies. As these soaps can be a bit drying, you might find you need to moisturise skin afterwards.

SULPHUR SOAPS are very drying and suited to acne-prone and greasy skins only.

DEODORANT/ANTI-BACTERIAL SOAPS There is a certain amount of controversy among dermatologists over the manufacture of these soaps because of the chemical additives which can have harsh, drying effects on the skin, even though these soaps may otherwise fulfil their claims. Anti-bacterial soaps can interfere with the natural bacteria balance of the skin, so leaving it more prone to skin infections. It should be noted that there is no substitute for a good underarm deodorant/ anti-perspirant!

TRIPLE MILLED/HARD MILLED SOAPS These impressive-sounding terms simply mean that, in the manufacturing, the soaps have been processed more often so that they become very hard and will therefore last longer.

WASH CREAMS contain either the mildest detergent or none at all. They are made up from plant, herb, vegetable, bran or wheatgerm extract and are particularly useful for highly sensitive and dry skins. Available from health-food stores and large chemists.

Bath additives

Bath additives are fun: they make you smell good and boost your morale but, used incorrectly, they can cause skin allergies, excessive dryness and become a problem instead of a body-pampering luxury. To help you understand their functions so you can assess their suitability for your skin, these are the categories:

SALTS AND CRYSTALS are effective as water softeners and add slight scent and colour. They can have a drying effect on some skins. If you live in a hard water area and have dry skin, add a little oil to the water.

BUBBLE BATHS are basically cleansing agents with added scent, colour and chemicals—plus a stabiliser that prevents foam disappearing after thirty seconds! They are best suited to greasy skins. Many brands have a high chemical content and could cause reactions in sensitive skins. If you have a dry skin, but like bubbles, use only a small amount of bubble bath in the water.

GELS are cleansing agents with chemicals added to make the jelly-like consistency. They are quite mild, and suited to most skins.

MILKS are water softeners and cleansers. Many brands actually contain powdered milk, and these are good for dry skins. Greasy, spotty skins may find that milks aggravate the condition. Sensitive skins should be cautious of heavily scented brands produced by some perfume houses.

ESSENCES simply scent the water, and are generally either alcohol or oil-based. Greasy skins are best suited to the alcohol-based variety, and dry skins to oil-based essences. Like milks, they can be heavily scented.

OILS are ideally suited to dry skins as they are specifically designed to moisturise and lubricate skin. There are two main types: *floating* which remain on the water's surface and cling to the body as it emerges from the bath water, and *emulsified* which disperse in the water, and are slightly less oily.

Make your own bath range

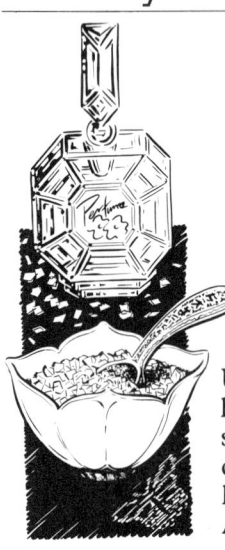

Using soaps and bath additives that you have made yourself is satisfying, money-saving, and you have the advantage of choosing the fragrance you would most like to match up with your perfume.
All of the following are simple to make:

BATH SALTS Epsom salts are renowned for easing muscular tensions, and are the base for this recipe for fragrant, prettily tinted bath salts: pound a few drops of food colouring, and the same amount of your favourite scent or essential oil, with a large pack of Epsom salts. For a pretty marbled effect, pound the fragrance in first and fold the colour through. Keep in a bowl by your bath; they lose their colour when stoppered in a jar. Try mixing blue and red colouring with lavender oil; green colouring with refreshing pine essence.

BATH OIL Any vegetable oil base is suitable for making bath oil; do not use baby oil as it will "sit" on the surface of the water, and not be properly absorbed by the skin. The finest oil you can use is almond oil. Mix three-quarters of one cup oil

with one quarter of a cup aromatic oil, eg, jasmine, mint (very invigorating) or perhaps lemon; alternatively, you can mix several aromatic oils together with the vegetable oil for your own special bath oil recipe. A large range of aromatic oils is available from Baldwin's, 173 Walworth Rd, London SE17; enclose an SAE for list and prices. If you prefer, you can make your own aromatic oil (see page 105).

SOAP Making your own soap, when there are so many cheap, good brands available, is a false economy, especially as the process involved is rather laborious. However, you can be very thrifty and melt down old soap scraps in a saucepan, with a little water, though be sure the fragrances blend! You can then shape the soap, when cool enough to handle, into balls, and roll them in oatmeal for a very professional finish that will benefit your skin, too.

SOAPLESS FACE AND BODY CLEANSER The Swiss use muslin bags stuffed with dry bran to clean their bodies! When left to soak for an hour or so, the bran emits a milky substance which makes a mild, non-lathering cleanser, specially suited to delicate, sensitive and allergy-prone skins. The principle is used in commercial products: look for bran wash creams at your local health-food stores, or make your own with squares of cheesecloth or muslin, and a handful of bran.

BUBBLE BATH This recipe for bubble bath is non-drying and will leave skin feeling soft. The following is enough for one bath; make a fresh mixture every time. Pine oil is refreshing and reviving, but you could substitute with any favourite aromatic oil.

1 egg
½ cup clear, cheap shampoo
5 ml (1 tsp) gelatine
4 drops pine oil (or other aromatic oil)
2 drops green colouring (or other appropriate colouring)
Mix ingredients together with an electric beater. Pour under running water and watch the bubbles rise!

Baths as beauty treatments

A long soak in the bath *can* be good for you—providing you have added rather special ingredients to the water. From therapeutic mud baths to fragrant pick-up baths, here is a selection of treatment baths which you can try at home—plus some advice on how to take the waters, seriously.

Therapeutic baths

Therapeutic bathing may evoke some far from appealing visions of spartan sitz-baths at naturopathic clinics, but baths with medically formulated additives have long been known to relieve muscular—as well as mental—tensions. These baths are treatments and *not* substitutes for cleansing baths. You soak for approximately fifteen minutes to allow curative powers to take effect, before wrapping up in a warm towel.

SEAWEED BATH helps relieve aches and pains, reduces swellings and sprains. It is claimed by many beauty therapists that seaweed helps combat cellulite. You can buy it ready prepared from health-food stores, or fill a muslin bag with seaweed and let it soak for ten minutes before use. The temperature of the water should not be too hot, as the seaweed bath is quite strong, and can make you feel light-headed.

SEA SALT BATH makes the body perspire and thus draws out impurities from the skin; it acts in a similar way to a sauna, and is specially beneficial for oily skins. You can buy prepared sea salt baths, with added herbs and minerals, from health-food stores, or make your own, using two cups of sea salt per bath. Add some powdered kelp (dried seaweed) from health-food stores, for a real sea bath that will ease muscular tensions, too.

MUD BATH You don't have to go to a special spa for these: packs of dried earth of volcanic origin and rich in minerals, can be bought from health-food stores. In fine powder form, they turn the bath-water cloudy, not muddy! They help unclog pores and clear spotty backs. Do not be tempted to shower afterwards as the therapeutic effects last twenty-four hours.

VINEGAR BATH reduces drying and alkaline effects of soap and water, and is soothing for dry, itchy skin. Simply add a cup of cider vinegar to the bath water.

MUSTARD BATH is very invigorating when you feel cold, or stiff in the joints. You can buy prepared mustard baths, or just add a little powdered mustard to the bath!

Beautifying baths

The beautifying bath can soften, moisturise, scent or even tan the skin! Here are three basic recipes you might like to try:

MILK BATH is a skin-softening treatment that feels lovely. Add 568 ml (1 pt) milk to the bath water, or one cupful of powdered milk. Add a little almond oil, as Beverly Sassoon does, for a milk-and-almond bath that is extra softening; or a

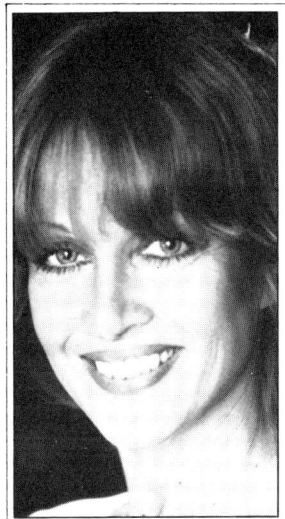

ANOUSKA HEMPEL, *actress who runs her own hotel, Blakes, in London: "I pour Fenjal and baby oil into the bath to moisturise my skin; I soak for a while, then soap it all off. After I've dried myself I rub masses of Orlane's B21 Crème Fluide For Body And Bust all over my body, very vigorously. I'm sure this helps fight cellulite and stops skin from being too greasy after all the bath oil. I wear a tracksuit to work every day and keep fit by running absolutely everywhere."*

spoonful of clear honey for a moisturising, soothing milk-and-honey bath.

HERBAL BATH smells marvellous and is relaxing for mind and body. Sprinkle your choice of herbs on the bath water or, to avoid messy tide-marks, gather the herbs in a muslin bag and tie to the bath taps so the water flows through it, or just leave the sachet in the bath. You should be able to use it for several baths. Dried lavender flowers are easily obtainable and fill the air with their aroma; camomile flowers open pores and are good for problem skins; mint is refreshing and reviving. Try mixing kitchen herbs, too: thyme and rosemary are particularly good.

Take the waters seriously

Dermatologists agree that soaking in hot water is drying for the skin as it causes surface skin oils to disperse: the hotter the water, the more it will dissolve away the oil, even without the use of soap. If you have any doubts that water dehydrates the skin, see how the pads of your fingers "ridge" when you've emerged from a long hot soak!

Twenty minutes should be the maximum time you spend in any bath. The temperature of a bath is important: a comfortably warm bath is best. A hot bath is energy-draining, but can be useful for those who have trouble sleeping, as it is so relaxing. A cool bath is a good reviving mental and physical pick-up: cowards could try draining off half a warm bath after a few minutes, then turning on the cold tap.

Always moisturise skin well after your bath, when it is slightly damp and pores are open and therefore more receptive. HARD AND SOFT WATER are gauged by the quantity of minerals in the water: the higher the amount, the harder the water. Claims that hard water is bad for the skin are exaggerated:

the only real difference between hard and soft water is that soap does not lather so well in hard water. For softer water, add a few teaspoons of plain household starch.

Water therapy: Your most precious weapon against cellulite

Hydrotherapy, practised since ancient Greek and Roman times, is one of the simplest yet most effective ways of helping to break down the fatty deposits in connective tissue that we call *cellulite*. Methods vary from under-water massage to application of high-pressure water jets, and are outlined below; you'll see you don't need sophisticated equipment to benefit.

WATER PRESSURE TREATMENTS Many Californians relax in their own warm water "energy tubs" or "jacuzzis". Jets placed around the sides of a pool create a pulsating whirlpool that gives the body an invigorating work-out, stimulating circulation as well as soothing tired muscles. Larger beauty salons and some health farms now have jacuzzis. Similar individual whirlpool baths, called Aerotones, can be found at many public swimming-baths; check with your local council for the nearest available to you.

You can create your own hydro massage with a shower; buy the Boots Shampoo & Bath Spray, and unscrew the detachable head so you have a strong water current which you can direct at soft body tissue. This treatment is particularly good for firming the bosom.

Many health hydros have "impulse showers", strong needle jets of water with controlled changes of temperature. This contrast showering has the bonus of toning circulation by contracting and dilating capillaries as water changes from cold to hot. You can achieve a similar effect if you have a shower at home. The hardy could brave a hose-down in the back garden with the tap full on—though for optimum results the water should be stimulatingly cold! Hold the hose several inches from the body and work from the ankles upward. Spend about fifteen minutes on this slightly masochistic—but very beneficial—operation.

EXERCISING IN WATER Whether you swim in the sea or practise isometrics in the bath, you achieve more immediate results from exercise because you are pushing against the pressure of the water: as your movements meet resistance, so your muscles are required to work harder.

When your body is immersed in a warm bath, muscles are relaxed and breathing is natural and even. You are in an ideal comfortable physical and mental condition to work with your body. Joan Price of the Face Place salons suggests the following simple movements to follow at every bath:

To strengthen arm muscles, upper back and firm breasts: Lie back with arms by side, palms upward, and slowly push arms up through water as if trying to lift a great weight.

To trim waist and firm stomach: Lie back and slowly sit up, pushing against water with arms at side.

To stretch back of legs and spine and firm stomach: Lie back and lift legs until they are at right angles to body, holding on to feet all the time; lower legs slowly back into the water.

UNDERWATER MASSAGE Mrs Leida Costigan, Director of the Henlow Grange Beauty Farm believes that water is an additional help in breaking down fatty deposits while skin is pummelled into shape, and advocates the following method for clients to follow at home:

The bath water should be pleasantly warm. Rub body hard all over with palms of hands. Lift flab and massage using circular pinching and twisting movements. Put hands on waist; pinch and knead. Concentrate especially on the inner thighs and arms upwards from wrist.

SWIMMING POOL WORK-OUTS Swimming is the ideal exercise for working all the muscles of the body at the same time—without placing undue strain on one area. It is the least tiring form of exercise, as the body is supported by the water all the while. Breast stroke is particularly beneficial for firming upper arms and thighs; the crawl promotes more efficient

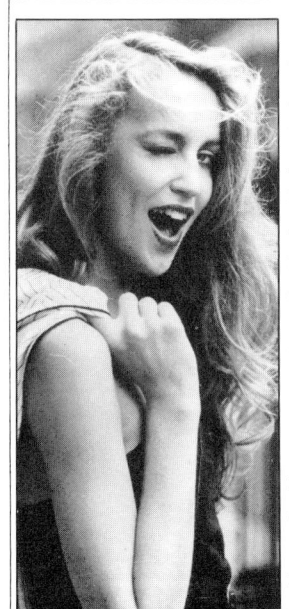

JERRY HALL, *model: "I use a mixture of natural sea salt, algae and kelp in the bath water, or German tonic salts, or pine extract. I exercise in the bath to keep my stomach firm and flat. First I breathe out very slowly, emptying my lungs. Then I breathe in and out ten times, very fast, so that I lift my abdomen up into my ribcage. It's best to do this in the bath when muscles are relaxed and warm. Sometimes, before going to bed, I cover my hands and legs with turtle cream from Mexico, then pull on thick socks and gloves. Next morning I wake up soft as a kitten!"*

breathing. Alan Hime, President of The British Swimming Coaches' Association and ex-Olympic coach, says: "The faster you swim, the faster the heart races, so in addition to improved muscular tone, the body builds up a healthy cardio-vascular system—and swimming gives you a wonderful feeling of well-being!"

Even if you are a non-swimmer you can try these simple but effective exercise in your local pool. They are devised by Nicole Ronsard, author of *Cellulite**. The water should be deep enough to reach your shoulders, and you will need to hold on to the pool-side railing or steps for support. The first two movements concentrate on firming the hip joint area and inner thighs; the last two, hips, buttocks and legs.

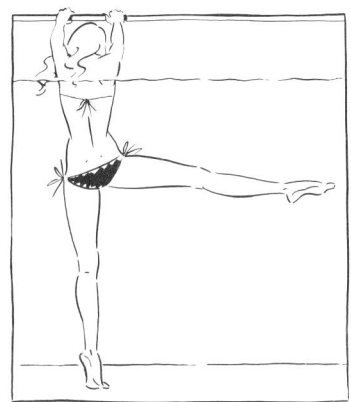

1 Face pool side. Feel secure as you hold the side. Raise right leg ten times, then left leg ten times, rising up on your toes.

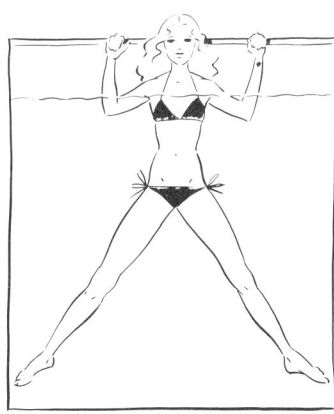

2 Back against pool side. Hold yourself firmly as you split your legs, knees stiff. As fast as you can, bring your legs together and split again, keeping legs perfectly straight. Repeat fifteen times.

*Copyright © 1973 by Beauty & Health Publishing Corp. Published by Transworld Publishers Ltd. as a Bantam Book at 85p.

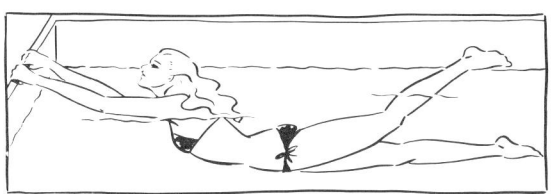

3 Hold side of pool firmly, arms extended as you float on your stomach. Kick. If you keep your knees stiff, you will feel movement all through the leg and hip area. Work as fast as is comfortable for you, counting to twenty or thirty.

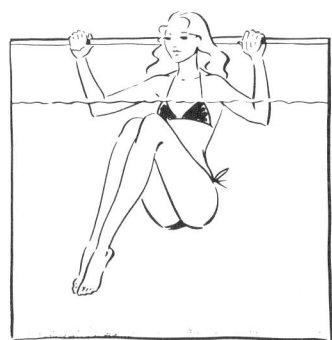

4 Back against pool side. Bend knees up to chest. Swing to the right, touching knees against the side, and then swing to the left. Repeat ten times on each side.

SEA WATER TREATMENTS Use the sea to firm flab: wade along the shoreline, where waves break against ankles, calves and thighs, for a sea-water massage; it is claimed that algae in the sea help break down cellulite pockets. Stand where waves are fiercest!

Saunas and steam baths

The purpose of any steam treatment on the body is the same: to induce relaxation of muscles and mind, and to increase perspiration so that grime is sweated from the pores. Whether you choose the fierce dry heat of the sauna, or the milder steam rooms of the Turkish baths (or simply the steamy atmosphere of your own bathroom!), you should be aware of the changes that take place in the body during the process: these treatments can be marvellous for mind and body—but can be harmful if abused.

SAUNA The dry heat sauna originated in Finland, where taking a sauna is a serious ritual which involves slapping the skin with birch branches as the heat grows stronger, and plunging into cold water—or snow! Though less drastic, the principle of our sauna bath remains the same. The sauna room

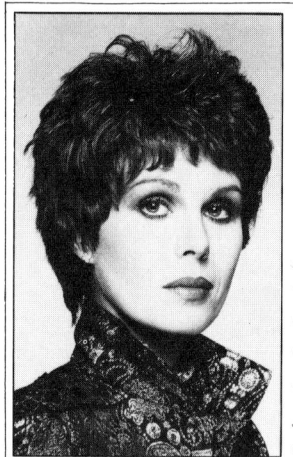

JOANNA LUMLEY, *actress:* "*I usually just put a little baby oil in the bath, which makes my skin nice and soft — and the bath easier to clean. I have a pumice stone which I have had for about 114 years but I have occasional fits of attacking myself with it on my feet, elbows, thighs, tops of my arms. I don't spend a lot of money on keeping myself beautiful. I use Vaseline as a face and body moisturiser, on my legs after shaving, and on my hair during the summer when I swim! I'm anti-sunbathing because I believe the sun is bad for the skin, and people who sunbathe all day are usually boring. All the money I save on cosmetics now, I shall put to good use when I'm fifty by having everything pulled, tucked, lifted and cut. Anything worth doing, I'll do it!*"

has benches on two levels: the higher one is hotter; and not for first-timers. Average temperature varies between 65° and 82°C (150°F to 180°F) but can be hotter; take it slowly at first, and if you feel faint, leave the sauna. Within a few minutes of entering the sauna, the body and skin temperatures rise, blood vessels under the skin dilate and the heart beats faster, thus increasing circulation.

A stay in a sauna should not exceed twenty minutes, and should always be supervised: it is easy to nod off in the relaxing atmosphere! Afterwards, a cool shower should be taken, preferably accompanied by a scrub-down with a bristle brush or friction mitt, to rid skin of loosened grime and dead skin.

Watchpoints

Spend no more than ten minutes in a sauna for the first time.
Wait at least one hour after a large meal before taking a sauna.
Do not take a sauna if:

- you are fasting, or on a strict diet
- you have a heart or respiratory condition
- you have high or low blood pressure
- you are pregnant
- you have had recent major surgery

Incidentally, if you have any ideas of weight-loss connected with the sauna, forget them. Although you can lose a couple of pounds in a half-hour session, the loss is all water and is returned immediately after the session, when you find you have a raging thirst! You should note that the sauna depletes fluids—not excess fats!

STEAM CABINETS which you can try at health farms and beauty salons, are similar in effect to saunas. Some prefer the steam cabinet to the sauna because you are seated in a cabinet with your head outside. However, the same precautions as for the sauna apply to the steam cabinet.

TURKISH BATHS are similar in principle to a sauna, though because you wander through rooms of varying heat, you can spend longer indulging in these enjoyable steam treatments. It is usual to proceeed from a dry warm room to a dry hotter room, then to a warm or hot steam room. You are given a massage and scrub-down on a marble slab: it's very satisfying to see dirt literally roll off the skin! There are cold plunge pools, sometimes cold showers, and the advantage of the Turkish bath is that you can choose the pace, and the temperature. Again, you should observe the same watchpoints for a Turkish bath as you would for a sauna.

Hair you can live without: What to do about it

"Superfluous hair" is the term we apply to body hair we would rather not have. It is for you to decide whether hairs on your body bother you enough for you to remove them, though current thinking dictates it is a sign of bad grooming to have visible hair on legs, and it is certainly unhygienic to have hair growth under the arms where sweat is easily trapped.

Body hair is most common on legs, arms and upper lips but may also occur on the chin, neck, breasts, stomach and back; it is these latter areas which cause most worry and make women fear they have an abnormal hair growth. This is rarely the case; hair growth is usually hereditary, though in rare cases when growth is exceptionally heavy, can be due to a hormonal imbalance, or a side-effect of the pill. If you are worried, do check with your GP.

The different ways of dealing with unwanted hair are outlined below; whichever method you choose, note that skin where hair has just been removed will be more sensitive than usual and, in the case of waxing, chemical depilation and shaving, could be quite sore. A slathering of scent-free moisturiser will soothe, and counteract any drying effects. Always wait twenty-four hours before applying deodorant after shaving or using chemical depilatory on underarms.

METHOD	HOW IT WORKS	WHERE TO USE	EFFECTIVENESS	COMMENTS
Abrading	Hair is "sand-papered" down with an abrasive pad, using circular rubbing movements.	On fine hair-growth only. Some women use abrasive pads from knee to thigh, where they find hair growth is lighter than from ankle to knee.	Cheap and easy method of hair removal, though care must be taken not to rub pad too vigorously, or redness may result.	Advantageous for those whose skins react badly to alternative methods of depilation. Abrasive pads are often called "hair removing gloves" as they are shaped like mitts, so hand can slip in between papers for easy use.
Bleaching	Commercial bleaching cream is applied to the area and left on for stipulated time, to lighten hairs. It is then rinsed off. The cream will not remove hairs, though continuous bleaching damages the hair and thus may cause it to break off. It is important to do a patch test.	Particularly suited to peach-fuzz "moustaches" which are not heavy enough to warrant removal. Also useful for light-growth hair which would not be noticeable if blonde.	Painless and harmless if directions adhered to, though rather a laborious process on large areas.	Ideal for hair that is growing back—but needs more length—for waxing.
Electrolysis	A fine needle is inserted into the hair follicle; a tiny electric current is passed down the follicle to kill the root.	Theoretically, electrolysis can be used on any part of the body where permanent hair removal is required, but because of the time and expense involved it is most often used on small areas, such as the face.	This is the only reliable method of permanently removing hair. However, all hairs cannot be removed in one session because, as some are shed in the normal cycle, their roots are impossible to locate. The main disadvantage is expense: a fifteen-minute session costs, on average, £2.50, and an upper lip that has been subject to temporary measures such as plucking or shaving could need numerous sessions before all hairs have been destroyed. It must be stressed that electrolysis does not affect the *cause* of the problem: if the hair growth is caused by an hormonal imbalance, hair will reappear.	Performed by a *skilled* electrolysist, this is a safe and most satisfactory method of hair removal. (For a list of registered members of the British Association of Electrolysists in your area, write to Christine Holdship, 22 Burnett Rd, Trowbridge, Wilts, enclosing an SAE). Most electrolysists give a free preliminary consultation, but if you are in any doubt as to the advisability of the treatment, particularly on a sensitive areas ask the advice of your GP. Electrolysis can be painful, though most people report only an uncomfortable pricking sensation; a slight swelling and redness should not last more than a few hours. If there is intense, prolonged irritation, or any sign of infection, a doctor should be consulted immediately. Never attempt any kind of do-it-yourself electrolysis; misuse of electrolysis "pencils", for example, can lead to permanent scarring.
Tweezer epilation	Each hair is grasped with electronic tweezers and a radio frequency current is passed down the hair shaft to destroy the root.	As for electrolysis.	An alternative to electrolysis, but hospital tests have shown that it is no more successful than plucking with ordinary tweezers. Permanent removal cannot be guaranteed and in some cases, regrowth may be even stronger.	The most expensive method of hair removal, the cost does not appear to be justified by results.

METHOD	HOW IT WORKS	WHERE TO USE	EFFECTIVENESS	COMMENTS
Shaving	Using an electric or safety razor, the hair is cut close to the skin.	Underarms and legs.	Shaving is the quickest way to remove hair, though as only the surface hair is removed, for many women hair "breaks through" as soon as twenty-four hours later.	Shaving with a safety razor can, for many, be a messy business— cut legs are as unattractive as hairy ones! Shaving does not, as is commonly believed, cause a stronger and thicker regrowth. It only gives this impression because it leaves the hair with a blunt as opposed to tapered end, which feels coarser to the touch. For this reason, facial hair should never be shaved.
Waxing	Hot beeswax is applied with a spatula. The wax then "sets" in a matter of seconds. The strips are pulled off: the force of the pull—similar in feel to ripping off a plaster—takes the hair out at the roots. A similar method, using a honey-based mix, incorporates the use of muslin or paper strips which are pressed on the wax, and then ripped off, taking wax and hair with them.	Arms, underarms, legs and "bikini line".	Hair is removed by the root, so regrowth is slower, from four to eight weeks. Continued waxing may cause hair to grow back finer and weaker, though this is not always the case. Waxing is the most effective method of hair removal for legs and underarms, and ideal for "bikini line" depilation just before a holiday.	Waxing can be quite painful. Those with sensitive skins are advised to have a patch test twenty-four hours beforehand, to be sure of no skin reactions. It is a fairly skilful procedure and wax has to be at a certain temperature to be effective without burning, so it is advisable to have waxing done professionally at a beauty salon. The real disadvantage of waxing is that the hairs must be long enough for the wax to be able to grip, so you have to allow for adequate regrowth before your next waxing session. Cold wax kits—wax pre-spread on muslin strips—are available for home use, though they are not very effective and can be very messy.
Plucking	Using eyebrow tweezers, hairs are removed individually by the root.	Suitable only for eyebrows, as it is such a lengthy process, though the patient have been known to pluck out hairs on legs: you could pluck out odd strays left after waxing, for instance. It is inadvisable to pluck hair from the face because it can distort hair follicles and thus make electrolysis, should you decide to undergo it in the future, a difficult and lengthy process.	Plucking is the best way to remove individual hairs, so it is ideal for shaping brows. Eyebrows need to be plucked every day as growth is cyclical, ie, hairs do not emerge simultaneously and therefore cannot be removed in one operation.	Always pluck eyebrows from underneath and in the direction of growth. Before plucking, wring out cotton wool in hot water and press against brows to open pores so the process is easier and not painful.
Chemical depilation	Depilatory creams contain a chemical which dissolves the hair shaft, but leaves the root intact. Cream is applied with a spatula, left on for stipulated time, then scraped off with a spatula, taking hairs with it. Used just before bathing.	Mainly for use on body areas although there are special formulations for the face.	Easier to use than wax and, though less convenient than shaving, area remains hair-free longer. On average, chemical depilatories need to be used every ten days to three weeks.	Always make a patch test first, as the chemicals can cause irritation. Follow the instructions accurately, and *never* leave on longer than stipulated: use a clock or watch. These chemicals can quite literally burn the skin, if left on for too long, so do be careful.

Deodorants:
What they can and can't do

The loose term we use for the product that helps check underarm perspiration is "deodorant". Nowadays, most deodorants have incorporated anti-perspirants, and it is this part of the formulation which helps prevent wetness. The deodorant merely masks odour with its own fragrance!

The apocrine glands are situated in the armpits and the groin; elsewhere on the body, we perspire freely with no odour, but the apocrine glands contain certain organic matter which, when combined with skin bacteria, result in the social disease we call BO: body odour. An anti-perspirant—which usually contains a chemical called aluminium chloride—has the effect of contracting these sweat pores with an astringent action. You may have heard that it is harmful and unnatural, but this is untrue; the perspiration is simply "rerouted" to the alternative eccrine glands elsewhere in the body.

Do not expect too much from your deodorant/anti-perspirant: if you are having bad skin reactions, or poor results, check the following points for maximum efficiency:

1 Never apply deodorant/anti-perspirant after shaving or using a depilatory; the chances are that if you have done in the past, your underarms have stung and soreness has developed. Some new products are claimed by the manufacturers to be suited for use directly after hair removal, but you should still check with a patch test—and be extra wary if your skin is sensitive.

2 The best time to apply your deodorant/anti-perspirant is at least thirty minutes after your bath. Tests prove that pores leading to the perspiration ducts close after bathing, so that the chemicals from the product cannot work thoroughly. Also, any dampness will dilute the product and decrease its efficiency: underarms should be quite dry (as well as clean!) before applying.

3 If you develop an allergy to your usual deodorant/anti-perspirant, change it. You can suddenly become allergic to a cosmetic product you have been happy with for a long time for no apparent reason.

4 If you have found a product that works for you, stay with it. There is no evidence to support the theory that deodorants/anti-perspirants lose their effectiveness with repeated use; if you have felt this to be true in the past, perhaps it was because you began to grow careless about application?

5 Make sure you are using the variety that is best for you. Roll-ons are no less effective than creams or lotions; the formulation, not the product presentation, is what is important.

If you have a perspiration problem, there are special deodorants/anti-perspirants that are heavy duty, and need only be applied every three days.

6 If you are allergic to *everything*, try Clinique's unperfumed allergy-tested anti-perspirant.

Oils and unguents
to make your body beautiful

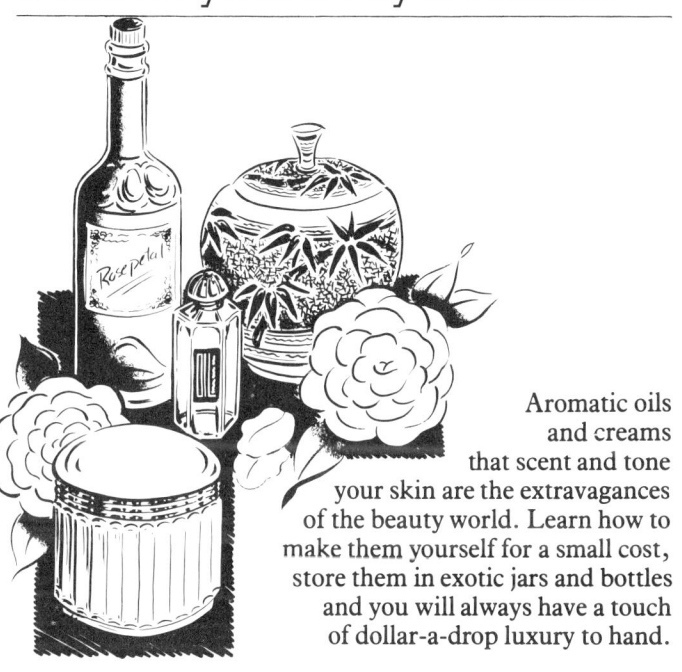

Aromatic oils and creams that scent and tone your skin are the extravagances of the beauty world. Learn how to make them yourself for a small cost, store them in exotic jars and bottles and you will always have a touch of dollar-a-drop luxury to hand.

AROMATIC OILS are excellent for home aromatherapy and massage sessions; in their more concentrated strength, you can use them as perfumes, or add a drop or two to your daily bath. You can use any herbs or flowers, fresh or dried, singly or in a bouquet of several. Those particularly recommended by Clare Maxwell-Hudson, the beauty therapist who devised these recipes, are: rosemary, lavender, rose petals, basil.
Steep 45 ml (3 tbsp) of chosen crushed herb or flower in 300 ml (½ pt) sunflower or corn oil; add 15 ml (1 tbsp) vodka or vinegar. Place in bottle, cork, and store in sunlight or a warm place such as the top of a storage heater or radiator: shake bottle daily. Leave for a week and strain; repeat process until desired strength is reached. For a really concentrated scent, you might have to repeat the process up to half a dozen times.

LEMON BODY TREATMENT CREAM This cream has a rich texture, a slightly greasy consistency and is readily absorbed, leaving rough patches on elbows, knees and hands smooth—and rich with the fragrance of lemons! Lanolin and almond oil nourish and lubricate skin; petroleum jelly protects hands, castor oil nourishes nails and lemon juice keeps the hands white.

15 ml (1 tbsp) lanolin
5 ml (1 tsp) castor oil
10 ml (2 tsp) almond oil
5 ml (1 tsp) Vaseline
5 ml (1 tsp) vegetable fat, eg, Trex
15 ml (1 tbsp) lemon juice
5 ml (1 tsp) glycerine
A few drops lemon verbena oil for fragrance (optional)

Melt all the oils together in a double boiler or over a water bath. When oils are melted, remove from heat and then slowly add lemon juice and glycerine, stirring all the time. Beat until mixture cools and thickens, using either a wooden spoon or lowest speed on kitchen mixer. A few drops of lemon verbena oil may be added to scent the cream.

LAVENDER BODY LOTION The ingredients will give you a cup of light, fluffy white cream, which is very easy to apply and leaves the skin with a lovely sheen. As it is non-greasy, it can be applied after the bath and immediately before dressing, and it will not leave sticky marks on clothes! You can buy or order ingredients from a good chemist.

Oil phase:
30 ml (2 tbsp) stearic acid
15 ml (1 tbsp) emulsifying wax
60 ml (4 tbsp) almond oil
Water phase:
Half a cup boiled water or heated mineral/distilled water
5 ml (1 tsp) glycerine
4 drops lavender oil

Melt the waxes and oil together in a bowl over a water bath and heat the water with the glycerine separately. Take the bowls off the heat and, stirring all the time, add the water to the oil. Beat the mixture either with a wooden spoon or with an electric beater on medium speed. Continue beating until the cream begins to thicken, then add the lavender oil. Beat the cream until it is cool.

Massage: Marvellous for mind as well as body

To be given a good body massage is both a pleasurable and therapeutic experience. Massage is one of the most ancient forms of natural healing; it stems from man's natural instinct to rub a part of the body that has been hurt. Depending on the massage movements used, and the strength with which they are applied, massage can soothe and relax, improve circulation of the blood and lymph drainage system — and not least, induce a feeling of well-being.

The most popular form of massage in this country is the European or Swedish massage. To be treated by a professional masseur or masseuse is obviously the ideal, but there are basic movements employed in this method of massage that you can learn to use on yourself (or a fortunate friend!) Accustom yourself to these movements first, then begin to adapt them. Arthur Mason, a masseur whose clients have included Marilyn Monroe, Aristotle Onassis and Liberace, believes: "The trademark of a good masseur is improvisation: massage is basically the art of developing the sense of touch. One should be able to sense with one's fingers the tenseness in certain muscles, and, with practice, the remedial movements come naturally."

Use massage every day. For instance, when you have a headache learn to massage the back of your neck and head instead of reaching for the aspirin; massage aching feet by rotating ankles, pulling and pressing each toe and pressing thumbs on soles of feet.

The basic professional massage movements

Massage movements can be divided, with the exception of finger kneading, into three categories: *effleurage*, gentle soothing movements; *petrissage*, pinching, wringing or rolling movements and *tapotement*, stimulating springy movements.

Effleurage Effleurage is used for applying oil at the start of a body massage, to soothe nerves and improve circulation. Flowing, stroking, smoothing movements with the flat of the hand.

Petrissage Stimulates circulation, helps relax contracted muscles, breaks down fatty tissues. Basic movements are:

1 Wringing: Pinching skin between thumbs and fingers, wringing in opposite directions, as one would a wet towel.

2 Rolling: Holding skin between thumbs and fingers using both hands, and slowly pinching so that skin "rolls" out from under thumbs.

Tapotement Performed correctly, these movements help break down fatty tissue, counteract cellulite formation and tone muscles. Basic movements are:

1 Hacking: A light, fast, chopping action, using sides of hands in alternating movements; it is essential to keep the fingers relaxed.

2 Clapping: Slapping gently with cupped hands.

3 Beating: Hitting gently with fists half closed.

4 Pounding: Pounding gently with sides of clenched fists.

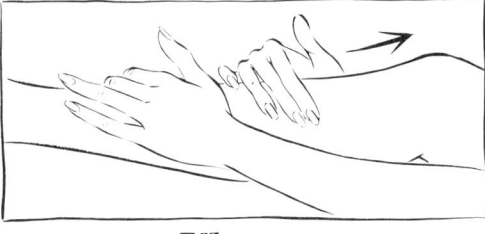

Effleurage

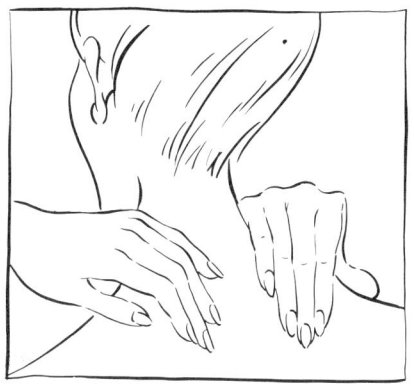

Finger kneading

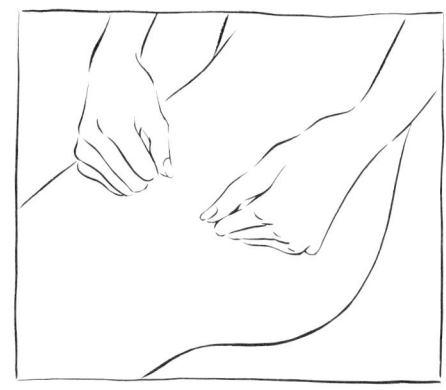

Beating and pounding

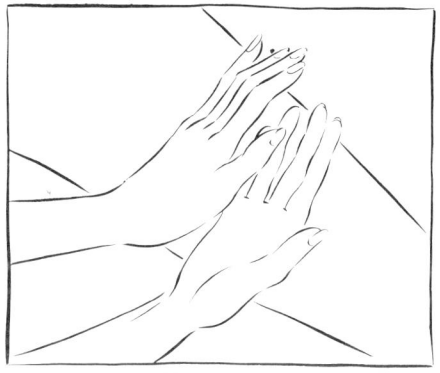

Hacking

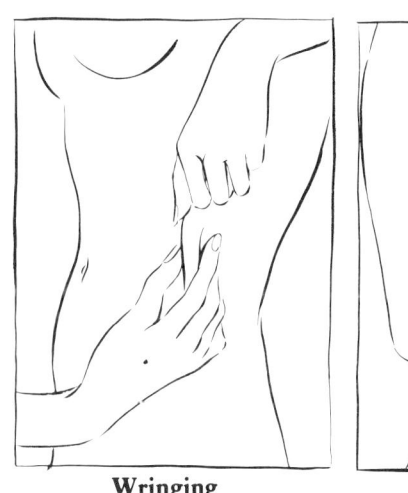

Wringing

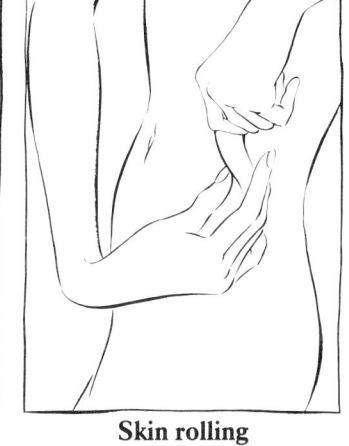

Skin rolling

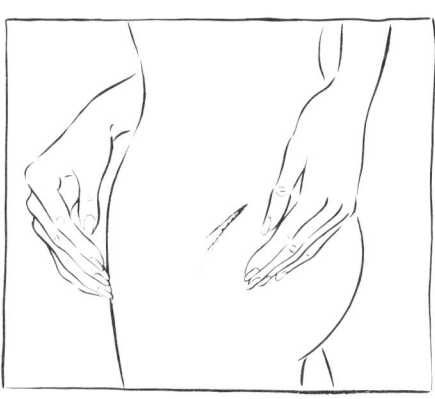

Clapping

How to give yourself a body massage

Your body should be warm and you should be feeling as relaxed as possible; after a bath is an ideal time to give yourself a leisurely massage. Aways use a body lotion or oil that will allow your hands to glide over your skin (and give you a moisturising treatment at the same time!). Vegetable oil with a drop or two of perfume added is fine. You could make your own aromatic massage oil (see page 105 for instructions) or buy an oil that is made specially for massage, such as Weleda's Silver Birch Oil, used in health farms and beauty salons. Birch leaves are renowned for relieving aching and tense muscles; other ingredients include camomile, an antiseptic, marigold, which has healing properties and lavender, which stimulates circulation. You can buy the oil from health-food stores or write to Weleda (UK) Ltd, Henor Rd, Ilkeston, Derbyshire, for details on direct mail order.

Teresa Leach, massage specialist at the Elizabeth Arden salon in London, suggests the following self-massage programme using the movements outlined above. Begin with your neck and shoulders, as these are the areas where tension gathers. Place a hand with palms down on each side of the neck. Then perform *finger kneading* movements at the back of your neck on both sides of your neckbone, working downwards from top to base of neck. Repeat until you feel relaxed. Another way to release tension is to apply strong *effleurage*, beginning at the nape and gliding down to your shoulders.

Now move down to your waist. Use the *wringing* movement on flab by starting at top of waist and working down to the hips, taking a strip of skin at a time and repeating until entire area is tingling. The *rolling* movement, applied afterwards, would be effective too.

To aid the digestive process, there is a special "colon movement" which may be performed on the stomach. It is a variation of effleurage, but traces the position of the colon in the abdomen. Start by stroking the right side of the stomach and then across the torso under the ribs.

To tone hips and thighs, use the hacking movement, starting on your right hip and moving slowly from the top of your hip down to the thigh; vary with *beating*, *pounding* and *clapping*. Repeat process for your left side.

Move to the feet: *finger kneading*, working your way from toes to ankles, will relax. Practise *effleurage* from ankle to knee to encourage flow of blood to heart; this last movement is particularly beneficial for those who suffer from swollen ankles or varicose veins.

How to give a friend a body massage
The advantage of giving a massage — or being given one — is that as the central nervous system is located in the back, many aches and pains can be eased through massage of the spine. It is important that the person to be massaged is warm and feels relaxed; any nervousness creates tension in the muscles and impedes relaxation. He or she should lie face down on the floor or on a firm mattress, feet slightly raised on pillows, arms bent and head lying on hands in a comfortable position. Below, Arthur Mason suggests a simple home massage for amateurs; with practice, you will be able to vary movements depending on whether a stimulating or simply relaxing massage is required.

1 Wring out hand towel in very hot water. Fan it over the body then press it gently on the back, massaging through the towel. This process should be repeated once.

2 To warm the oil, rub in hands.

3 Apply oil with effleurage: long sweeping movements in the direction of the heart.

4 From the bottom of the spine, "walk" the thumbs over each other from the base of the spine to the neck, and then down again. Repeat, this time with the fingers spread over the sides of the back.

5 Locate any pain spots: place left hand on top of pain spot and gently beat right fist over left hand.

6 Follow with petrissage and tapotement all over back and neck, concentrating on any areas where muscles seem knotted.

7 Finish with effleurage.

DO'S AND DONT'S OF HOME MASSAGE
- Never massage "naked" skin, ie, skin that has no covering of oil or lotion.
- Always massage in the direction of the heart.
- Never massage an inflamed area.
- Never massage anyone with a temperature.
- *Never* attempt any back or neck manipulation.

Shiatsu: The pressure point massage

This type of massage has been practised for centuries in the East. It is based on the principle that energy collects and stagnates in the body's known 365 pressure points, and that by applying pressure on these points with finger or thumb the life force, or T'Chi, can flow freely once more. A shiatsu massage can be painful but very beneficial, and is an excellent way of unknotting muscles, reducing tensions and banishing aches and pains in the head and back. Devotees include Margot Fonteyn, Martha Graham and Jackie Onassis. Shiatsu is becoming increasingly popular in this country, though it is difficult to find a good shiatsu practitioner.

The shiatsu philosophy is: If you have a pain, locate the area and rub it in order to heal the pain. Follow these basic shiatsu techniques devised by Yukiko Irwin, author and expert on shiatsu; they show you the pressure points to massage for improved eye and skin health, digestion, and relief from headaches:

Basic shiatsu techniques
Whether you use your thumb, middle finger, or two or three fingers together will depend on the spot being massaged. On small surface areas — around eyes, for instance — use only thumb or middle finger; on shoulders, back, buttocks you can use three fingers. You may not hit precisely the right pressure point the first time, so don't hesitate to poke around a bit (use a circular motion for probing). When you *do* locate the spot, you'll feel a tingly sensation. The greater the tension in that area, the more pronounced the tingling will be — and yes, it *can* be rather painful. (Good — it means you really *need* shiatsu!) You may use light, medium, or heavy pressure . . . again, the area being massaged will determine which. Press each spot indicated in the sketches for about three seconds . . . release pressure . . . repeat once or twice, or until you feel relief.

EYES Use ball of thumb or middle finger, apply medium pressure to points along eyebrow and at each temple. Use light pressure above eyesocket and below eyes. Heavier pressure — with two or three fingers — is needed for spots on top of head, base of skull, shoulders and back.

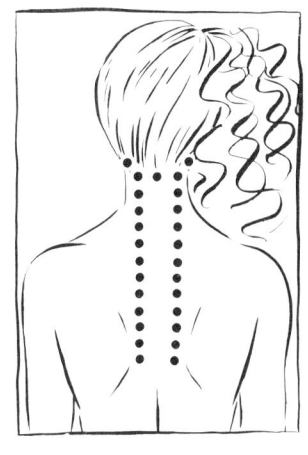

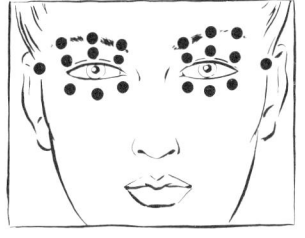

SKIN Massage all pressure points for eyes (above), plus the ones shown here.

Use heavy pressure on sides of neck, light pressure for two lines on front of throat, medium pressure under chin (right) and at base of throat. Massage abdomen (below left) down to the pubic bone; extend shoulder-blade area massage (below right) as far down the back as you can reach; heavy pressure on spots above buttocks will stimulate adrenal glands and kidneys, both beneficial to skin tone.

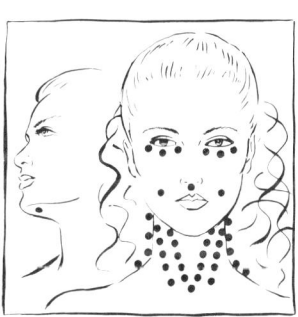

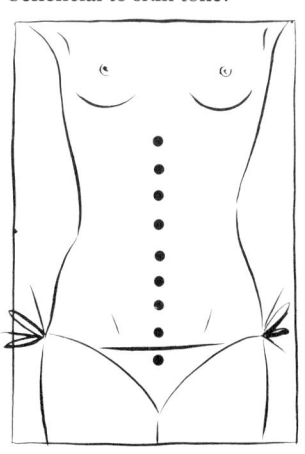

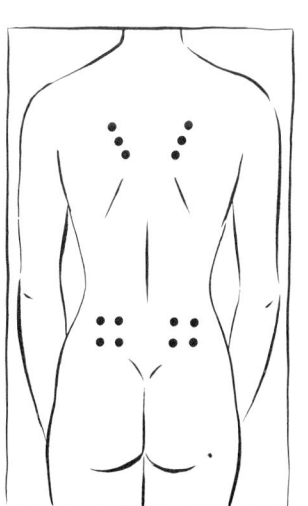

DIGESTION "Nervous" stomach due to tension can cause both diarrhoea and constipation. Stimulation of the abdominal area — especially the major artery running down the middle — can relieve and prevent it. First, massage all points in neck and back shown already in skin sketches; then use light-to-medium pressure on abdomen. Start massage directly under rib-cage, continue down to pubic bone (right).

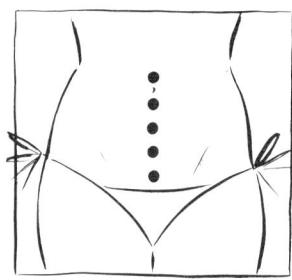

HOW TO GET RID OF A HEADACHE First, massage all pressure points shown above for eyes. Then work on top of head, starting at hairline and moving back to crown. Use heavy pressure here. Shiatsu spot at base of skull is very important; don't overlook! Extend shoulder massage as far down as you can reach . . . then work on ankles (yes, they really do affect the head!) Three vital shiatsu sites are located in a curve around anklebone on each side; press both sides at once, encircling Achilles tendon with your hand and using a pinching pressure. Repeat on other ankle. Keep this massage up until your headache starts to fade away.

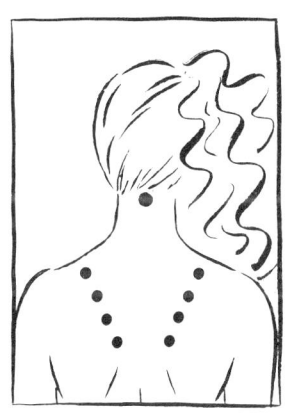

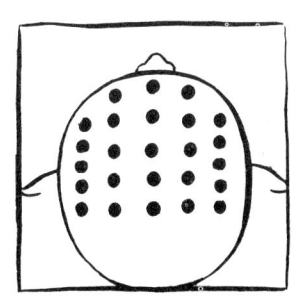

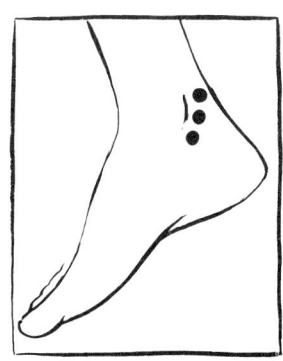

109

Aromatherapy: The essential oil treatment

Aromatherapy is the massage and inhalation of the essential oils of herbs, grasses, fruits and flowers. It is probably the most luxurious of all beauty treatments: a soothing, relaxing body massage performed with fragrant oils. Of over a hundred oils available, it is said that each has a different function: lavender is cleansing and antiseptic, rosemary is an astringent, sage a circulation stimulant; basil, an antibiotic; rose, neroli, marjoram, anti-depressants.

Essential oils are claimed to help break down cellulite deposits, lessen sinus problems and even improve acne. Instead of acting as carriers for massage movements, these lightweight oils are said to penetrate the body's organs to further well-being. Whether you believe this or not, aromatherapy is at least a highly sensual experience which benefits skin tissue and relaxes muscles and mind.

Daniele Ryman is the leading authority in the aromatherapy field in England and pupil of the late Margeurite Maury who pioneered the treatment in Europe. Daniele mixes her own essential oils and is amused by cynics who scoff at this "back to nature" treatment: "We go beyond the pure and natural movement — to chemistry! For example, Listerine is made from ingredients found in many plants: phenol, thymol." Daniele is realistic about the rejuvenating powers of aromatherapy. "I cannot make people of sixty look thirty, but if they have aromatherapy treatments at forty they should be able to look that age for some time."

The massage used is a combination of acupressure and European massage and is highly technical, but you can buy the essential oils from Daniele and use them for your own self-massage. Use them on the base of the back, neck and face; on the breasts, to firm them; and in circular movements on the stomach — particularly beneficial if you are pregnant and want to avoid stretch marks. For more details on Daniele's oils and treatments, send an sae to: Margeurite Maury Aromatherapy, Suite 101, Park Lane Hotel, Park Lane, London W1.

Breasts: They can be improved – here's how

Short of plastic surgery, there is no known beauty treatment that will drastically reduce a large bust, or increase a small bust. Adipose—fat—tissues surrounding the mammary glands determine the shape and size of your breasts, but there are methods by which you can *improve* the shape of your breasts, and make them firmer.

Exercises

Exercises work by strengthening the underlying muscles which support the breasts. You can perform these classic exercises sitting at your desk, watching TV, or any time:

● This exercise is recommended for expectant mothers to prevent sagging breasts after pregnancy, but you don't need to be pregnant to benefit. Grasp forearms with hands as though pushing up sleeves. Push, relax. See breasts lift as muscles tighten. Repeat five times. Move arms to eye level, repeat five times; move arms above head, repeat five times.

● Sit upright on a stool or edge of chair so you have enough room behind you for your elbows to swing back without hitting the chair back. Place palms of hands a few inches away from bosom, fingers touching and level with breastbone, elbows out at sides. With short, jerky movements, pull elbows back to try and meet behind your back.

Note For the best breast-improving exercise of all, take up swimming: it is marvellous for firming up supportive muscles of breasts and upper arms.

These exercises devised by expert Naja Cori of New York are designed not only to firm up breasts but to improve posture and thus show your breasts to advantage:

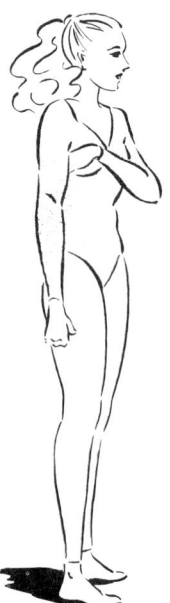

1 Before you exercise the pectoral muscles, you should know where this area is located and how it feels when it responds to exercise. Imagine you have a very heavy suitcase in you right hand. Place your left hand in the right armpit, pressing the heel of your hand against your breast. (That's the pectoral area.) Lift your right shoulder, then press down, imagining the weight of the suitcase. You should feel the tightening of the pectoral muscle. Now place your right hand in your left armpit and repeat.

2 To feel proper shoulder position, clasp your hands behind your back and keep them pressed against buttocks. Press your shoulders down and feel the pectoral muscles tensing. Without lifting your shoulders, bring the rounded part of each shoulder forward in front of your collarbone. Then push shoulders as far back as you can. In good posture the rounded part of the shoulder should extend behind the collarbone — never in front of it.

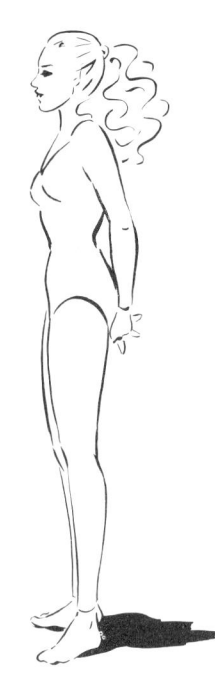

4 Lie on your back with your knees bent. The palms of your hands and soles of your feet should be flat on the floor. Lift up and arch your back. Rotate shoulders and arms so palms are face up. Lift your chest as high as possible. Your chin should meet your chest. Lower your body to the floor.

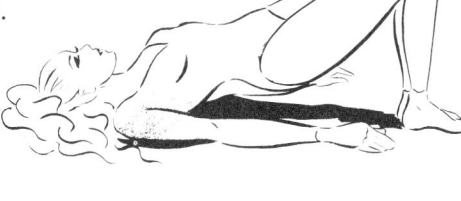

5 Sit cross-legged. Keep your back straight and clasp your knees with your hands. Arch your back and rotate your elbows inward. Then rotate elbows outward. Curve your spine, and bring your chin to your chest. Your shoulders should be back and down.

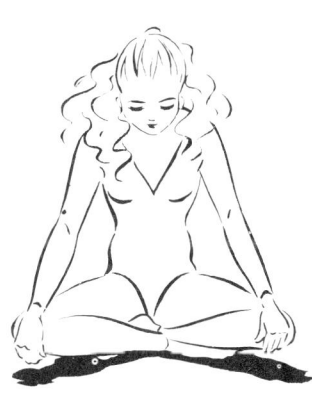

3 Lie on your stomach with your nipples just touching the floor. Place your hands apart and in front of shoulders. Straighten your arms and rotate elbows inward. Push your shoulders back and down — really exaggerate this movement. Then bend elbows outward as you return to original position. This exercise should feel like a stretch from the nipples all the way to the shoulders.

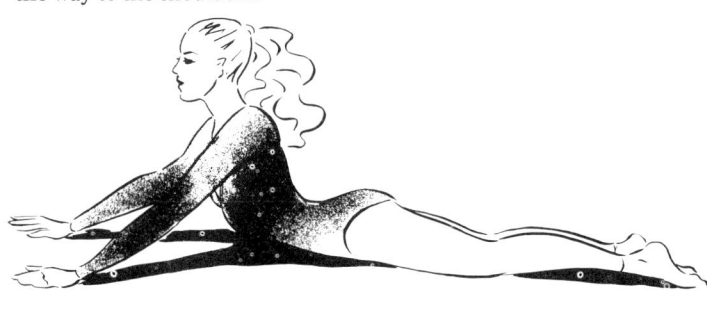

6 Proper breathing will help you maintain the good posture vital to a high, round bustline. Sit with legs crossed. Keep a vertical spine, shoulders back and down. You should feel a little curve under your shoulder blades — not your spine. Place your hands on your ribcage. Your ribs should expand as you inhale, contract as you exhale. Chest and shoulders should not move at all. Repeat exercise ten times.

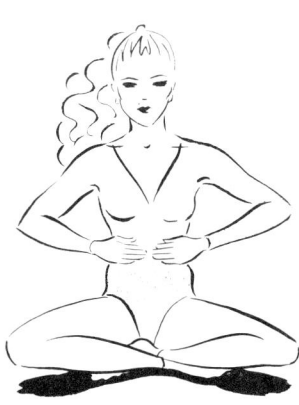

Hydrotherapy

Continuous water pressure applied to the breasts can show genuine improvement in the shape of the bosom. Icy cold water should be sprayed or splashed on to each breast for a couple of minutes every day; the temperature and pressure of the water both help to break down fatty deposits in the breast tissue and firm underlying chest muscles. Dedicated French-women even rub ice cubes on their breasts (though effectiveness of this cannot be guaranteed!). A strong shower jet is ideal for some hydrotherapy, otherwise patience is required to splash cold water on the breasts for a full two minutes.

Massage

Massaging the breasts helps increase circulation and thus hopefully improve breast size. Used with a specialised breast treatment cream or oil, massage can show effective results in a short space of time. Always use circular movements in gentle, sweeping but firm strokes. Daniele Ryman, aromatherapy expert (see page 110) claims that daily massaging of breasts with certain essential oils can develop mammary glands and thus enlarge breasts. Clarins' bust treatment range of milks and oils, based on plant extracts which are claimed to firm, tone, develop or reduce the bust, contain no hormones and are widely used in beauty salons and health farms. For more details, send an sae to Clarins, 85 Pennine Drive, London NW2.

Why wear a bra?

There are few women whose bust- line cannot be improved by the wearing of a good bra. It should be unconstricting yet supportive and leave no marks on shoulders or breasts. Perhaps if you have small upright breasts you feel you do not need a bra, but unless you are *constantly* exercising pectoral muscles, breasts will sag to some degree. Says Lotte Berk, exercise and body expert: "Age has nothing to do with it: the muscles need help to support the breasts." Bright idea from the bra manufacturers are exercise bras, especially designed to be worn for jogging and other strenuous activities. They offer extra support for the bosom yet are light and unconstricting.

Factors that can affect your breasts

● Bad posture: Rounded back and hollowed chest do not improve the bustline! Stand sideways on to a full-length mirror and check your back is straight, your shoulders back. If you have been standing incorrectly, you will notice an enormous difference.

● Hormonal changes within the body: Most evident of these is the pill; many women report breast growth when taking the pill, and in some cases the increase remains when they are taken off the pill.

● Steam cabinet sessions, saunas: These can make breasts sag a little; to prevent this, soak a towel in cold water and wrap it around the bosom in sauna or steam sessions.

● Frequent hot baths: These can make breasts sag.

● One pregnancy closely followed by another, breast feeding: Both these can have a detrimental effect on the breasts. Pre and post-natal exercises help avoid this as does the wearing of a good bra.

● Drastic weight loss: Sudden weight loss after illness or intensive dieting can result in breasts sagging, as can a diet high in carbohydrates and low in protein.

Developers—or disasters?

Over the years there have been many different aids for bust improvement on the market; most have been proved to be ineffective and some, dangerous. One gadget consisting of plastic tubes containing a spring compressed between two plungers is supposed to enlarge the breasts; the Federal Drugs Association in the USA has proved this to be untrue. The original bust developer involved placing a cup, attached to a rubber bulb, over each breast and pumping to create a vacuum, which caused a temporary swelling of the breast; unfortunately these devices are still on the market and are medically unsafe.

One form of bust apparatus which is to be recommended, however, is based on hydrotherapy and massages each breast with high pressure water; it can be used to firm the bust, develop or reduce and has had promising results. A good and cheap version of this is the Aqua-Maid, available from the Aqua-Maid Company, 227 Putney Bridge Rd, London SW15; write to them enclosing an sae for further details.

Liquid injections of silicone to enlarge breasts are dangerous, have caused suffering and in some cases, even death. The *safe* method of introducing silicone into breasts for augmentation is in plastic sacs.

Cosmetic surgery

This should only be considered as a final resort, and then only in extreme cases. Though many women are happy with the results of their breast reductions or augmentations, it should be pointed out that the success rate is not 100 percent, and once done, the operation cannot be reversed. Augmentation involves the insertion of sacs of silicone into the breast; reduction involves making an incision into the breast and re-siting the nipple. For more details on cosmetic breast surgery, please turn to page 174.

Instant improvement ideas for breasts

● Try the cover girls' tape trick for a stunning cleavage: Cut several lengths of Sellotape; with one hand, hold breast in desired position; with other hand, attach lengths to skin just below breast until you feel the breast has adequate support.

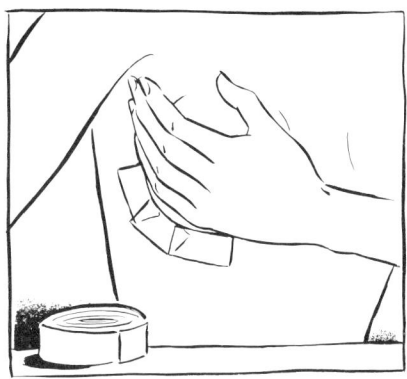

This is particularly good for plunge-front dresses as the tape is needed only around the *outer* curves of the breast, to push them together.

- Even out skin blotches and cover imperfections when you wear a low-necked dress by smoothing face foundation over exposed skin; always use a damp sponge to apply for a light, natural look.

- You can improve on a cleavage, or create one, with the subtle use of your blusher. Use a tawny or rose-wine shade and brush lightly between breasts, increasing colour gradually until a realistic effect is achieved.

- Emphasise a pretty cleavage with a dusting of translucent powder in a frosted or metallic finish, or dip your blusher brush in gold shadow; apply sparingly to highlight on curves of breasts.

Shape up your legs

If you have recently taken up swimming, bicycling, exercise classes or even disco dancing you may have noticed an appreciable difference in the shape of your legs. It is encouraging to know that exercise *can* improve the look of your legs. Below, you will discover specialised leg exercises, plus advice and tips on the many different ways you can make the best of your legs. Incidentally, there's no need to worry you'll end up with bulging calves: you'd have to exercise as much as an Olympic athlete for that to happen!

Exercise: How to give your legs curves in all the right places

Follow these quick, simple and effective exercises to improve shape and tone of legs; with daily perseverance you will see encouraging results.

Curvier calves

- A hundred *relevés* a day — up and down on your toes continuously – will firm and shape calves.

- With balls of feet on a telephone directory, heels extending

over edge, rise up and down as many times as you can manage.

- On tips of toes, walk up one stair and then step back again, walk up, step back, repeat for a couple of minutes.

Thinner thighs

- Draw knee up while standing and slowly unfold leg in front of body, right to tips of toes. Feel muscle tighten in thigh. Repeat four times each side.

Slimmer ankles

- Although thick ankles can never become slim, this classic exercise, which you can do any time, will help: Sit down and cross legs. Point toe of top leg and describe ten slow clockwise circles in the air; do the same counterclockwise ten times. Repeat. Change legs and rotate other ankle.

Note The more you exercise, the more developed leg muscles become; if you have heavy legs, avoid excessive exercise, especially bicycling, a super calf-developer! Heavily-muscled legs cannot be made less so, although massage will help smooth out bunched-up muscles.

Six super slimming leg exercises

The problem flab area on legs is from knee to thigh; here are half a dozen spot reducing exercises that are designed to whittle down pudgy outer thighs and firm up inner thighs:

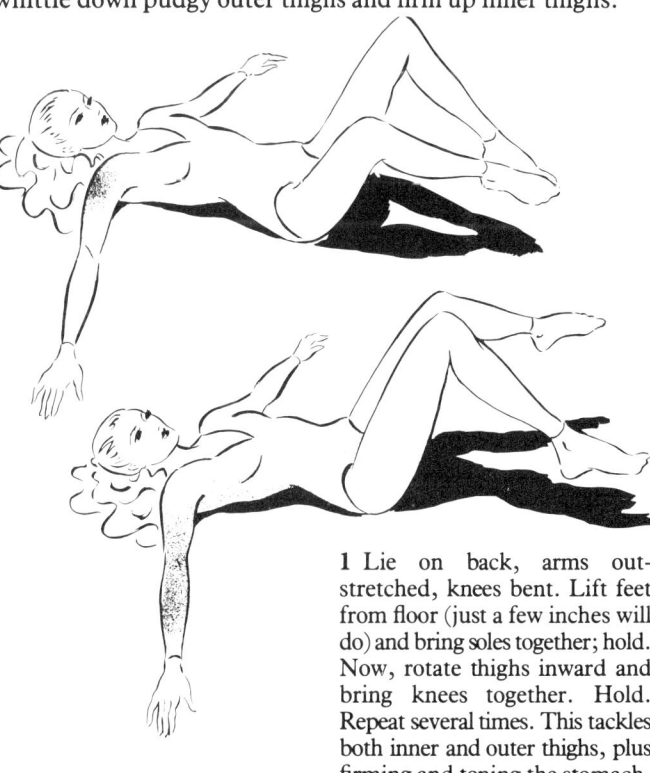

1 Lie on back, arms outstretched, knees bent. Lift feet from floor (just a few inches will do) and bring soles together; hold. Now, rotate thighs inward and bring knees together. Hold. Repeat several times. This tackles both inner and outer thighs, plus firming and toning the stomach.

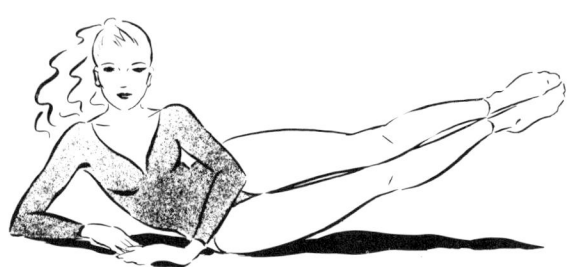

2 Side leg lift is especially beneficial for inner thighs. Lie on side. Support weight on elbow; keep legs straight, top one resting on lower one. Tighten buttocks; slowly lift and lower legs ten times. Do the same on other side.

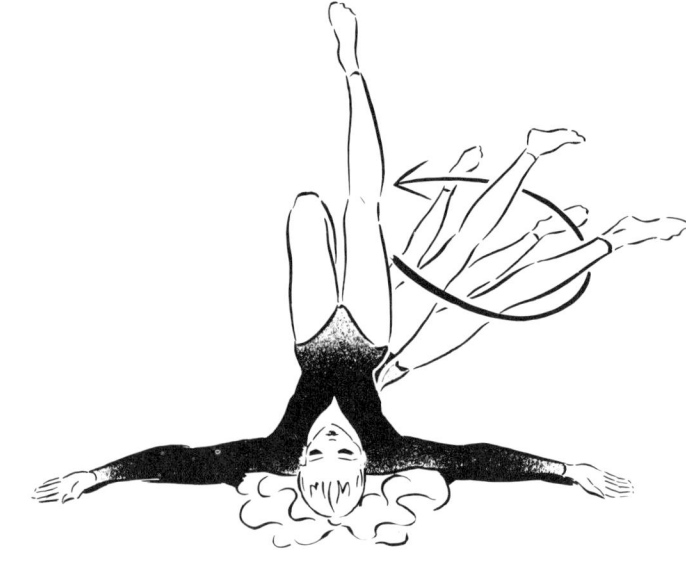

4 Leg circles benefit the entire thigh as well as hips. Lie on back, arms out, one knee bent. Lift other leg — knee straight — and make a sweeping circle with it. The wider the circle the better, but do not touch the floor. Do ten circles, then reverse direction. Repeat with other leg.

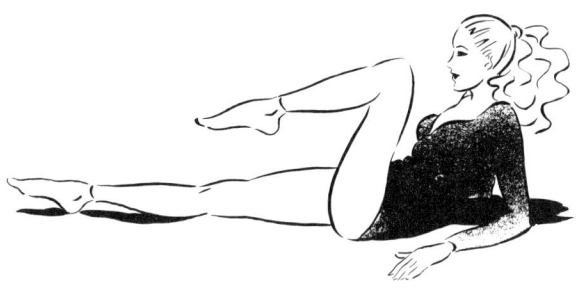

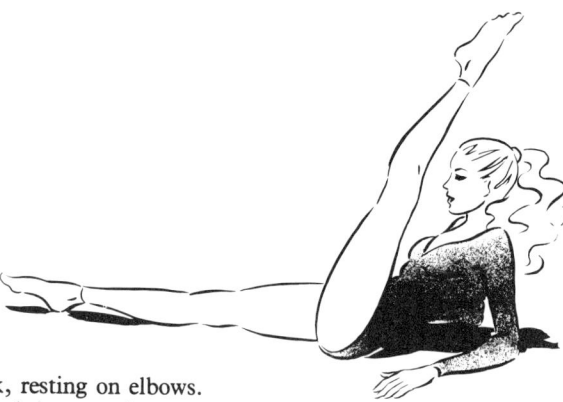

3 Lie back, resting on elbows. Point toes; bring one knee as close to your nose as you can, keeping other leg on floor. Now straighten leg, trying to keep it close to face. Repeat eight times with each leg. This strong stretch firms backs of thighs.

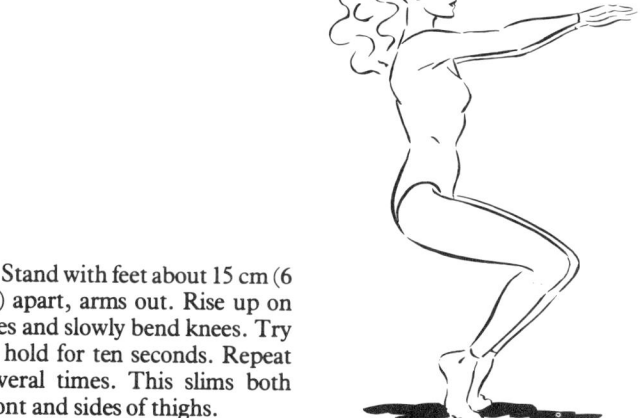

5 Stand with feet about 15 cm (6 in) apart, arms out. Rise up on toes and slowly bend knees. Try to hold for ten seconds. Repeat several times. This slims both front and sides of thighs.

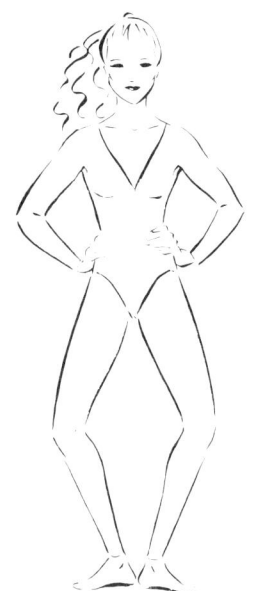

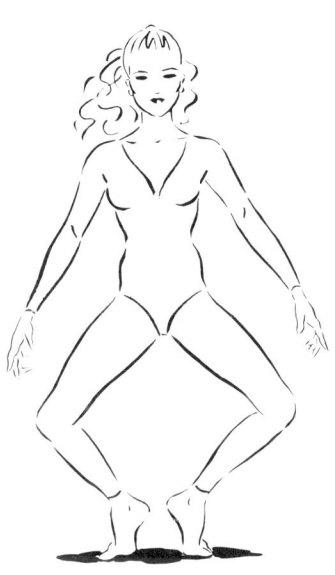

6 Simple ballet *pliés* work wonders on fat thighs. Place feet with heels together at a forty-five degree angle; bend knees, keeping feet flat on floor. Lift heels and go into a *deep* knee bend, hold. Lower heels; straighten legs again.

Ten tips for silky, sensuous legs

1 Use moisturising lotion or hand cream after every bath, applying when skin is still damp; stroke on in sweeping movements from ankle to knee, from knee to mid-thigh.

2 If you have rough, bumpy knees, try The Golden Door improvement programme, p 97, or a softening paraffin wax treatment, p 96.

3 Keep legs hair-free with daily shaving or weekly use of a cream depilatory; hair growth above knees is usually light enough to be left alone, bleached, or "sanded away" with an abrasive glove.

4 Use a pumice or loofah on obstinate "chicken skin" on thighs; for more intensive treatment, try Marina Andrews' bath-soak programme, p 96.

5 White legs seldom look attractive and brown legs always look slimmer: when the weather warms up use an overnight tanning cream. Apply with a damp sponge and dilute slightly around ankles, backs and fronts of knees to avoid a patchy effect.

6 Show legs to advantage when you sit down; the slimmest thighs spread and look unsightly when pressed on to a chair! Keep weight on buttocks, cross legs lightly high on thigh and align shins so they are parallel and vertical.

7 Make the most of your leg length by adjusting your step to suit your height: if you are tall, take large, confident strides; if you have fairly short legs, strides should be smaller.

8 Legs look best when you walk *properly*. Whether you are wearing high heels or jogging shoes, keep feet parallel and toes pointed forward. Heels should touch ground a second before ball of foot.

9 Unless you are trying to camouflage marks on legs, wear the sheerest tights or stockings, look for ten or fifteen denier, but handle carefully. Choose them with a slight sparkle or sheen for ultimate flattery to legs.

10 When legs are bare, you can improve their look with your face contour and highlighter cream or powder: sweep highlighter up shinbone, or ankle bone; fine down heavy ankles and calves with strategic use of contour make-up.

Lumps, bumps and veins: How to treat them

● Cellulite bulges and dimples are difficult to banish; they benefit from a five-point improvement programme of high-pressure water therapy (swimming can be helpful, especially in sea water), a healthy low-carbohydrate diet, increased water intake, daily massage and exercise. You could also try slimming creams that contain plant and herbal extracts, for example ivy, seaweed and horse-chestnut, which are reputed to have reducing and firming properties. Although they do not work miracles overnight, continuous daily application with firm massage movements will produce an improvement in the condition. Both Clarins and Biotherm make good slenderising creams.

● Five million women in this country suffer from varicose veins; unfortunately the causes are generally hereditary. Varicose veins are aggravated by overweight, which puts extra pressure on them, or restricting tights or hosiery of any kind. Ankle-strap shoes should be avoided, too. Sufferers should rest legs whenever possible and avoid standing for long periods (though walking is fine). Elastic or support hose used to compress and conceal veins can be helpful. In severe cases medical treatment may be necessary, and involves either a series of injections, or surgery.

● Broken surface capillaries which take the form of spidery purplish veins can be treated by sclerotherapy, the injecting of a chemical into the veins to dry up the blood. In milder cases, camouflage make-up may be enough to disguise the condition. Some doctors believe that increased intake of vitamin C may help by strengthening the capillary walls and thus prevent further rupturing.

Treats for feet

No part of your body *deserves* more tender loving care than your feet. We squeeze them into shoes that are the wrong shape, stand on them for hours at a time and generally give them a very rough deal. Read how you can lavish a little luxury on your much-maligned feet — and help prevent any troublesome foot problems at the same time.

Foot therapies

● Give your feet a reviving massage after you have been standing or walking for any length of time. Using thumb or finger, press firmly over entire sole of foot. Spend two or three minutes on each foot. According to the ancient theory of foot reflexology, nerve endings in the soles of the feet control all the body's vital organs, so that massaging soles *might* tone up the rest of your body!

● Give your soles a massage that is more therapeutic than relaxing: fill a pair of flat walking shoes with dried peas or round beans. Walk in the bean-filled shoes for as long as you can bear: the beans will massage every inch of your soles.

● Toes benefit from a work-out, too: on the beach, try picking up pebbles or tiny seashells with your toes.

● Keep a stock of products especially for feet. Foot powder, anti-perspirant spray and foot refresher spray are all designed to keep feet cool and healthy. A plant mist spray filled with chilled water and a little cologne makes a good substitute for foot refresher spray.

● The best exercise for your feet is to walk barefoot in the sand or on a good springy lawn; every muscle and ligament is toned. Walk around the house barefoot whenever you can. The time to keep your shoes *on* is on the dance class or disco floor, ground or pavement: these hard surfaces are dangerous, and skin will quickly toughen.

Foot problems: Causes and cures

● Corns are a build-up of hard dead skin that appear on toe joints and on soles of feet. They are a result of ill-fitting shoes: pointed toes are often to blame. Corns should be removed professionally by a qualified chiropodist.

● Bunions are a thickening of the skin at the head of a metatarsal bone; they form a painful, obtrusive lump at the side of the foot. The causes are too-tight shoes, tight stockings and pointed toes on shoes. They should be treated by a specialist; do not hope they will go away — they won't!

● Callouses are areas of hard, flattened skin, caused by badly fitting shoes and walking barefoot on hard ground. If they are not too severe they can be treated at home with gradual abrasion, otherwise a chiropodist should treat them.

● Veruccas are a viral infection. They manifest themselves in the shape of inward-growing warts. They must be removed professionally with the use of acid pastes or liquids, freezing or, as a last resort, surgery.

● Athlete's foot is a highly contagious fungal infection which thrives on damp warm areas of the skin, especially between toes. The skin scales and splits and is accompanied by an itchy rash. You can buy a good home treatment, such as Mycil.

● Ingrowing toenails are caused by cutting the nail down at the sides, instead of straight across. The nail grows into the flesh and is very painful. This condition should be treated professionally as soon as possible as it can be difficult to remedy if left too late. Do not be tempted to ease or cut the nail free yourself.

Note For the address of your nearest State Registered Chiropodist, write to The Society of Chiropodists, 8 Wimpole St, London W1M 8BX. They will also send foot health leaflets on request.

Feet pick-ups and perk-ups

● Tired feet will benefit from a whirlpool foot bath. Make your own by sitting on the edge of the bath with feet under taps on at full pressure; start with warm water, increase to hot then gradually turn to cold.

● Hot, swollen feet and ankles can be soothed and depuffed by rubbing an ice-cube over them.

● Try an old-fashioned foot bath to relieve aches and pains: throw a handful of baking soda into a bowl of hot water, or add a few drops of reviving, fragrant lavender oil to the water instead. For extra self-indulgence, follow with a spirit rub and massage.

● Use a tingling mint gel mask on tired, puffy feet; a honey and egg mask on dry feet.

● Give your feet a friction rub to tone and refresh them, with your favourite light cologne.

● Relieve tired feet by lying with feet higher than head for ten minutes; this mini-treatment is ideal before you go out for the evening.

● Soften feet with a hot-oil treatment: massage hot sesame or sweet almond oil into feet; remove excess with non-alcohol-based toner.

- Feet need frequent abrasion to prevent formation of tough, horny skin and callouses: use pumice stone, loofah daily in bath and give feet a once-weekly sloughing treatment with vegetable oil and coarse sea salt. Rub well in before entering the bath.
- Try the super-softening paraffin wax treatment outlined on page 96.

The perfect pedicure

You'll need: moisturising cream or lotion, nail clippers, an orange stick, emery board, cotton wool, tissues, a pumice stone or abrasive paste, nail enamel remover, nail enamel, basecoat and sealer, towel. After every use, clean dead skin from instruments and dip wood and metal into antiseptic lotion, before storing in a bag. If you cut yourself, apply a little hydrogen peroxide to the area.

1 Remove old nail enamel. Cut toenails straight across with clipper; rounded shape encourages ingrown toenails. Never allow free edge of nail to extend beyond tip of toe. Gently file smooth any rough edges with an emery board.

2 Soak feet in a basin of warm soapy water (or sit at the edge of the bath) to which you have added a handful of softening Epsom salts.

3 Use a pumice stone or abrasive paste to fine down thickened skin areas or callouses.

4 Rinse and dry feet; massage in moisturising lotion or cream.

5 Wind a wisp of cotton wool around an orange stick and dampen; use to work around cuticles to clean nails.

6 Before painting nails, twist a tissue into a narrow strip and weave in and out of toes to prevent enamel smudging. Apply base coat. Apply two coats of nail enamel, allowing coats to dry between applications, and follow with sealer. Keep feet free from tights or shoes for a minimum of one hour, as stockings and shoes leave imprints on enamel if replaced too quickly.

Six tips for fabulous feet

1 After every bath, use fine side of emery board on feet to smooth away any rough spots that could snag tights. Follow with moisturising lotion and a light dusting of talc.

2 Never buy shoes that feel too tight or generally uncomfortable. It is a fallacy that you will "break them in". The best time to buy shoes is late afternoon when feet are at their largest; if your feet are inclined to swell in summer, try sandals on when feet are swollen, or buy half a size larger.

3 To avoid foot trouble, buy shoes that provide good support under the instep and heel, and with enough room for the feet to spread inside the shoes.

4 High heels may look smart but throw the body's alignment off-balance; wear them as little as possible!

5 Never wear the same pair of shoes two days in succession.

6 Dry your feet well after bathing, particularly between the toes; damp feet provide the perfect environment for foot infections.

How to have show-off hands and nails

There is much more to lovely hands and nails than the occasional dollop of hand cream and the right shade of nail enamel. Here, from experts, models and cosmetic houses, we have gleaned tips and tricks that will make you look as if you have a manicurist permanently on call!

Nail-care kit

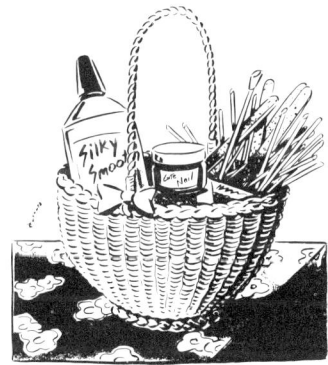

Keep the following basics stored in a pretty basket by your bedside — and *use* them:
  Orange sticks
  Cotton buds
  Cuticle cream
  Hand cream
  Wooden emery boards (metal files are too harsh)
  Hoof stick (wooden stick with rubber pad at end for pushing down cuticles)

Top nail tips

- Keep nails fashionably short; they are easier to look after and you will have fewer breakage problems, especially if you type.
- The most common cause of soft, breaking nails is exposure to detergents and household cleansers: wear rubber gloves when washing.

- Preserve nails by using a pencil to make 'phone calls, using knuckles whenever possible to press lift buttons, etc, and never use nails to prise open compacts or untie string.
- Check the habit of peeling off old enamel; you will also peel off protective layer of nail and weaken it. Use proper enamel remover *always*.
- Nail enamel acts as a protector against scuffs to nails but constant application, especially without basecoat, may, in time, cause yellowing of nails. Once in a while, leave nails free of enamel.

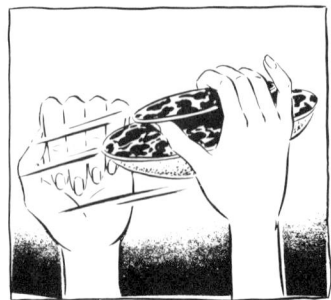

- Healthy nails look best buffed to a high shine: a chamois leather buffer will stimulate circulation and strengthen nails.
- Apple cider vinegar, applied straight to nails, is said to strengthen them: a treatment worth trying if your nails are soft and pliable.
- Nails and cuticles, where the new nail grows, benefit from a hot oil soak. Heat almond, castor, wheatgerm or baby oil in Pyrex container and soak nails for ten minutes.
- Use a cuticle cream nightly to "feed" growing nail bed; Vaseline is fine, or you could decant any of the above oils into a dropper bottle. Massage in well to stimulate growth.
- Although cuticle scissors can be bought at chemists, they are best left for professional use only. It is easy to nip skin when using them, and thus provoke an infection. You should not need cuticle scissors if you regularly push back cuticles with a towel after every hand-wash and give your nails regular cream or oil massage treatments, pushing back afterwards with hoof stick.
- Smoking discolours fingers and nails. The best remedy is, of course, to stop smoking, but stains can be bleached by applying freshly squeezed lemon juice with a brush to nails.
- Avoid "mini" size emery boards; they may be more convenient to carry around with you but you need the length of a longer board for extra manoeuvrability. Wooden boards are more pliable than metal, and less likely to "shred" nail.
- Cut nails with special nail scissors only when they are soft, ie after a warm bath, or oil soak. Scissors should be kept very sharp for a clean edge to nails.

- Use a nail whitener pencil for a pretty effect on natural nails: pencil on under free edge of nail in back and forth strokes.
- Don't be tempted to use straight acetone on nails because it is cheaper than nail enamel remover; it will dry and split nails. Removers have special oils added to the formulation to prevent adverse effects on nails.
- Shape nails by filing into smooth, rounded ovals but leave growth up side so nails don't ingrow and cause infection. File one way only, from sides to centre; back and forth "sawing" shreds nail fibres. Always use the *fine* side of an emery board.
- Typing, playing the piano, knitting — and becoming pregnant — all help boost nail growth! Frequent shaking out of hands increases circulation to fingertips to stimulate growth of nails.
- Use remover dabbed on *surgical* cotton wool; it is the smoothest type of cotton wool and works quickest at removing nail enamel. Tissues are less economical.

How to have lovely hands

- Detergents, soaps and household cleansers all have adverse drying effects on the skin. Wear rubber gloves for all housework; for a conditioning benefit while you work, massage in a little hand cream and wear fine cotton gloves *under* your rubber gloves.
- Keep a tube or pot of hand cream by your kitchen sink, washbasin and in your office drawer. Use after *every* time you wash your hands.
- To bleach and soften hands, rub a cut lemon half over skin. (To be economical, use a squeezed lemon!)

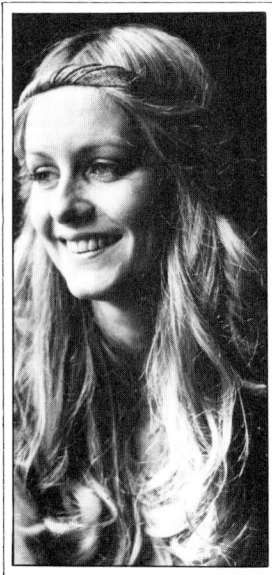

TWIGGY, *actress and model: "I learnt this very useful nail-mending trick in Los Angeles. Use coffee filter papers, which have a smooth, round curve, to fake nail edges. Tear off a piece of the paper a little bigger than the broken nail, paint nail with nail mender glue and stick on the paper so the curve protrudes above nail. Paint back of new 'nail' with clear nail varnish and push the sides down neatly with an orange stick. The 'nail' dries like papier mâché, and can be painted. If you bang your 'nail' it's not affected at all. As the 'nail' grows out, change paper every three weeks."*

- For a special softening treat, mash ripe banana with olive oil; smooth on and massage in well. Rinse off with lukewarm water and follow with hand lotion.
- The massaging action of applying hand cream is as beneficial to the hands as the cream itself; the vigorous action stimulates circulation and encourages healthy skin. The right way to massage in hand cream: Warm hands first by shaking them to increase blood flow. Massage cream in palm to palm, then rub into backs of hands. Imagine you are putting on a pair of gloves, and work down each finger slowly, rubbing well around joints and in between fingers. Massage with downward movements from fingers to wrists.
- Blue-toned hands are due to poor circulation. Keep hands warm in cold weather with gloves; massage frequently.
- Quick relief from red, raw hands advocated by The Golden Door spa: mix the juice of one orange with one spoonful of honey and apply to hands.
- Your favourite moisturising mask can be used on your hands, too; or try a softening, nourishing paraffin wax treatment, p 96.
- Dermatitis on hands indicates an allergy or sensitivity and should be treated by your doctor.

Nail problems: Causes and cures

- Alleviate nail problems due to poor health by eating the right foods. Follow a diet rich in protein. Additional diet helpers for split, breaking nails: calcium tablets (or lots of milk), a tablespoon of powdered gelatine daily, brewer's yeast tablets.
- White patches on nails are caused by previous injury to the growing nail bed; they will grow out in time.
- Cracks on edge of free nail result from filing nails too far down sides, which weakens them. Patch nail with a commercial nail mender to seal split until it grows out.
- If you catch a nail in a door or drawer, a black spot of blood will appear under nail. Apply cold compresses and keep hand elevated for a short while.
- Hangnails are caused by cutting away cuticles. Instead, release cuticles from nails by pushing them back with towel every time you dry them, and regularly apply cuticle cream and push back cuticles with hoof stick. Hangnails should be carefully and neatly cut.
- Nylon and acrylic in nail protectors makes nails more resilient to cracks and breaks, but does not change nail structure. Use as a preventive measure, especially if your nails are weak and soft.
- Splitting, brittle nails indicate dryness due to overuse of nail enamel, remover or soap, etc. Correct damage by feeding the matrix — root of nail — with oil or cream massages.

- Horizontal ridges in nails are due to uneven growth rate. This can be caused by injury to nail at nail base, while it was growing, or illness one month earlier. Leave to grow out and prevent further ridges by treating cuticles gently.
- If you bite your nails, shame yourself into stopping: paint them bright red to bring attention to them! Have a professional manicure once a month to encourage you, use an emery board to smooth tempting rough edges, and paint white iodine on nails twice daily to harden them, and make biting less rewarding.

Putting on the polish

The best-manicured hands can be spoilt by badly-applied nail enamel. Follow these points for best results:

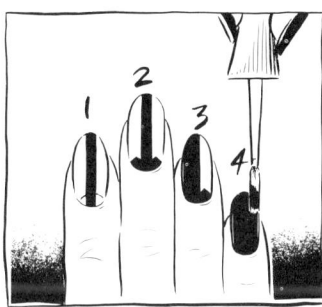

- Apply colour to nail in four swift strokes: from root to tip along nail centre, around nail bed in one smooth arc, from root to tip on either side of centre strip.
- After application, work lightly round tip of each nail with thumb of other hand to remove bulk of enamel; this "freeing" of nail edge prevents chipping.
- Remove any traces of enamel on surrounding skin with cotton bud dipped in nail enamel remover.
- Always use a topcoat for longer-lasting colour, protection and high shine.
- The final coat *after* topcoat for impatient fingers is a quick-dry spray or gloss, which makes immediate touch-work possible.
- Apply nail enamel, ideally, before bedtime so that nail enamel can dry hard overnight.
- Never apply nail enamel near a fan heater, or in a draught as "bubbling" of enamel may result.
- For the illusion of longer, slimmer nails, leave a slight space at either side of nail when painting.
- Pale, creamy colours and deep harsh reds are difficult to wear unless nails are perfectly shaped. The most flattering enamel shades are the mid-tones of corals and pinks.
- Thin old, thickening nail enamel with a drop or two of remover; add drops until correct consistency is reached.

- Leaving half-moons exposed looks stylish but is tricky. Only the steady-handed should attempt this: the first brush stroke should be taken from one side of the moon edge to the other.
- Mix nail colour with clear varnish for a coloured gloss that looks pretty with a tan.

The professional manicure

Follow Revlon's expert manicure, taught to professional manicurists. You will need to set aside one hour, but as you become more expert, you will be able to do the operation in less time. Try and fit in a manicure once weekly.

1 Dissolve old nail enamel with remover on cotton wool: hold on each nail for a few seconds then wipe nail clean.
2 Use the fine side of an emery board to shape nails into an attractive oval shape. File from side to centre in one direction, being careful not to file too low at the corners of the nails; this prevents nail breakages and gives an illusion of extra length.

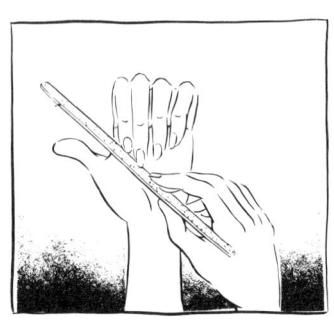

3 Massage cuticle cream or oil around each cuticle.
4 Immerse fingers in a bowl of warm, soapy water to soften cuticles; leave for three to five minutes.
5 Dry hands with towel.

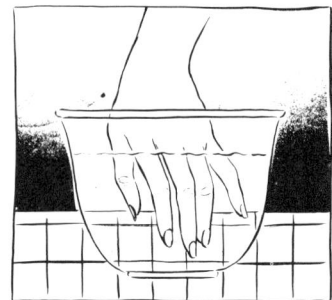

6 Gently push back cuticles in circular movements with an orange stick, covering up with wisp of cotton wool, or use a cotton bud.
7 Wipe away any residue of cuticle massage cream with cotton wool and warm water.
8 Apply cuticle remover around cuticle wall and under free edge of nails: Revlon's cuticle remover helps to bleach stains.

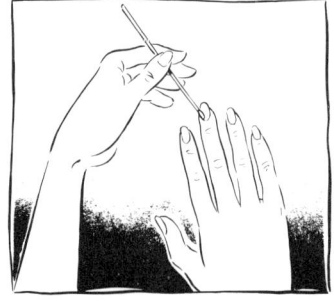

9 Gently work with circular movements around cuticles to remove tissue, using cuticle stick protected with a wisp of cotton wool.
10 Massage nourishing cream into hands with firm movements from fingers to wrist, one finger at a time.
11 Wash away traces of cuticle remover with warm soapy water; dry hands.

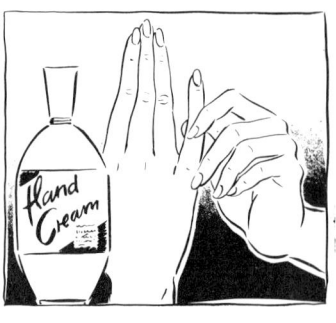

12 Bevel rough edges by gently flicking nail with fine side of file. with smooth side of file.
13 Wash nails with soapy water and nail brush to eliminate traces of oil or cream so that base coat adheres; dry nails.
14 Apply base coat. Always start on little finger to avoid smudging.
15 Apply two to three coats of enamel. Leave space at bottom of nail so as not to "flood" cuticle.
16 Apply top "sealer" coat.

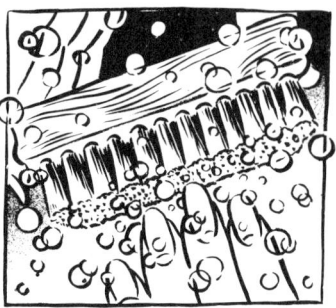

Nails: True or false?

Fake nails can be marvellous for nail-biters, and for covering bad splits or breakages, but should only ever be considered as a temporary measure — and should only be used on healthy nails. The following kinds of fake nails are currently available:
STICK-ON FALSE NAILS are made of flame-retardant cellulose acetate. They can be applied at home with special fixative and can look very natural if the right size is chosen.
BRUSH-ON ACRYLIC NAILS are a comparatively new treatment first introduced in the USA. Though home kits are available they should always be applied by an expert in a beauty salon as the process is a tricky one. The nail surface is first roughened so that the false nail can adhere, and foil or paper horseshoe-shaped moulds are placed under free edge of nail. The acrylic chemical is painted on the nail, allowed to harden and the mould removed. The nail can then be styled to any shape or length, and painted. The false nail binds easily to the natural nail and looks very effective. This type of false nail has to grow out naturally with your own nail, and cannot be removed.
NAIL EXTENSIONS are made of plastic and are bonded to your nails with a special nail glue. They grow out naturally and can be filed.

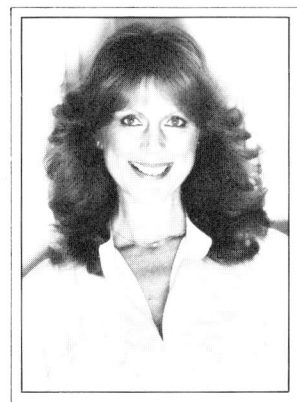

PAULENE STONE, *model: "I haven't worn nail varnish for months. I suddenly went off it, and discovered my nails had become very yellow underneath. After a while they actually started aching, as if they were crying out for varnish, rather like withdrawal symptoms! I stuck through this phase, and now my nails are not discoloured at all, and in far better condition."*

NAIL WRAPPING can be used to re-attach a broken nail tip or to extend nail length. Fast-drying glue fluid and fine tissue papers are used to build a "fake" bond for nail. Unless you have a steady hand and patience, this treatment is best left to a professional.

Salon treatments: The ones that work

Throughout this section we have concentrated on treatments you can give yourself. There are of course treatments which, because of the techniques and machinery involved, can only be administered by experts in a salon. Below is a breakdown of the most popular salon treatments that are worth trying, and produce results. An added advantage of the salon treatment is that you just lie back and enjoy it!

VACUUM SUCTION is a slimming treatment particularly effective on parts of the body prone to fatty deposits, ie, hips, thighs and upper arms, which are hard to slim down by exercise or massage. The treatment is electrical and performed by means of a box-like unit, to which are attached eight to ten rubber tubes, with clear plastic cups on the ends. The unit is switched on and an alternating current which stops and starts at regular intervals flows into the cups which are then placed on the body. This current enables the cups to act as a suction pump, sucking up the flesh for a few seconds, then releasing it. This is a strong (but absolutely painless) treatment which helps break down the fat and so endorses the theory of lymphatic drainage, ie, the re-absorption and elimination of fat and waste matter. Each treatment lasts for an hour and the cups can be constantly moved about to cover any area of the body except the stomach, where the internal organs are too near the skin's surface. Vacuum suction is a cumulative process and for full benefits a course of twelve treatments is recommended.

BODY WRAP This is another slimming treatment, particularly beneficial for improving slack skin due to loss of elasticity through ageing, rigorous dieting, pregnancy, cellulite, etc. The ultimate effect is said to be diuretic in that it eliminates waste tissue. A minimum of three treatments is advised for best results. The process is as follows: After a steam bath to open pores, a warm herb gel is applied to the whole body, or the specific areas to be treated. Bandages are wrapped over the treated areas and left for an hour and a half while the client relaxes. The bandages are then removed, and the gel will have been absorbed.

G5 is the most versatile of all salon treatments for the body, because it is effected by a vibratory machine with five different attachments. Each attachment is applied to the body by a beautician, who decides which attachment or "head" is needed. These vary from a rubber mat with rubber spikes used for dermabrasion and stimulation of blood and skin, to a soft rubber crescent shape which is rotated over the stomach to stimulate the flow of digestive juices and aid the digestive process. G5 is ideal if you like several treatments in the same session!

GALVANIC, HIGH FREQUENCY AND FARADIC CURRENTS Specialised electrical treatments in salons are often used in conjunction with three types of electric current. Facials which involve electricity use the *galvanic* and *high frequency* currents because these cause chemical reactions on the skin when used in conjunction with the specially prepared gels and creams made by René Guinot. These currents also aid the skin's reception and absorption of the particular treatments applied. For body-exercise treatments, the *Faradic* current is preferable as it provides vigorous stimulation of muscles.

The most popular facial using electricity is *Cathiodermie* which is a skin cell rejuvenation process and therefore considered to be beneficial to acne sufferers.

The treatment is as follows: After cleansing the skin of all make-up, a solution is applied with massage by the beautician which helps overcome the skin's natural resistance to electric currents. Then a thick gel is smoothed over the face. This contains ions which conduct electricity. The galvanic current is then switched on and transferred to the skin through metal rollers and a two-pronged fork which are lightly rubbed over the face. This equipment is operated by a beautician specially trained in the Cathiodermie process. The electric currents are generated from a unit to which the beautician's hand sets are connected by flexes. While the beautician works, the client holds an electrode (metal rod) which completes the electrical circuit. The galvanic current enables the gel to absorb all the oil and debris from the pores and become opaque; at this point a cream is applied, which releases oxygen when mixed with the gel — this activates the cell regeneration process. The face is then covered with fine gauze and the high frequency current switched on; this is transferred to the face through a glass bulb which is lightly rubbed over the gauze. The high frequency current stimulates nerve fibres and blood vessels so they reject all the debris, and the cream helps this process. Again, the client holds an electrode, but apart from the high frequency treatment when a mild tingling sensation may be experienced, no pain or discomfort will be felt at any time. The gauze is then removed and the pores closed by smoothing a solution over the skin followed by a cold compress. Finally, a nourishing mask is applied for twenty minutes, then wiped off. The whole treatment lasts for at least an hour and a quarter. Afterwards, the skin should be kept clean of make-up for at least five hours.

Cathiodermie is thought to have the most beneficial effects when used as a cumulative process. For instance, a bad acne sufferer may require three or four treatments a month, but if skin improves, the treatment may be reduced to once a month to keep it clear.

SLENDERTONE is a slimming treatment used in conjunction with the *Faradic* current, which works on the principle of vigorous muscle exercise. The current is conducted from a large unit by sixteen to twenty rubber tubes. At the end of the tubes are rubber pads which are fastened over certain muscles with straps. The client lies down on a bed and the equipment is fastened on. When the unit is activated, the current sends impulses to the muscles, so they work involuntarily, alternately contracting and relaxing very quickly. It is said that one hourly session with *Slendertone* is equivalent to a thousand vigorous exercises, and like most slimming treatments should be part of a course of treatments for lasting effects. *Slendertone* is also used simply to tone slack muscles. Mohammed Ali has used this treatment before a fight!

SOLARIUM. Infra-red and ultra-violet rays are transmitted through a giant lamp suspended over the body. It is, in fact, concentrated sunlight — and heat — without the sun. Solariums are ideal for those with very fair skins that burn easily and for those who wish to prepare their skins for the sun, so they tan more readily. A solarium course prepares and conditions the skin so that you can, when you go into the sun (with all the usual precautions), tan without burning.

Initially, a solarium treatment involves a one, or two-minute, exposure to the lamp. The client strips and lies underneath the solarium on a bed. By the end of a series of treatments the client should be able to remain for up to twenty minutes under the lamp. Although the skin will not actually tan, it will acquire a healthy colour. The solarium is widely accepted by beauticians as the skin's best sun preparation.

Solariums are also used for the treatment of skin conditions: acne, psoriasis, eczema, etc, all respond to the rays' healing and antiseptic properties. The heat from the lamp is also used for treatment of muscle ailments such as arthritis and lumbago. *Note* A new sun preparation on the market, available at selected salons, is the UVA lamp. This lamp is claimed to filter off the harmful burning rays, known as UVB, so only the gentler tanning rays, UVA, reach the body. This treatment is for those who want to go brown and cannot get away to the sun, or for those who normally cannot go brown in the sun because they burn.

STEAM CABINETS are similar to Turkish baths, except that the client lies in a tub full of steam with a plastic cover zipped up to the neck, leaving the head free. Hot steam swirls around the body, deep-cleansing the skin and relaxing muscles. A small weight-loss will also occur, due to profuse sweating, but the weight is replaced as soon as a drink is taken. Try this treatment if your skin needs a deep cleanse, or you simply want to unwind.

Have yourself a free health farm weekend

The next best thing to spending time (and a lot of money!) at a health farm is to recreate one at home. Using this chapter — and the entire book — as a reference, work out a tailor-made health and beauty weekend that suits *your* needs and tastes.

Spend one whole weekend on a self-indulgent, pampering programme that incorporates all the beauty treatments you've always wanted to try but have never allowed yourself the time for, or never known how to do. If you can share your weekend with a friend, so much the better; you can take turns to give one another a body massage, or facial, etc. Most health farms offer approximately six treatments a day, some even more; the benefit of being your own beautician is that you can concentrate on your priorities. Fill in your own regime on the chart on page 124.

Whether you decide on paraffin waxes, a deep hair conditioning, a manicure or whatever else for your more sybaritic treatments, be sure to incorporate a walk in the fresh air, a body massage and some form of exercise in your daily programme. Remember that the most important treatment a health farm offers is the total relaxation of mind and body: a gradual slowing-down of the system. You can help achieve this by cutting out social engagements, taking the 'phone off the hook and having three nights (the night before your health farm weekend, too!) of natural sleep. Before bedtime, soak in a fragrant bath; if you have trouble getting to sleep, sip a cup of camomile tea instead of reaching for a pill. In the evening, read a book or play soothing classical music instead of watching

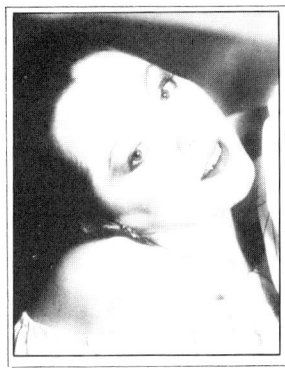

DULCIE HUSTON, actress: "Once a year without fail I go to a health farm for a week to recover from the rigours of London life! It really sets me up: I have massages, steam baths, lots of exercise and fresh air. I follow a purifying programme for the digestive system, drinking only hot water and lemon, and eating only salads.

television! Be deliciously lazy: live in a tracksuit or leotard, and give your skin a rest by wearing no make-up.

You might find that you enjoy your health farm weekend so much that you will want to incorporate some of these suggestions into your daily lifestyle. Promise to treat yourself to a health farm weekend every six weeks — you deserve it!

Because your health farm weekend will be fairly active, you need quite a high energy intake: the fasting that some health farms advocate needs to be accompanied by totally sedentary activities! For your first health farm day, follow the purifying regime from one of America's most exclusive health spas: The Golden Door's "Virtue-Making Day". This includes a liquid diet which leaves you feeling satisfied because it provides blood-sugar builders every two-and-a-half hours. Prepare the "meals" the night before so you need waste no time in the kitchen! The second day, adopt the less stringent, more flexible regime recommended by one of this country's top health farms, Stobo Castle in Scotland. It allows you up to 800 calories a day. First thing in the morning, drink a glass of hot water with a slice of lemon; it really does help to cleanse the system and is a habit worth following every morning of your life.

Diet for the golden door virtue-making day

Note: With the exception of almond milk, with each serving of liquid eat 13 g (1½ oz) sunflower seeds and three pine nuts.
8.00 am Grapefruit juice.
100 ml (4 oz) freshly squeezed grapefuit juice
50 ml (2 oz) water
Mix and serve.
10.30 am Almond milk.
6 whole almonds, blanched and peeled
½ medium-sized ripe banana
½ cup water
2 ice cubes
few drops fresh lemon juice
pinch nutmeg
pinch vanilla
Place in blender; liquidise and serve.

1.00 pm Gazpacho
1 medium tomato, peeled and diced
¼ large cucumber, peeled and chopped
1 slice onion
2 sprigs parsley
Place in blender; liquidise and serve.
3.30 pm Pineapple-cucumber juice
75 g (3 oz) cucumber, peeled
25 g (1 oz) fresh pineapple
2 sprigs parsley
50 ml (2 oz) apple juice
Place in blender; liquidise and serve.
6.00 pm Almond milk.
8.30 pm Carrot-apple juice
50 ml (2 oz) carrot juice
50 ml (2 oz) apple juice
⅓ apple, peeled
Place in blender; liquidise and serve.

Diet notes

This regime is recommended for people in average good health, but is not advised for sufferers from diabetes, hypoglycaemia or any condition requiring medical care. If in doubt, check with your doctor.
1 No coffee or tea is allowed; instead, drink freshly squeezed, unsweetened lemon juice, herb teas and bottled spring water, as much and as often as you like.
2 You must drink all liquids slowly, using a teaspoon. Nibble the sunflower seeds slowly; they should be hulled, raw and eaten unsalted.

Stobo castle's high-protein daily regime

All juices should be fresh. If you are weight-watching, note that a glass of fresh tomato juice, using four tomatoes, contains about thirty-two calories; a glass of fresh grapefruit juice, using one to two grapefruits, contains about sixty calories, and a glass of fresh orange juice, using two oranges, contains about eighty calories. To make Stobo's tomato juice cocktail, skin four tomatoes by pouring boiling water on them and peeling off skin with a sharp knife. Liquidise in blender, then strain. Add salt, pepper, and Worcestershire sauce to taste.
BREAKFAST Two slices of crispbread with honey or marmalade, or non-dieters could have a boiled egg and whole-meal toast, no butter; glass fresh juice; coffee or tea.
MID-MORNING JUICE BREAK Glass fresh juice.
LUNCH Large mixed salad of fresh raw vegetables; protein in the form of cheese, egg or fish. Piece fresh fruit or fruit yogurt.
MID-AFTERNOON JUICE BREAK Glass fresh juice.
DINNER Protein in the form of fish or meat; mixed salad of fresh raw vegetables or two varieties of cooked vegetables. Piece fresh fruit or fruit yogurt, or low-calorie dessert.

Your Personal Health Farm Chart

Fill in your own programme on the chart below—and keep to it!

	SATURDAY	SUNDAY
	Cleansing drink	Cleansing drink
Exercise:		
	8.00 am liquid break	Breakfast
Treatment:		
	10.30 am liquid break	Juice break
Treatment:		
	1.00 pm liquid break	Lunch
Treatment:		
Treatment:		
	3.30 pm liquid break	Juice break
Treatment:		
Exercise:		
	6.00 pm liquid break	Dinner
Treatment:		
	8.30 pm liquid break	
	Bath and bed	Bath and bed

Note: Make Friday a relaxing evening and early night!

HAIR

If you've ever wanted to have glossier, healthier hair (and who hasn't?) you'll find here all the tricks and tips from the world's top hairstylists. And if you've always wanted to colour or perm your hair but never dared, learn about the pluses — and the pitfalls — from the experts. All the right products and equipment — even the right diet — needed for maintaining healthy hair are outlined on these pages, plus professional treatments for you to copy at home to keep your hair looking its shiny, swinging best.

The right hair-care equipment

To be your own successful hairstylist, you need the correct tools that will improve and enhance the condition, and appearance, of your hair. Many hair problems are caused by using the wrong tools, eg, too-harsh dryers, combs that snag the hair, but the choice is so vast that it is easy to become confused and make mistakes. Follow this guide for the very best (and not necessarily the most expensive) equipment you can use on your hair. Some are essentials, others optional extras you might like to try.

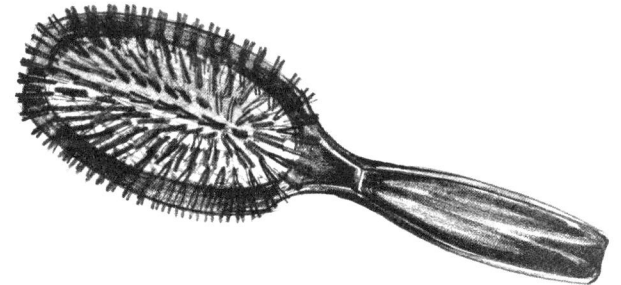

BASIC HAIRBRUSH should have quills with rounded ends. Any quills that feel harsh to the palm of your hand will feel equally harsh on your scalp and can be harmful. Many trichologists prefer a natural bristle (hog or boar) brush, but nylon or plastic is acceptable as long as quills are rounded and not sharp. Brushes with rubber bases are useful as they cut down on static and can be taken apart for easy cleaning. *Used for:* Brushing through hair daily to remove dust and distribute natural oils along hair from roots to ends.

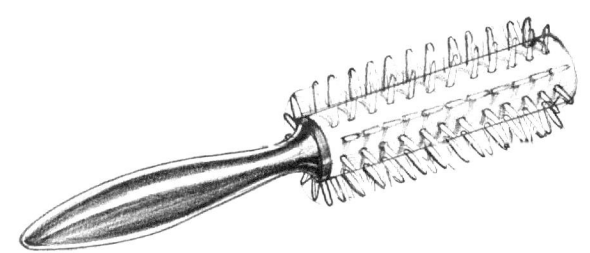

DRESSING/STYLING BRUSH can be full or half radial (quills totally or partially covering base), in varying sizes and with quills of different lengths. As these brushes are simply used to style the hair, nylon quills are fine, but if they feel too sharp, they can easily be smoothed on an abrasive surface. Quills placed evenly and widely apart are useful when used in conjunction with a hairdryer, as they allow hot air to flow freely between bristles for speedier drying. *Used for:* Dressing the hair into a style; with a hairdryer, to pull the hair straight, or to hold in a curl. The larger the brush, the larger the curl or wave; a small, full radial brush with narrow quills is ideal for short, curly hair. Some have "twist" handles which facilitate blow-drying.

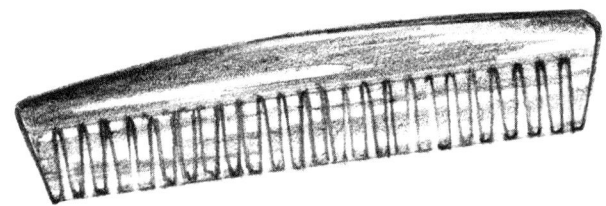

COMB According to Philip Kingsley, top trichologist, the ideal hair comb is saw-cut, that is to say the edges of teeth are machine-cut and flat, therefore will not snag or harm hair. He suggests you look for a comb made of vulcanite, a form of hard rubber; bone, ivory or tortoiseshell are fine, too, but far more expensive. *Used for:* Wide-toothed comb essential for combing through wet hair so it does not pull at hair and weaken it; narrow-toothed comb for styling hair. Save money by buying a two-in-one comb with narrow and wide teeth at opposite ends.

To clean brushes and combs

Prepare brushes first by drawing comb through quills to remove hairs, surface dust, etc. Wash in warm, soapy water, scrubbing a soft-bristled nail brush gently against quills to remove grease.

Drying and styling accessories

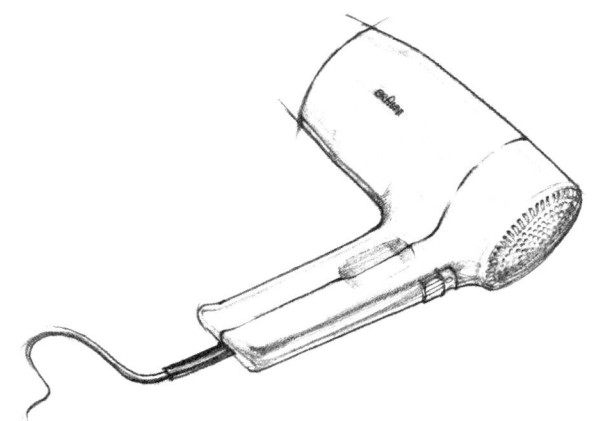

HAIRDRYER should not be stronger than 1000 watts. There is no doubt that excessive use of hairdryers is damaging to hair; a hair-care company recently discovered that a high-speed hairdryer took only thirty minutes to bake a small sponge cake! Choose a dryer that is *not* the most powerful on the market,

does not overheat in the hand and, if you travel, one that is dual-voltage. Use your dryer sensibly: in short bursts, and never close to the hair. Wave it back and forth across the section you are drying. Switch to the lower heat setting on your dryer: hair will take a little longer to dry, but it is worth the extra time! Many hairdryers have attachments that style the hair as it dries: these include curling wands, combs and brushes to make waves, curls or straighten hair. They are useful and fun to use, but are not essential if you have the relevant styling brushes; you can then blow-style hair yourself (see p 134). Hood salon dryers can be bought for the home but the obvious disadvantage is that they are cumbersome, though not as hot for the hair as the hand-held dryer.

HEATED ROLLERS are very handy to speedily restyle hair that has wilted. You can buy those which produce steam, as well as those which heat on electric rods; both work on the same principle of "heat setting" hair. Although electric rollers are thermostatically controlled to avoid overheating, use of any kind of heated rollers should be limited to two or three times a week, as overuse can result in dry, damaged hair. Some heated rollers, with the addition of a special solution, condition hair while they set it, which is a useful precaution against over-drying. You could further protect your hair by copying a trick of many hair salons: cover your heated rollers with a fine layer of foam, cut to size and stitched along a seam, or wrap tissue around them. For best results, use heated rollers on damp hair, and allow hair to cool after you remove rollers, before brushing through.

CURLING RODS/WANDS style hair by heat-setting the shape with steam or electricity. Steam wands are easier for beginners to manage and are a little gentler on hair; electric wands have thermostats to prevent overheating. Both types need careful handling so hair does not burn! Fine curling rods are useful to curl; thicker ones to straighten, or introduce body into hair. It is sensible to buy a curling rod with a stand, so the hot rod does not burn any surface it rests on.

CRIMPING IRON is similar to the above. It looks rather like a waffle iron, and heat-sets corrugations into the hair for a pretty, rippling effect. Again, care is needed not to burn hair.

ULTRA-VIOLET HEAT LAMPS have become popular as a means of drying hair without disturbing the natural style, as they have no air flow. Heat is gentler than the average hair-dryer, but there is a misconception that these lamps cannot harm the hair; of course, if you hold the lamp too close, your hair can be damaged. Many salons have "octopus lamps" which are multiple U-V lamps on one base that dry hair from all angles. You can also achieve "static" drying by fixing a type of mesh screen over certain models of hairdryers; this screen cuts out the harsh airflow, but not the heat.

Useful extras

PLANT MISTER filled with warm water. *Used for:* Livening a wash 'n' wear hairstyle when you don't need to shampoo; damping hair for restyling; spraying on final rinse to hair after shampooing, eg, herbal infusion or lemon juice and water.

TERRY TOWELLING MITTS easy to make from squares of thick, soft towelling. *Used for:* Speedy drying of wash 'n' wear hair.

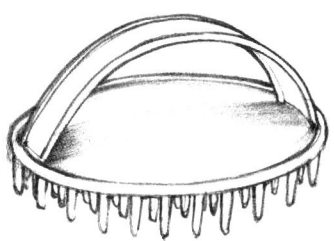

CIRCULAR MASSAGE BRUSH made of rubber; by Denman. *Used for:* A stimulating shampoo; scalp massage.

Recognise your hair type – and know how to look after it

Before your hair can benefit from any treatment, you have to know your hair type so you can treat it accordingly. Here, hair types are broken down into their simplest categories, dry and greasy, but under each heading you will see the many combinations involved. Normal hair is fortunate enough to need a minimum of special care and can be recognised by its naturally healthy sheen, and body, though those lucky enough to have normal hair should still maintain upkeep with regular conditioning treatments, appropriate shampoos, etc.

Hair type is generally decided by heredity: sebaceous glands attached to the follicle at the root of each hair produce natural oils. If hair is greasy, too much oil is produced; if hair is dry, too little oil, and if hair is normal, the amount of sebum (oil) flow lubricates hair to just the right degree. However, it is important to note that outside factors such as stress, illness, chemical treatments, can alter structure and texture of all types of hair. Therefore if naturally greasy hair becomes dry for whatever reason, it should be treated as for dry hair; if hair is greasy at the roots and dry at the ends, the two types should be treated separately, ie, hair would need to be degreased at roots and conditioned at ends only.

Greasy hair

It looks lank, lifeless and, due to over-production of sebum glands in the scalp, is greasy rather than shiny. Oil in the hair attracts dust and debris, so that greasy hair gets dirty quickly. It will not hold a style for long. Although the rate of oil secretion is hereditary, this rate can be intensified by stress, which is known to trigger the hormones that affect oil glands.

How you can help

● Brush hair as little as possible, more to style than to distribute oil.

● Keep brushes, combs — and your pillowcase — scrupulously clean at all times.

● Use a shampoo suited to greasy hair, but not one that is too harsh and will strip the hair's natural oils. Otherwise, use a very mild shampoo. Lather once only. Keep water cool, as hot water steps up oil-flow.

● Be sure to shampoo scalp with pads of fingers so that scalp, and not just hair, is degreased.

● If you feel you need a conditioner to "tame" hair, use the mild variety that detangles only and does not leave a film on the hair; you may be able to use conditioner on the ends of your hair only.

● Try a final rinse to restore hair's normal acid balance (and remove any last traces of shampoo): six parts vinegar to one part water, or equal parts lemon juice and water.

● Avoid the "heat insulators" that trap heat and encourage grease-flow: hats, scarves, turbans.

● A short, simple hairstyle is more practical for greasy hair, and will be easier to wash every day.

Dry hair

Dry hair appears dull, lacking in shine, is often brittle and splits at ends and, in extreme cases, breaks off. It is often frizzy, high in static and generally difficult to control. When hair is naturally dry, the scalp is dry, but in many cases dry hair is a temporary condition, a result of abuse of electrical hair-care equipment and/or over-processing through perming, tinting etc, so that you may have a greasy scalp and dry hair.

How you can help

● Brush hair daily from roots to tips to distribute oil-flow evenly along hair shaft. A few drops of rosemary oil on your hairbrush will add lustre at the same time.

● Cut down on use of electrical appliances: keep hairdryer on lowest setting if you must use one; restrict use of tongs, heated rollers, etc to twice weekly. Instead use conventional rollers or alternative methods of setting hair (see p 136).

● Treat your hair to regular conditioning packs. Protein packs are particularly good for your hair type, or make your own simple, effective treatments (see p 130). Wrap treated hair with a towel: the warmth aids penetration.

• Always use a shampoo that is especially formulated for your hair type: those with protein, egg, lanolin or coconut oil are all suitable. You could improvise by adding a beaten egg to any ordinary shampoo (rinse off with cool water!) or add a spoonful of any kitchen oil instead. Do not wait until hair is really dirty to shampoo, but when you wash use one lather only.

• Follow shampoo with a conditioner that coats hair with a fine protective layer.

• Keep hair covered in the sun, either with a scarf or hat or with a sun block in lotion or gel form, designed for the hair.

• Avoid dehydrating atmospheres such as saunas or intensely heated rooms. Both will contribute to "drying out" your hair.

• The worst offenders for dry hair are perms, straightening treatments and permanent colourants. Chemicals used in these treatments can damage and greatly dry hair. If your hair has been harmed by any of these treatments, stop using them; substitute a semi-permanent rinse for a tint! Prevention is better than cure: badly permed and/or tinted hair can become so dry it has to be cut off.

• Rinse hair well after swimming, as both sea and chlorinated pool water dry hair and encourage frizzing.

• Have hair trimmed regularly, so any split ends can be checked and not travel further up the hair shaft to do more damage.

• A weekly scalp massage will help stimulate oil glands and thus increase sebum flow. For extra benefits, use an aromatic oil (see p 133 for scalp massage how-to).

All about hair-care products: What they can and can't do

Claims for hair-care products become ever more extravagant: one American manufacturer describes his hair conditioner as a "nucleic hair rectifier pH modulator"! If the shampoo shelves baffle you with science, this simple what's what in the world of hair-care should set you straight.

SHAMPOOS contain cleansing agents, water, foaming agents, thickeners, colouring, fragrance, and varying additives that make a shampoo "specialised". It is widely believed that so-called "detergent shampoos" are too harsh for the hair, and that soap-based shampoo is preferable. This is untrue as detergent is simply another word for any kind of cleansing agent, including soap: what is being referred to is the *synthetic* detergent contained in all shampoos today. This is fine for all types of hair, unless an allergy should result; see p 132 for how to make a super-mild shampoo from soap flakes. The big advantage of using a modern shampoo rather than soap-based

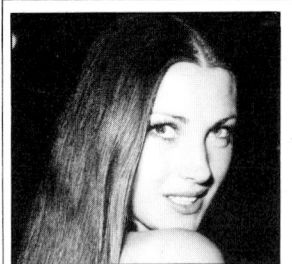

JANE SEYMOUR, *actress: "I wash my hair every morning with a shampoo made from seeds of the jojoba plant★ which grows in the desert. I break all the rules, like brushing my hair when it's wet — but I always use a Mason Pearson brush!"*

is that it is geared to working with today's hard water, and rinses out far more easily than soap. The foaming agent in shampoo facilitates easy rinsing, too, though a shampoo will work equally well without any lather; foaming agents are added to reassure us that the shampoo is doing its work well!

The most popular additives in shampoo are conditioners, which add body to hair by coating it with protein, but more effective results may be gained by using a good conditioner after shampoo.

Many manufacturers make proud claims on their labels that their shampoos are pH or acid-balanced, and therefore gentlest and best for hair; in fact most shampoos are naturally acid-balanced. The strongest alkaline shampoo sold today is milder than an average bar of soap! The shampoo most suited to your hair can best be found by trying several: you may even discover that a shampoo formulated for a hair type different to your own works best on you. Mild shampoos are always best for hair, but don't reach for the baby shampoos: these are not necessarily the mildest. Economy size shampoos are not always the bargain they appear to be, as sometimes extra water is added to thin down the product, so more has to be used to make it effective.

What a shampoo should do for your hair

• Remove dirt, scalp debris and grease (not natural oils) from your hair. Too harsh a shampoo will strip hair of *all* natural oils, creating a dull finish and leaving hair matted.

• Rinse out easily.

• Leave hair manageable, glossy and not tangled.

CONDITIONERS in cream or lotion form are used after shampooing to help hair retain its natural condition. They are designed to impart lustre to hair, add body, detangle, and, in some cases, restore body and actually help repair damaged hair. All conditioners smooth down rough scales along each hair so hair looks shiny and soft, but if you have that result from shampoo only, you don't need conditioner!

The mildest form of conditioner is called a "creme rinse". This is sometimes designed to do little more than separate each hair and thus make hair easier to brush or comb. Many conditioners coat hairs with protein, which adds body and seals in

★ *Jojoba oil shampoo available from The Body Shop, 1 Crane Street, Chichester, West Sussex, and branches: write for mail order details, including an SAE.*

moisture; a smoothing ingredient, such as glycerine, does the same job. Proteins used in conditioners include balsam, an oily substance from the tree of the same name, gelatine, milk, egg and animal placenta. Heavy-duty conditioners contain protein which is broken down into molecules so small that they fill in gaps in the hair shaft and bond it, making hair less porous, stronger and resistant to damage; they often need to be left on the hair for some time for maximum penetration. As with shampoo, trial and error is the best method of discovering which conditioners are most suited to your hair. Normal or dry hair benefits from a heavy-duty conditioning pack at least once a fortnight.

HAIRDRESSINGS otherwise known as "brilliantines", are used to tame dry, unruly hair between shampoos, provide a shine without greasiness, and to enable hair to be brushed easily into a style. In cream or spray-on form, they should be used very sparingly so the hair does not become greasy. Many dressings contain mineral oil or beeswax, and in fact a smear of Vaseline or a few drops of olive oil mixed with perfume and combed through the hair will have the same effect as commercial varieties. Hairstylist and salon-owner Ricci Burns firmly believes in hair dressings: "It's like putting moisturiser on your skin. I can never understand why people pile conditioner on their hair when they wash it, yet never put anything on their hair when it's dry!"

LACQUER HAIRSPRAYS hold a hairstyle in place, and are useful to keep "flyaway ends" of chignon styles etc, in check. With today's simple, easy-to-care-for styles, regular use of a hairspray should not be necessary. If you must use a hairspray, use one that is a lesser strength than you think you need, and brush it out as soon as possible: the chemicals used in hairsprays are strong, and can have drying effects on the hair. (Hence the heavy perfumes of many sprays, which are simply used to mask the smell of chemicals!) The aerosol spray cans are being replaced by ecologically-safe "pump" dispenser sprays; these are easier to control, and there is less danger of lacquer that has been sprayed in atmosphere stinging eyes.

SETTING LOTIONS AND GELS contain the same basics as used in hairsprays. They will hold curl only until the hair gets wet, and are a preferable method to lacquer of keeping a style in place. Some setting lotions offer protection against hairdryer heat by leaving a thin moisturising film on each hair. Good home alternatives to commercial setting lotions are beer (although it smells awful!), fresh milk, lemon juice (more suited to greasy hair), or a little sugar dissolved in boiling water and left to cool. For even dispersal, pour into a plastic spray bottle.

ENVIRONMENTAL PROTECTORS deposit a film on hair which helps protect against the elements. They are parti-cularly useful for seaside holidays, where hair can frizz and dry out from seawater, sun, etc. Some protectors do contain sun blocks, though it should be noted that, in very strong sun, there is no better protection for your hair — or head — than a large hat! Protectors are available in lotion or gel form; the more occlusive the product, the more effective.

How to wash hair properly

There is a definite technique, if not an art, in washing hair for optimum results. Follow this step-by-step guide to make sure that, at each shampoo session, you are giving your hair every opportunity to look its best.

● If you do not have a shower, buy an attachment. They are cheap, and do a far more efficient rinsing job than pouring jugs of water over your head!

● Before commencing shampoo, comb through hair to rid it of any tangles: remove snags by holding clump of snagged hair with one hand, and working comb through hair from end to root.

● Rinse hair very, very well; not just to wet hair for shampoo, but to rid hair of surface dirt. Use warm water for your whole shampoo: hot water can dull and dry hair. Incidentally, Leonard, top London hairstylist, advises purists not to waste their time collecting tubs of rainwater; he points out that city rainwater is polluted!

● Use about a tablespoon of shampoo; less for short hair, perhaps more if hair is exceptionally long. Note that extra shampoo won't result in cleaner hair. For even distribution, dissolve shampoo in a little warm water before applying. Always apply from hands, not the shampoo bottle or tube.

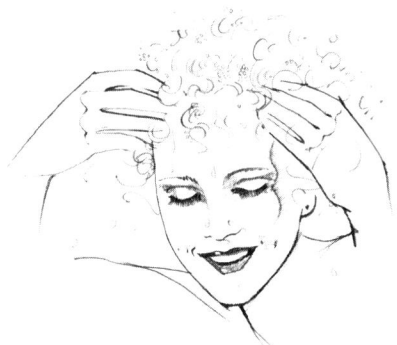

● Use pads of fingers, not nails, to massage shampoo into scalp. Work through to ends of hair. Unless hair is very dirty or greasy, one application should be enough: over-shampooing removes hair's natural oils.

- Rinse hair very thoroughly; rinse again to check there is no shampoo still in hair. Any residue left can dull hair. If hair is "squeaky clean", that indicates shampoo was too harsh.
- Squeeze out excess moisture gently with hands. Rub a small amount of conditioner between hands before massaging on to hair, not scalp. Greasy hair may require conditioner on ends only. Comb conditioner through to ends and leave on for stipulated time.
- Rinse conditioner out of hair. Do not be afraid to rinse thoroughly: a tiny amount of conditioner will cling to every hair, no matter how much you rinse!

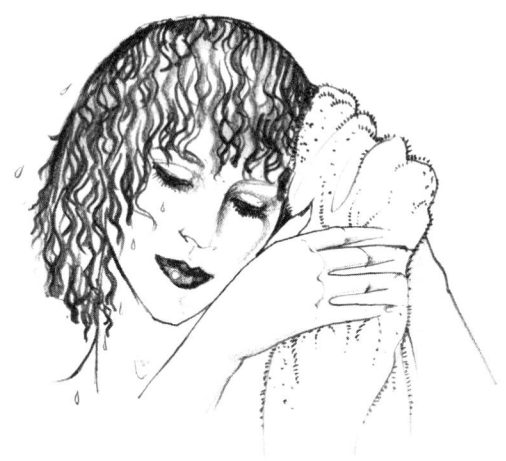

- Blot hair with dry, fluffy towel; never rub, as hair is at its weakest when wet. Use a second towel to wrap around hair. Leave for a few minutes to absorb excess moisture. Comb hair through and follow usual drying procedure.

How often should you wash your hair?

Vidal Sassoon, who has his own excellent range of hair-care products, believes in "washing your hair every day — just as you do your body — provided the shampoo is mild". A short, sporty cut that is left to dry naturally is easily shampooed in the shower every morning; long, waist-length hair is more of a problem to wash daily! As a general rule, wash at least every two/three days with a mild shampoo, and never wait until hair looks, or feels, dirty.

Home hair treatments: Ten of the best

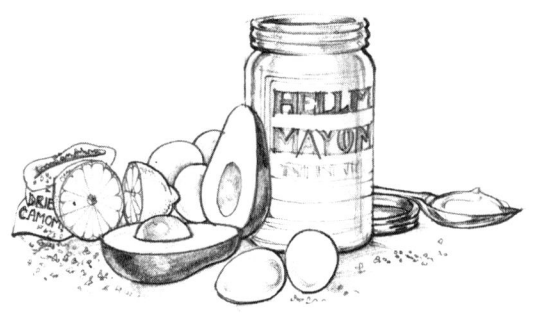

All of the following hair-care "recipes" are fun to follow, ingredients are inexpensive and, most important, results are effective. If you can't afford a conditioning treatment in a hair salon (or would like to save yourself some cash), choose from one of several below. And once you're sold on the idea of making your own hair-care products, try a home-made shampoo or brightening finishing rinse!

BONE MARROW HAIR REVIVER Some of the chicest and priciest Parisian hair salons have a bone marrow conditioning treatment which is left on the hair for the rich protein to penetrate. It may not be the pleasantest treatment you'll ever give your hair — but it could be the most beneficial! Scoop out the marrow from a large bone, heat it until warm and massage well into the scalp. The paste should be left on for a minimum of thirty minutes, keep the head covered with a warm towel. Shampoo out afterwards.

CLASSIC HOT OIL TREATMENT Everyone has their favourite oil to use as a hair conditioner: Vidal Sassoon prefers cold-pressed almond oil, or plain kitchen corn oil; Harry King, top New York hair stylist, likes coconut oil. Castor oil is widely used in hair salons; olive oil is considered too greasy and heavy. The hot oil treatment is a marvellous method of introducing shine and bounce to the hair. Warm oil and massage well into hair; if you have a dry scalp, massage with pads of fingers into scalp. Wrap head in a hot, damp towel and leave oil on hair for at least thirty minutes, or ideally overnight. Care must be taken to shampoo the oil out very well afterwards: at least two latherings will be necessary. Follow with conditioner as usual.

SKIMMED MILK COCKTAIL CONDITIONER This hard-working conditioner from Richard Stein Haircutting, New York, sounds like a health drink, but all the goodness in the ingredients is as good for your hair as it is for your body!

2 cups skimmed milk
30 ml (2 tbsp) bran
15 ml (1 tbsp) wheatgerm
15 ml (1 tbsp) lecithin
Liquid from 2 capsules wheatgerm oil
1 egg yolk

Blend all ingredients together in a liquidiser. Work half the mixture through hair and leave on for ten minutes. Wash three times with a shampoo that is seven parts water to one part shampoo. You can keep the remainder of the Cocktail Conditioner in the 'fridge for up to two weeks.

HENNA HAIR SHINER You may have tried using henna not as a colourant, but as a great conditioner. Next time you buy some neutral henna, try this recipe which makes henna even better for your hair.

150 g (6 oz) neutral henna, mixed to a paste with warm water
1 egg yolk
½ small carton yogurt

Leave on hair for thirty minutes. Rinse well and shampoo.

EGG FLIP Egg yolks are a strong source of protein and are often used in hair-care treatments. American hair expert Georgette Briand uses them with castor oil for double conditioning benefits.

75 ml (5 tbsp) castor oil
1 egg yolk

Mix both ingredients well together. Apply to dry hair; cover head with paper towels and a shower cap. Leave on for two hours. Shampoo twice, and rinse very well.

The following five hair-care recipes were formulated by Anita Roddick, owner of The Body Shops and Mark Constantine, herbalist and trichologist. All herbs etc mentioned are available from The Body Shop, 1 Crane Street, Chichester, West Sussex and all The Body Shop branches; send an SAE for product catalogue, mail order details and price list.

PURE SOAP SHAMPOO This shampoo is ideal for people who are allergic to the synthetic detergents in commercial shampoos; even if you are not, try this Pure Soap Shampoo for its beneficial properties. Use immediately after making.

25 g (1 oz) Boots' pure soap flakes, crushed to a powder
25 g (1 oz) Sedra (a crushed Persian herb, used as a conditioner)
120 ml (4 fl oz) rosewater

Mix crushed soap flakes with Sedra. Heat rosewater, add to mixture and blend to form a paste. Use two applications on hair; rinse well.

HEAVY DUTY HERBAL CONDITIONER Pure herbs make this an ideal treatment for dry hair with split ends.

13 g (½ oz) rosemary spikes (available from grocer), ground into a fine powder

13 g (½ oz) camomile flowers
13 g (½ oz) Sedra
Juice of half a lemon

Mix all ingredients together with 75 ml (3 fl oz) boiling water to form a frothy paste. Rub well into hair. Pull a polythene bag over hair and cover with a towel. Leave on hair for thirty minutes before rinsing.

AVOCADO AND MAYONNAISE PROTEIN PACK Two of the biggest boosters for glossy, healthy hair — avocado and mayonnaise — combine with rosemary spikes to combat a dry scalp and dry, damaged hair.

½ cup Hellmann's mayonnaise
½ ripe avocado
300 ml (½ pt) rosemary infusion — steep 25 g (1 oz) rosemary spikes in boiling water; strain

Blend mayonnaise and avocado together. Wet hair and massage paste into scalp, as well as hair. Wrap head in an old silk scarf which has been wrung out in the rosemary infusion. Cover with plastic bag or foil for a couple of hours. Rinse in warm or tepid water; follow usual shampoo programme.

FINISHING RINSE FOR LIGHT HAIR Use after regular shampoo and conditioner as a final rinse to add lights to hair.

25 g (1 oz) camomile flowers
25 g (1 oz) marigold flowers

Make an infusion by pouring 300 ml (½ pt) boiling water over flowers; leave to stand for three hours, covering with a cloth. Strain into a bottle. Pour over clean, wet hair, allowing excess to drip back into a pot for re-use. Do not rinse out, and let hair dry naturally.

FINISHING RINSE FOR DARK HAIR Use after regular shampoo and conditioner to add shine and lustre.

13 g (½ oz) rosemary spikes
13 g (½ oz) camomile flowers
13 g (½ oz) marigold flowers
13 g (½ oz) Persian henna

Method, as above.

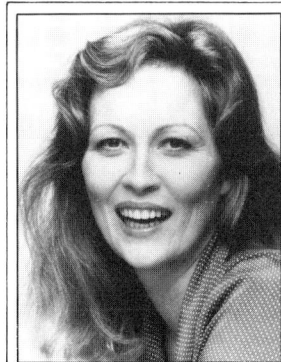

FAYE DUNAWAY, *actress:*
"The first thing I do each morning is brush my hair. This wakes me up, is wonderful for my scalp, and is also an easy way to exercise. I bend down, throw my hair forward and brush vigorously from the nape of the neck forward for about ten minutes, always with a Kent hairbrush."

News from the top

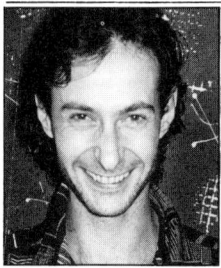

Harry King is the New York hairstylist who has styled or cut the hair of many of the world's most celebrated women: Charlotte Rampling, Sophia Loren, Jackie Bissett, Diana Ross, to name a few. Here he offers his sound, specialist advice on two subjects which perplex many women! **Harry King on: Choosing the right hairstyle . . .**

"The old rules about choosing a style to suit your face shape or whatever are just that: old rules. The function of a good hairstyle, like a good make-up, is to accentuate your best features. If you have beautiful eyes, your haircut should be designed to show them off. Don't go by what suits a model in a magazine: go by what suits you. A good haircut has to fit your lifestyle: it should be practical, and above all, not too serious!"

. . . and choosing the right hairdresser

"Find someone who makes you feel relaxed. If your hairdresser intimidates you at all, find another. Going to a hair salon should be a pleasurable experience, not like going to the dentist! How to find a good hairdresser? By word of mouth, by the names you read in the magazines, by haircuts you see he does. Don't go with preconceived ideas. Just because you've made up your mind what you want, doesn't mean you're right; it's not always possible to see yourself in a positive way. Never become a slave to a hair salon. You should be given a good haircut and be able to wash it yourself — so you can get on with other things in life!"

How to cut hair yourself

There is no substitute for a good, professional haircut. However, if you are broke, have an enormous amount of patience and a bit of nerve, here are a few good alternatives!

You will need:

● Professional stainless steel haircutting scissors 15 cm (6 in) long, from J & T Gorney, 16 Oakwell Mount, Leeds 8, Yorkshire; write to them enclosing an SAE for mail order details.

● A well-lit room where you can get comfortably close to the mirror, either sitting or standing; a good comb and brush.

● Freshly shampooed and conditioned hair. Know your hair texture (fine, medium, thick) and how much you plan to cut. Have a mental picture of the look you wish to achieve *before* you start to cut.

Note The following cut is for one-length hair only:

Photograph by David Cloud

132

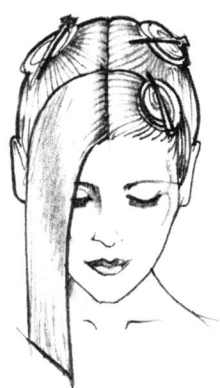

1 Comb through wet hair. Separate into four sections, starting with centre parting (down to nape of neck); then bisect parting from ear to ear. Pin up three sections so they are out of the way.

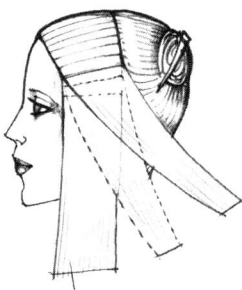

2 Loose section will be cut in several steps, by subsectioning into many tiny strands. The illustration shows roughly how many subsections you will have to make.

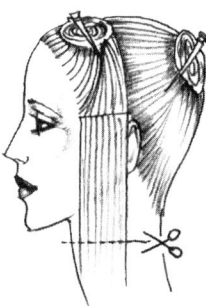

3 Start subsectioning at bottom: Separate out one strand and pin up rest. This strand is your Guide Strand, to measure all the rest by.

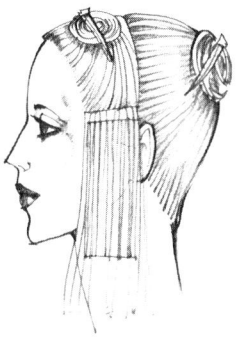

4 Section another strand and comb it over the Guide. (Again, pin up remaining hair.) Trim, flush with Guide Strand. Continue until all hair in quadrant is cut. Repeat on other side.

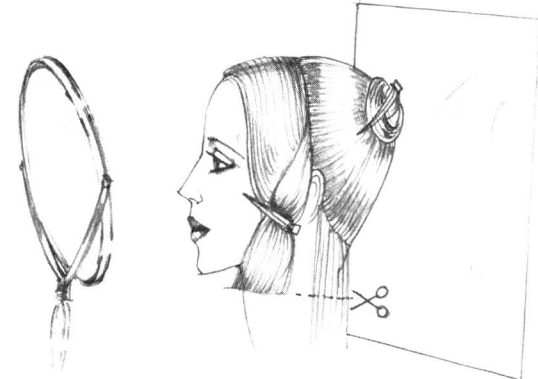

5´ Back sections are a bit trickier, although method is the same. You'll need two mirrors, one in front of you and one behind, so you can see what you are doing.

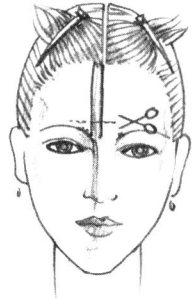

6 Fringe can be trimmed with a variant of the basic section method: Part hair in centre; clip fringe to either side. Section off a tiny Guide Strand, then trim other sections to match it.

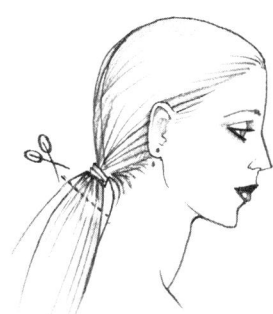

Quick trick for a blunt cut that's slightly longer at the sides than the back: Pull hair to the nape in a ponytail; cut just below the rubber band.

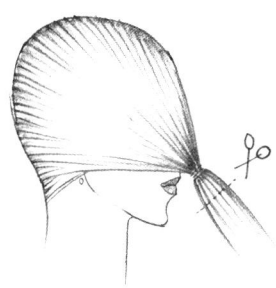

For a pageboy blunt cut, longer in the back than at the sides, part hair to nape, pull it into ponytail just below nose and cut below rubber band. (You can even out both ponytail cuts by the section method, if necessary.)

The super scalp massage

This is wonderfully relaxing, loosens a taut scalp and, most important, improves the circulation, which stimulates healthy new hair growth. Top trichologist Philip Kingsley believes that, in ninety percent of cases, thin hair can be improved with regular massage. You can massage your head whenever you have a spare moment or, for greater benefit, use a little aromatic oil to scent and condition hair at the same time. Here's how:

Use the pads of your fingers, not your nails (which would scratch and irritate scalp) to massage your scalp. Make small, circular movements all over your head, using fingers and thumbs of both hands. It is important that you move the scalp, and not your fingers, as you massage. You might find, if you are particularly tense, that you want to concentrate especially on the base of the neck. Spend time massaging your scalp where it feels best, but cover every inch, taking as little, or as much, time as you choose. It should be an enjoyable, as well as a beneficial treatment!

How to blow-dry hair like the experts

Whether you want to tame frizzy hair into a sleek bob or convert straight hair into a mass of curls, follow the professionals' tips for best results:
- Towel-dry hair before you blow dry. Comb through hair in preparation for drying.
- Use warmer temperature and higher speed to dry off hair to just-damp; switch to cooler and slower setting for blow-styling. *Note* If you are not sure whether heat setting is too hot for hair, test on back of hand. You can reduce temperature, too, by holding dryer further away from hair. Never hold dryer closer than 15 cm (6 in) to head.
- Direct air current at hair, not scalp. Keep dryer in constant motion; never focus on one spot.
- To blow-style, always work with small sections of hair as they are easier to control. Clip hair you are not working on out of the way; giant metal clips are the most practical.
- Use larger brushes for sleek, bouncy styles, smaller for curlier styles; the same applies to brush attachments on dryers.
- For sleek, smooth hair: Brush downward from crown with long strokes while directing air flow from *above*.

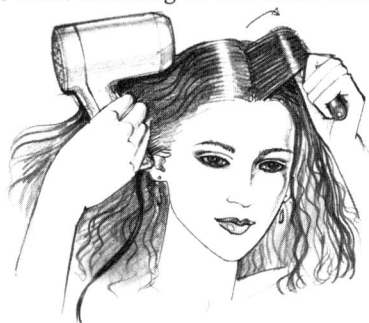

- To add bounce at roots: Hold section of hair at right angles to head while you apply air flow to hair on brush.
- To straighten wavy or frizzy hair: Take section of hair and grasp ends with bristles of brush. Twist brush so hair is pulled taut, then pull downward and outward, directing air flow across top of hair.
- For a straight, thick, full effect (ideal for a chunky, layered

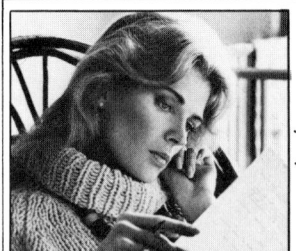

cut): Dry and brush hair from *underneath*. Let hair fall forward over face — it's easier!
- To curl hair: Use your brush as you would a roller, wrapping hair around, section by section. Direct air to hair on brush.
- To give short, layered hair a feathery effect: Blow air current *across* hair. Use brush like a rake to separate sections.

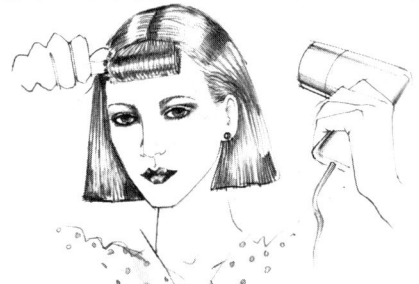

- To make a fringe look sleek and bouncy: Brush fringe backwards first, blowing dry as you brush. Twirl hair forwards around brush. Let air current dry hair completely. Turn off dryer and hold brush until air cools if you want fringe to curl slightly under. For straighter fringe, brush hair backwards while drying; when almost dry, reverse and brush fringe flat on to forehead.
- Always leave "styled" blow-dried hair to cool before brushing through.

Vidal Sassoon's method of drying one-length hair super-straight

Vidal Sassoon advocates this method of drying long, one-length hair and suggests it as a preferable alternative to chemically straightening frizzy hair. It's also a safer bet than ironing your hair straight!

Place one large foam-covered roller in the crown of hair. Wrap all the rest of your hair around your head in one direction. Put in pins to secure, and blow-dry for thirty minutes. Take out pins and wrap hair in the other direction around your head. Pin it, and blow-dry for ten minutes. When hair is completely dry, take out the pins and brush your hair.

Help your hair to better health

You can apply protein treatments to the hair to improve the condition, but the only way you can improve the quality of the hair shaft as it emerges from the scalp — or accelerate hair growth — is by nourishing hair from within. If you are in good health, you should have a healthy head of hair. If you are ill or are lacking in a good diet your hair will suffer as a result. Scan the lists below to see which foods you should eat — and those you should avoid — for healthy, lustrous hair. It is interesting to note that they read like a well-balanced diet plan for a healthy body, too!

What healthy hair needs

- Hair *is* protein, so plenty of protein intake — fish, meat — is one of the most important nutrients for your hair.
- Iron in the form of red meat.
- Fresh vegetables, preferably raw or cooked to a minimum: be sure to eat one large, raw mixed salad daily.
- Cottage cheese or hard cheeses.
- Wholewheat bread; wheatgerm.
- Vegetable oils.
- Six glasses of water daily.
- Several fresh fruits daily, including citrus fruit for vitamin C content.
- Natural low-fat yogurt.

What healthy hair can do without

- Crash diets or diets that aren't nutritionally balanced. Even a purely calorific deficiency will result in dull, brittle hair.
- Sugar.
- Preserves (except honey).
- Chocolates, sweet desserts, pastries etc.
- Salt sprinkled on food.
- Animal fats: milk in excess, butter, cream.

The big hair boosters

Even the healthiest hair will benefit from extra helpers: Philip Kingsley, leading trichologist, recommends the following to his clients; all are designed to make hair look its shining best.

Brewer's yeast is the easiest form of vitamin B for the body to assimilate. Vitamin B controls your nervous system, which in turn affects your skin and scalp. Regular intake of brewer's yeast will make your hair look glossier and also improve the condition. Take 3 tbsp (45 ml) powdered brewer's yeast blended with any liquid, or in tablet form (dosage depends on strength: you may need as many as twelve daily!).

Dessicated liver tablets are rich in iron, and are particularly beneficial if you are anaemic. They are preferable to iron pills, as they do not adversely affect the digestive system. Take between four and eight tablets a day.

Molasses contains lots of valuable minerals, as it is unrefined. Helps keep system regular, which in turn benefits skin and scalp. Take four capsules (preferable to liquid form) at night.

Gelatine is a protein which enters the system immediately to go to work on improving hair; combined with brewer's yeast, gelatine has an even better effect, and is marvellous for nails, too! Take 1 tbsp (15 ml) unflavoured gelatine daily.

Problem hair: Causes and cures

Many minor hair complaints are connected with the sufferer's general health and are corrected when health or diet improve. However, stress is a key factor in more serious disorders of hair and scalp, particularly hair loss, which is on the increase among women as they take on more stress-related jobs at higher executive levels.

If you have any hair or scalp problem which you cannot treat yourself, seek professional help from a trichologist, a specialist of the hair and scalp. If you are in London, you can go to The Scalp and Hair Hospital, 228 Stockwell Road, Brixton SW9 9SU; 01-733 2056, or write to them enclosing an SAE for your nearest practising trichologist and/or a free leaflet on hair-care.

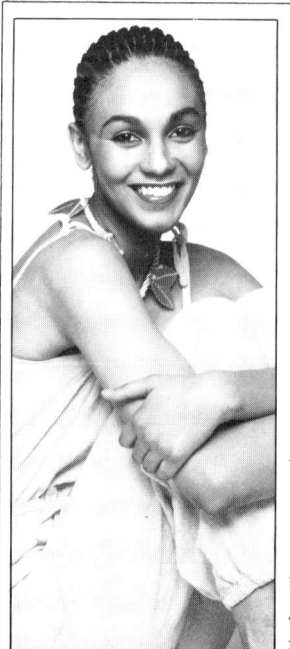

MOUCHETTE O'CONNOR, *model: "My hair is plaited into two dozen cornrows by my sister! It takes at least two hours but when it's done they stay for six weeks. I keep my hair in cornrows when I shampoo and even when I give it a hot oil treatment. I use Coromist spray for an instant shine and stroke on Vitapointe cream to tame and condition between washes. A special Afro comb — you can buy them at Boots now — prevents snarls but I comb my hair as little as possible because the more I leave it, the better it grows. I can never understand why black girls straighten their hair. Why not make the best of what you have?"*

CONDITION	CAUSES	CURES
Traction alopecia Hair is literally pulled out from scalp by mistreatment.	Scraping hair back too tightly in rubber bands; pulling hair out with harsh brush. In rare cases the hair is unconsciously pulled out by the sufferer: a result of tension.	If you must wear hair pulled back, loosen ponytail or knot; ease pressure by wearing a fabric-covered stretch band. Hair must be treated very gently to give it a chance to grow back.
Dull, thinning hair	Anaemia: iron deficiency.	Increased iron intake in form of capsules and more iron in diet, eg liver, spinach.
Weak, damaged hair: breaks off easily	Overtreatment from chemicals in dyes or perms; drying out from excess use of hairdryers, etc.	Cut hair; a club cut makes thin hair look fuller. Commence intensive re-conditioning treatment; use mild shampoos. Stop any chemical processing; limit blow-drying.
Alopecia Hair loss: varies from bald spots on head to total fall-out.	Cause is not always definable; most common cause is tension or shock: blood fails to circulate properly and hair follicle dies. Sometimes hormonal or metabolic change can induce hair loss; it is not uncommon during and after pregnancy.	If the cause is stress-related, prevention is better — and easier — than cure. With massage and special treatments from a trichologist, hair grows back in most cases, and initially can be white or grey, although colour eventually returns.
Premature greying	Shock and stress, which affect formation of pigment in hair. This is a gradual process; hair *cannot* turn grey overnight.	Best cure is to relax; massive doses of brewer's yeast have slowed down greying process and restored colour in new hair.
Dandruff White flakes in the hair are scalp cells which are sloughing off faster than normal; this condition is easily confused with shampoo deposit forming crust on scalp through inadequate rinsing.	Causes are diverse and not easily diagnosed: chiefly stress, bad diet or wrong hair-care.	Specialised dandruff shampoo; try several if condition persists as, like all medicaments, effectiveness decreases with regular use. These shampoos are fairly harsh on hair so always follow with conditioner. In some cases, treatment with UV lamp, just a couple of minutes daily, has proved successful. Watch diet. In severe or recurrent cases, see specialist.

New ways to make waves

These are the exciting new alternatives to hairdryers, heated rollers, etc: natural ways of introducing anything from loose waves to tight curls into wet or damp hair. They can be left to dry naturally, and so are better for your hair. Experiment with each until you find the methods that work best for you — everyone's hair reacts differently!

USE GIANT SILVER METAL CLIPS to make a sleek, shoulder-length bob. Divide wet hair into large sections all over the head; curl each section towards the face and secure with a large clip (not too close to scalp or the clip may leave an indent in hair). When hair is dry, remove clips and brush hair with a large, spiral styling brush to flip under at ends.

USE PIPE CLEANERS to make masses of curls. Twist a section of hair right to the end. (The smaller the section, the tighter the finished effect.) Take a pipe cleaner (or two twisted together for fatter curls) and wind twisted section along pipe cleaner so twists are flush with one another; twist up end of

pipe cleaner to secure. Repeat over entire head. When dry, carefully untwist hair from pipe cleaner and run fingers through hair or, for a looser effect, brush through from underneath.

USE YOUR FINGERS to form a head of loose, rippling waves. Twist section of hair into a "rope" until it forms a curl at roots; secure with a grip. Repeat over whole head. When hair is dry, unpin and brush through.

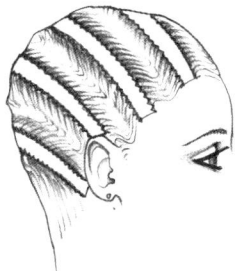

USE SCOTCH TAPE for a finger-waved, Thirties style. Press damp hair into finger waves, and use Scotch tape to anchor each one in place. When the style is dry, hold hair and gently ease tape off. If hair is very fine, or does not hold a set, apply a little setting lotion to hair before commencing.

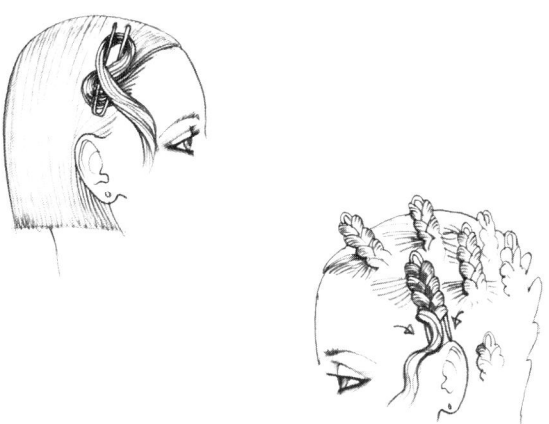

USE HAIR GRIPS AND PINS to make fine curls all over the head. Twist small sections of hair in figure-of-eights around flat *hair grips;* flip back ends to hold in place. Untwist when dry; brush through. Weave small sections of hair down the length of straight, large *hairpins*, flip back ends to secure. Untwist when dry and brush through.

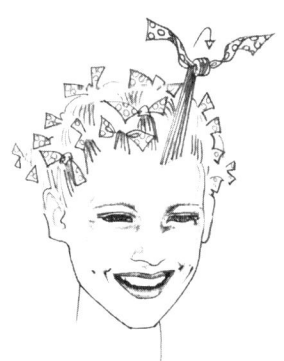

USE OLD-FASHIONED RAGS, comfortable enough to sleep in, for a head of undulating waves. Cut old sheeting or similar into strips each measuring 25 cm by 5 cm (10 in by 2 in) or, if hair is just damp, you could use folded tissues. Wind end of each hair section around rag, then roll up to root; tie ends of rag together. The more rags you use, the more waves! If you want a wave at ends of hair only, just twist ends around rags and leave length of hair free. In the morning, untie rags and brush through.

USE YOUR FINGERS for a crimped, Pre-Raphaelite effect. Plait sections of hair from crown to root; the smaller the sections and the firmer the plait, the tighter the "crimp". Undo when dry. Run fingers through hair or, for a looser look, brush hair through from underneath.

Hair-raising techniques

These are the big hair pickups. . .the simplest ways to twist and knot hair into exciting shapes. If you've ever wanted to put your hair up with just one big grip, like they do in the movies, you can learn now!
Note To hold wisps of hair that escape from knots etc, spray a little setting lotion on to a clean toothbrush, and stroke wisps into place.

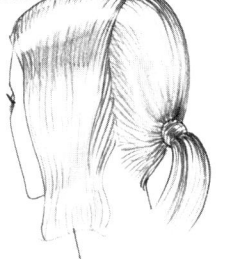 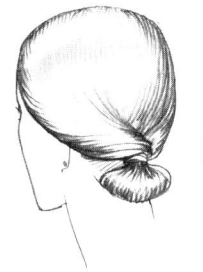

CLASSIC CHIGNON Make a parting across crown, and brush centre back section into a ponytail at nape of neck, securing with a fabric-covered band. Twist side sections alternately around band to cover it; secure with small pins. Tidy chignon by rolling over fingers, brushing and securing at base with hairpin.

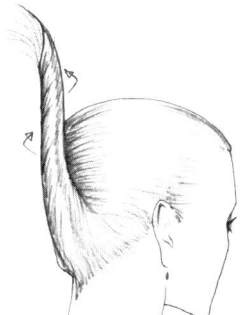 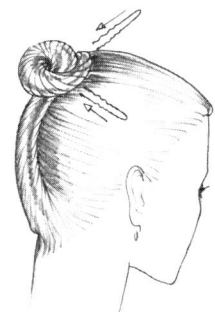

FRENCH TWIST Brush hair back as you would to make a ponytail, but twist ponytail upward toward crown. Twist remaining length at crown to form a knot; secure with hairpins.
TOP KNOT Brush hair toward crown to make a ponytail on top of head; secure with fabric-covered band. Twist ponytail around to form knot to cover band; fasten with pins.

How to use combs in hair

Hair combs are the most indispensable accessory for long hair: you can flip your hair up with just one large, curved comb, or you can sweep hair back off one side of face using just one decorative comb for an instant evening hairstyle. If combs fall out of your hair, chances are you are using them incorrectly. Here's how to make them grip: Use comb to smooth hair back. Insert in hair in the opposite direction you want comb to go, right side to head. Reverse so teeth grip hairs. Push in securely.

Emergency measures

If your hair is less-than-clean, and there's no time to shampoo, take your choice from these hair-savers.
- Cover bristles of your hairbrush with an old stocking. Brush well through hair. Much of the dirt and oil will be absorbed by the stocking.
- Talcum powder is just as effective as dry shampoo in absorbing dirt and debris in hair. Be sure to brush through hair well: the aim is to brush out powder along with grease, not leave it in to "fluff up" the hair!
- Make several partings in hair; secure with large pins. Rub cologne-soaked pads of cotton wool along partings to absorb oil and dirt; brush hair through.
- Save time by setting your hairstyle as you have your bath: wind hair around rollers and let steam "set" hair. This is a good alternative to using electrically-heated rollers.

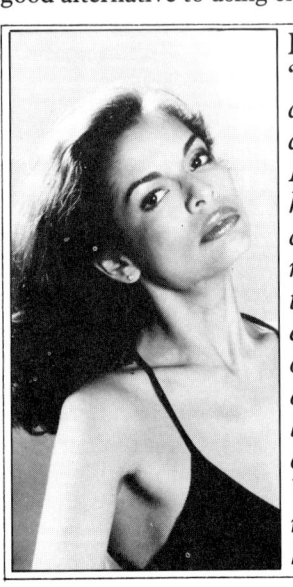

BIANCA JAGGER, *celebrity: "I like a very natural look for hair and never use rollers or blow-dryers because they are so drying. I sometimes have a colourless henna treatment at Leonard's to add a shine and on holiday I give my hair an almond or coconut oil treatment to counteract the drying effects of sun and sea. I heat the oil, comb it through, wrap a towel around my head and leave it for as long as possible. Then I wash the oil out with a mild shampoo. When I want a dressy look, I tuck real little white flowers into my hair."*

Ten experts give you hot tips for great hair

GREGOR OF SCHUMI "Colouring just the tips of layered hair, using any shade of red, give a marvellous glistening effect; molten gold on blonde hair looks terrific. The advantage is that the colour can be cut out when you're tired of it!"

CHRISTINE OF MANE LINE "Precision cutting is vital. Fine, English hair needs blunt cutting. Razor cutting is terrible for hair; it breaks the cuticle (outer layer). If you look at razor-cut hair under a microscope it's frightening! You can achieve the same effect as a razor cut, without the damage, by 'thinning' hair with points of scissors."

HARRY KING OF NEW YORK "If your hair is short, instead of setting it, apply setting lotion to wet hair, and comb through. Carry on with your make-up. When hair is dry, you'll find the lotion will have given your hair enough body to make it manageable. You can them 'mould' hair and push it around with your fingers to make a great shape."

MICHAEL OF MICHAELJOHN "Hair that looks shiny and healthy is essential, whatever the style. You should condition your hair after *every* shampoo, especially if it's been permed or coloured. Looking after your hair is as important as looking after your skin: you should take just as much time and trouble!"

SAM AT MOLTON BROWN "If you leave hair to dry naturally, towel-dry by gently pushing hair in an upward direction from roots to ends: that 'lifts' roots to add bounce. Drying hair from roots to ends will make it shinier, too. When hair is just damp, use the heat of your hands to curl hair in a more controlled way: squeeze hair with hands to coax it into the shape you want."

VIDAL SASSOON "Try this for glorious body and shine: Combine whipped egg whites, powdered skim milk and processed wheatgerm oil in sufficient quantities to make a paste. Apply to hair and leave on for thirty minutes before washing out."

SIMON AT SCHUMI "For a speedy, fun change of style use coloured fake hair swatches and plaits to match whatever you're wearing. Slick hair back from the face with Max Factor's Clear Gel Hair Dressing (for men). If your hair's long, tie it in a neat knot at the back; pin swatch on to cover ends. If hair's short, just comb through and pin the piece on anywhere you like!"

ELLIS OF ELLIS HELEN "Shampooing hair daily keeps it looking lively and bouncy. Why do people still seem to think that daily washing ruins hair? Shampoos today are so mild they won't dry out the hair. If you have a perm, or your hair goes 'flat' after sleeping on it, a quick shampoo in the morning will revive the style."

JOHN FRIEDA "Perms are a marvellous way of giving hair body and movement. Many women fight the idea because they think permed hair has a 'set' look, but now perms are so gentle and relaxed they can give the most natural-looking waves. Drying permed hair correctly is vital: Don't comb hair through, which separates curl and inclines hair to frizz; gently coax hair into shape, and when it's totally dry, brush through."

RICCI BURNS "Treat your hair to a wonderful cut and shampoo hair before you go out. Hair looks terrific when it's sparkling clean, simple and shiny; you can't improve on it. In summer, wear hair glossed with gel or pistachio wax; then you can add something amusing, like a flower."

Perming:
How to make it a success

Whether you want just more body, rippling waves or a full head of glorious curls, a permanent wave can supply them. The hair is literally restructured to a new shape with the use of chemical solutions and setting rollers, and the effect is irreversible until the perm grows out. It is strongly advised that you go to a professional who, apart from being able to tell which type of perm is best for your hair, can set your hair to the style you want: the way the rollers or perm rods are placed decrees just where the curl or waves will be.

The perming process

The hair is softened with a waving solution to make it receptive to its new shape. Special perming rods or rollers, sometimes together with fine papers applied to the ends of the hair to prevent frizz, are used to set hair; the size of the roller will govern the size of the curl or wave. The perming lotion is rinsed off and a second lotion — the neutralizer — is applied. This "refirms" the hair so it takes on the shape formed by the rollers.

Watchpoints

● Don't have a perm if: your hair has been overprocessed by tinting or bleaching; your hair or scalp are in bad condition. Your hairdresser will advise you if your hair is able to withstand perming. If he says no, don't traipse from salon to salon until you find one who agrees — perming damaged hair can result in break-offs and even hair falling out.

● Try to have a test first, on a small section of hair (nape of neck will not show), to see how a perm will take on your hair. Degree of curl varies with products, size of rollers, and your hair, so having a test lessens your chances of having an unsuccessful perm.

● Before a perm, treat your hair to a good conditioning treatment — and a good haircut.

● Even the mildest perm lifts colour on tinted hair. If you want to have both, and your hairdresser can tell you if it's possible on your hair, have the perm a few weeks *before* a tint.

● Think seriously before you decide to have a perm; it is important to realise that the structure of the hair is permanently changed, and that the effect is irreversible.

After-care

Permed hair is more vulnerable; you need to look after it well to keep it in good condition.

● Don't use a hairdryer for at least two days after your perm, as it will weaken the perm.

● Give hair regular conditioning treatments.

● Shampoo hair often to keep hair bouncy; no amount of shampooing can "wash out" perm!

Straightening hair

This process is simply a perm in reverse: large rollers slightly stretch the hair to straighten out curl. It is tricky to do and should *not* be attempted at home. Creams that are purported to straighten hair should be avoided, as they are extremely damaging. Instead of straightening hair, make the most of what you have: with the right cut and care, even the frizziest hair can look great.

HAIR COLOUR

Having your hair colour changed can be the biggest ego booster there is. whether you're a safe mouse not daring to change, a bleached-out blonde wondering what went wrong, or a redhead who's recently discovered henna, you'll want to know how you can make your hair colour one of your biggest beauty assets.

The chemical colourants:
Temporaries and tints

COLOUR RINSES are the mildest form of hair colourant: they coat each hair with colour, and do not alter the structure of the hair in any way, but simply wash out after each shampoo. Colour rinses are formulated as shampoos, setting lotions, or after-shampoo rinses. As they are so mild, the effect on the hair is very slight: they can add warmth to dark hair, bring out red lights, help mask grey hair or soften brassy tones.

Advantages   Easy to use at home
                  Easy to remove
                  You can experiment each time you wash hair

Disadvantages Can dull hair

Can rub off on to clothing and pillowslips

SEMI-PERMANENT COLOUR partially penetrates the hair cuticle — the hair's natural coating — and lasts for approximately six weeks. Colour change can be quite noticeable, but dark hair cannot be made lighter. The lotion or mousse is applied after shampooing and left on the hair for up to thirty minutes. You can use semi-permanent colour at home, but do be sure that it contains no peroxide; sometimes labels can be deceptive. Follow instructions accurately and wear rubber gloves; rub a barrier cream, like Vaseline, around the hairline before you begin so that the dye does not stain skin.

Advantages   A good way of experimenting with hair colour prior to tinting hair

Adds a sheen to hair

Can be used to liven tinted hair between root touch-ups

No regrowth: colour simply fades out

Disadvantages Cannot be used on damaged or porous hair, or patchy effect will result. (Test porosity of hair by pulling out one hair from head when wet; if hair stretches and doesn't break when pulled at either end, hair is porous.)

TINTS are permanent hair colours that penetrate the cuticle of the hair and so alter the hair's structure. It is true that tinted hair is more susceptible to damage, but with the right after-care, there should be no deterioration in the quality of the hair; in many cases, fine hair gains body and frizzy hair becomes less so! However, tinting is a serious step and should only be taken if you are prepared to spend time and money on regular touch-ups of root regrowth.

Although tinting hair can alter colour radically, it is never recommended to change from three or four shades lighter or darker than your natural colour; two or three shades lighter than your natural colouring is ideal. To help you decide on the colour that's right for you, look at women with similar complexions to yourself whose hair you admire; try on wigs, or use a semi-permanent first. Once you have decided to have your hair tinted, try to go to a professional. Although tinting is costly at a salon, your hairdresser will be able to tell you if your hair is in good enough condition for a tint. He will also help advise you on your colour choice, and is of course more of an expert than you in the tricky process of applying tint. Should you not be happy with the result, he is better equipped to deal with corrective treatment than you! When you have hair tinted, use daylight to look at colour rather than the artificial lights of a salon.

Prior to having hair tinted, a patch test for possible skin allergy is essential: you could be allergic to the perfume,

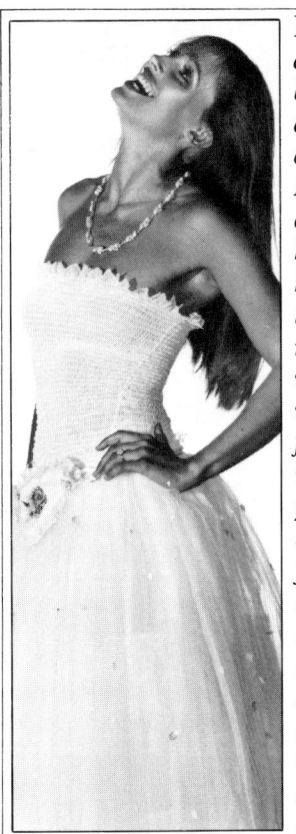

LYNDALL HOBBS, *celebrity and film director: "My hair is the bane of my life! It's long and fine and needs gentle treatment. Once every six weeks I go to Philip Kingsley, the trichologist, for a conditioning treatment, and I use his products at home. I also take his vitamin and brewer's yeast tablets to keep my hair strong. I never brush my hair, but use a wide-toothed tortoiseshell comb; when my hair's wet I just run my fingers through and leave to dry. If it gets tangled I apply conditioner, pile it all under a shower cap and do something vigorous — like frantic exercising — to heat the scalp! I cut my fringe with nail scissors and have a trim once in a blue moon because my hair grows so slowly. I am too terrified to do anything to the colour because when I was twelve I slapped on the peroxide and my hair turned orange!"*

peroxide or chemicals in the dye itself; serious skin eruptions can result in tint allergies. A small amount of tint is applied to a patch of skin behind the ear or in the crease of elbow, and should be left on for forty-eight hours. If there is no reaction, it is safe to go ahead. This process should be repeated after each retouch, as an allergy can suddenly develop to a tint you have been happily using for years. It is a good idea when you are first tested for allergic reaction to give the hairdresser a cutting of your hair for him to test with your chosen colour, within that forty-eight hour period.

The tinting process is as follows: Hydrogen peroxide is mixed with the required dye to activate the colour, which is then applied to the hair with a special tinting brush and left for a minimum of twenty minutes; heat speeds the process. The hair is then thoroughly shampooed. It is essential that all the tint is washed out, otherwise oxidisation will result, ie colour will alter on contact with the air. All hair tints oxidise to some extent and it is usually necessary to have the whole head retinted every few months to regain intensity of original colour.

Advantages   Can obtain total colour coverage

Disadvantages Needs considerable upkeep: mild, non-medicated shampoos, regular conditioning treatments; root regrowth needs to be tinted about once a month
Time-consuming

BLEACHING strips natural pigmentation from hair and so lightens it. High-volume peroxide is mixed with bleach and left on hair to "lift" colour. The process is not recommended by good hair salons as it results in a flat, bland colour; if you want to go blonde, consider highlights instead.

Advantages None
Disadvantages Hair colour lacking in depth; does not look natural
Weakens hair and makes it more vulnerable to breakage

HIGHLIGHTS/LOWLIGHTS Both of these colour processes are similar, in that small sections of hair are treated with tint to give the overall effect of streaked hair. For classic highlights, several strands of hair are picked out at a time, tinted, then wrapped with tinfoil to separate from untreated hair. The result is of finely-streaked hair that looks very natural: note that true blondes have many different colours in their hair! Lowlights use a lower volume peroxide and are used to enrich darker hair

Advantages Can achieve very natural effect
Hair only needs to be retreated every six/nine months, as there is no discernible regrowth
Less likely to damage hair than overall bleaching
Disadvantages The most expensive hair salon treatment
Very time-consuming: can take several hours to highlight a whole head

The natural colourants: Herbals and hennas

In the last five years herbs, flowers and, in particular, henna, have all gained favour in the hair colourants field. Their advantage is that they are "natural" sources of dye and so cannot harm hair as bleaching or tinting can; they add shine and lustre to the hair. Their disadvantages are that results cannot be accurately predicted, and, apart from henna, the colour effect on the hair is slight. The following are the most common that you can use at home. To make a herbal infusion, steep flower heads or herbs, fresh or dried, in boiling water for at least ten minutes before using as an after-shampooing final rinse.
CAMOMILE brings out highlights in light brown hair, and adds blonde highlights to fair hair; you can better see results after several applications.
MARIGOLDS give golden lights to blonde hair.

RHUBARB ROOT is probably the strongest herbal hair lightener. It lends golden tones to mousey hair, and chestnut tones to black. Add boiling water and boil root for up to an hour. Leave infusion to cool; use as final rinse.
ROSEMARY brings out rich lights in dark hair.
SAGE has a darkening effect on hair; it is particularly good for masking grey hair.
HENNA is a powder crushed from the leaves of the henna plant. Neutral henna, used solely for conditioning the hair, is from the first-year growth of the plant, while leaves are still colourless. It is scarcer than red henna and therefore more expensive. After the first year, the leaves yield the red dye which has become so popular as an at-home method of making hair warmer and redder in tone. Depending on colour of hair, and amount of time left on head, henna can turn hair fiery red if the hair is light brown, and make dark brown hair look marvellously rich and coppery. Henna is best on dark heads — and is definitely not for blondes, grey hair, bleached or tinted hair. It is sensible to test henna for colour response on a hair cutting first.

To apply, mix enough henna powder with hot water to form a malleable paste. Apply over entire head with tinting brush; leave out your front hairline, which is naturally lighter than rest of hair. Leave henna on hair for thirty minutes to one hour according to intensity desired, but apply to hairline in the last ten minutes. Shampoo out well. After first application, only reapply to roots. Be sure to keep henna off your face: it's used as a decorative skin stain in Morocco!

For henna highlights on dark hair (at a salon), Daniel Galvin suggests tinting strands with light blonde tint. Tint should not be washed off, but henna then applied to whole head and left as usual before shampooing out. The dark hair becomes chestnut, with coppery-chestnut overtones.

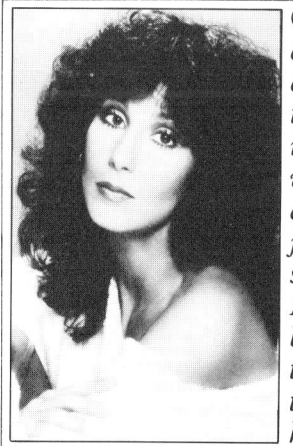

CHER, *singer: "The only thing I ever regretted in my whole life was cutting my hair. It went from over three feet in length to about an inch and a half! What happened was that I decided to shorten it and get a perm, and the result was just horrible. It made my hair like straw. So to get rid of all the perm, I had to cut down to the scalp. I've been wearing wigs now so I'm not too upset, but cutting off my hair is the only action in my life I wish I hadn't taken."*

Daniel Galvin, the world's top colour expert, answers your queries

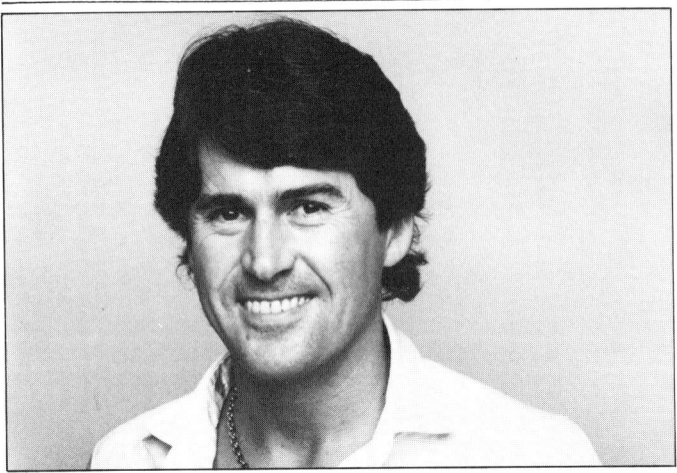

If there is a hair colour problem on a TV or film set, Daniel is the person flown in to solve it. He's dyed every celebrity's hair from Anouk Aimée to Zandra Rhodes, converted Albert Finney's hair from mouse to black in *Murder on the Orient Express* and even given a blue sheen to a black horse! Daniel has written a book for other hairdressers to learn from his techniques, and has the only hair salon in England that specialises in the colour and condition of hair*. Says Daniel on hair colour: "Most hair colour mistakes are made by clients 'leaving it to the hairdresser' and then wondering why the colour isn't the way they imagined it. You should know what the various colour processes involve so you can explain exactly what you want! Remember that hair was never intended by nature to be a beauty asset: *everyone* can have hair colouring more flattering and beautiful than nature ever intended." Here, Daniel answers the questions Cosmo readers most often ask about hair colour.

Q *How harmful is tint to hair?*
A As long as instructions are followed accurately, tint should do no harm to your hair. However manufacturers often state on home tinting packs that after the development time of tint — thirty to forty-five minutes, according to the product — the pigment stops working. They neglect to state that the *peroxide* in the tint carries on working all the time, however long the tint

is left on the head! So colour left too long on the hair creates what I call "burn out", where the pigment stops acting, but the peroxide continues: the result is brittle, damaged hair. Tint is also harmful to hair if applied to the whole head every time, and the colour is never even: for example, if mid-brown tint is used, the roots will be medium brown and the already tinted hair will be dark brown; this is called "build-up". Tint should be left on roots for twenty to thirty minutes, and then combed through to ends of hair for only ten to fifteen minutes.

Q *Is there a colour build-up with semi-permanent rinses?*
A Yes. At first, semi-permanent rinses are marvellous for the hair, but the colour is reapplied before previous application has faded out, so the colour eventually becomes deeper and brighter.

Q *Can I tint hair at home?*
A If you want to go only one shade darker or lighter, and you follow the manufacturer's instructions carefully, it should be fine. Beyond that, I'd advise you to go to a professional. Never shampoo in tint, because that way you cover entire head each time you colour, and build-up results. Instead, use the sectioning-off method with a tinting brush, and get a friend to help for the back of your hair!

Q *My hair has been overbleached. How can it be corrected?*
A The condition of the hair has to be improved before any colour correction is attempted. Hair can be so overbleached it literally falls apart: it's exceptionally stretchy when wet and feels slimy in texture when dry! Cut it off to as short as you can bear, and concentrate on intensive conditioning treatments to keep hair on the scalp. To temporarily veil the bad colour, apply water rinses at each shampoo. Only when the hair is in better condition can you apply anything stronger. It's best not to allow hair to get into this condition: never have your whole head bleached — highlights look far more effective.

Q *What can I do to disguise prematurely grey hair?*
A When hair develops a salt-and-pepper look the client invariably asks for a tint. This is unnecessary, because the salt and pepper streaks make natural lights in the hair: they just aren't the right shades! I prefer to use a semi-permanent rinse; for instance, if hair is medium brown, I use a light golden brown semi-permanent which will tone the grey hairs down to one shade lighter than rest of head, so result is attractive, gentle highlights. For a very small amount of greying hair, accompanied by a flat, natural colour on rest of head, I use tinted highlights in the *original natural* colour, which lifts the base colour and gives movement – so detracting from the grey hairs!

Q *My hair is bleached but when I go in the sun it becomes very brassy-looking. What can I do?*
A Let's say your hair was lightened with bleach to canary

The Daniel Galvin Colour Salon, 59 George Street, London W1; 01-486 8601

yellow, and then toned down with tint to beige/blonde; when you sit in the sun, the artificial pigmentation "lifts" rapidly, leaving the peroxide base! Sea water and chlorinated swimming-pool water have the same effect. I always tell clients with tinted hair to cover their hair with hats or scarves in the sun, and rinse hair thoroughly after sea or pool dips. Alternatively, sun shields which you slick through hair to protect it from UV rays are very effective.

Q *I thought that if I used a semi-permanent rinse stronger — by using twice as much and leaving it on for longer — it wouldn't fade so quickly. Why doesn't it work?*

A Using twice the amount of semi-permanent colouring won't make any difference at all. If you leave it on for twice the usual time you will add colour depth, but after thirty minutes it stops reacting. Leaving it on for the whole day won't give a stronger colour! Semi-permanents always fade in the same time lapse.

Q *I want to switch from my boring brown hair colour to blonde — what's the best way?*

A Your hair would have to be bleached to lift it to a blonde shade, but the result would be a matt blonde colour with no depth. It's important to consider your skin and eye colouring with such a dramatic change. If you have brown hair, you probably have brown eyes; it's rare to see the blue eyes of a blonde on a brunette. I've seen dyed blonde hair "drain" the colour of the skin and make the eyes look smaller; I'd suggest instead that you make hair only a couple of shades lighter, to complement your skin tone and make your eyes look larger. I don't advocate dyeing eyebrows in an effort to make hair colouring look more believable; it never works, and the process is risky on such a sensitive skin area.

Q *Will dryers, heated rollers, etc affect my hair colour?*

A Hand dryers, tongs and heated rollers alter hair colour only if they are used indiscriminately, ie if they are allowed to burn the hair. This results in the cuticle, the outer layer of hair which holds in the artificial pigment, stripping off in parts. Where there is no cuticle, the colour will not stay in the hair. Overbleaching and overperming hair can result in damaged cuticle, too.

Q *Is it safe for hair to be tinted and permed?*

A I don't believe the two go together, if you want to keep hair in prime condition. If the client has a perm, and wants a colour change, I would prefer to use vegetable colourants or low-lights, which will not affect the condition of the hair.

Q *How can I liven up naturally blonde hair that looks dull?*

A I'd recommend tinted highlights two shades lighter than your natural colour: in other words, the shade the ends of your hair turn in the sun! Be sure to have tinted lights, not bleached lights, that will emphasise your natural pigmentation. Go to a salon that uses silver foil for highlights; blonde hair is often fine and frail, and the alternative method of highlighting — pulling strands with a crochet hook through a tight rubber cap with holes in it — can be painful, and can easily split hair.

Another way you could enliven blonde hair that has turned a little drab is to use a semi-permanent rinse in a molten gold that will bring back the natural blonde colour of your childhood.

Q *I like the fun idea of "crazy colour" — but wonder if it is harmful to my hair?*

A Crazy Colour is now a readily available salon product — not so very different from the silk dyes I used in the 'Sixties to achieve vivid green hair! Usually clients ask for flashes of colour, or just tips of hair to be coloured. If the shade required is more pastel, eg pink or yellow, the hair is bleached first and the Crazy Colour is added afterwards in the same way as a semi-permanent. The hair is not harmed because it only has to be bleached once, then Crazy Colour is reapplied once every four to six weeks. When deeper shades of Crazy Colour are used on darker hair, I put golden-brown lights in hair, then shampoo Crazy Colour on the lights.

Q *I heard recently that henna isn't so great for hair after all — is that true?*

A Henna *is* good for the hair — provided it is used correctly. There are several watchpoints. First, henna should be applied on the whole head *for the first time only* (it needs heat to activate, too) and thereafter on roots only, just like a tint. I've seen very bad cases of henna build-up where the client was having henna reapplied all over the head every time: the colour had become a harsh blue/red tone, and the hair had become coarse. Neutral henna is a marvellous conditioner; it should be left on the hair for thirty minutes, and needs no heat.

Be wary of different coloured hennas: there is only one true henna colour, and that is red. I formulated a "black" henna which is in fact a mixture of red henna and rang, a herbal dye. Together they make a blackish/brown henna which is fine for hair; many salons have evolved their own similar formulas (henna and black coffee is popular). However, there are compound hennas on the market which have a metallic salts base which is *not* good for the hair. You can apply tint over pure henna, but if you put it on over any of the compound metallic hennas, the hair literally disintegrates!

Henna "lifts" artificial pigmentation, so if you decide to stop tinting hair red and you want to switch to henna, the paste should be applied to roots only, and the rest of hair tinted down to match the roots.

So, henna is great used the right way, and disastrous used incorrectly!

MAKE-UP

Adopt the professionals' make-up techniques which can convert mousey features to cover-girl status; discover the practicalities of looking good in five minutes flat; learn how to give a jaded face instant bloom with strategic brush strokes. Master craftswoman who will reveal these tricks and more is Yvonne Gold, at twenty-two already acknowledged as the Matisse of the make-up business. Yvonne has come a long way since the days when she removed her brows with hair-removing cream. In her six years as top *visagiste* she's travelled from Tokyo to New York to make up faces of the famous such as Lesley-Anne Down, dancer Lynn Seymour, Claire Bloom and Marie Helvin. Says Yvonne, "Knowing your face — and coming to terms with it — is all-important. *Everyone* has cheekbones; you just have to know where yours are, and how to accentuate them. Follow the lines and contours of your face, and don't fight them." Putting on a face, admits Yvonne, is the biggest confidence trick of all; below, we show you how to get away with it.

Basic equipment

You can use the cheapest cosmetics if you have the right tools. Store applicators in a tiered toolbox or divided cutlery tray (wicker ones look pretty) with all your make-up, and keep brushes in a jar. Label each for speedy identification. Your fingers are useful tools, too: use them to blend shadows, apply light liquid foundations, smudge on lip gloss. Learn to work with the pads of your fingertips in swift, light strokes and keep hands clean and cool; if they are hot, holding them under lukewarm, not cold, water for a few seconds is the most effective way of cooling them.

MAKE-UP SPONGES Stock up with several of the synthetic variety. Keep them moist and seal them in protective plastic bags. Clean regularly with hot water and a mild detergent, rinsing till water runs clean.

VELOURS POWDER PUFFS Again, have several; these are preferable to cotton-wool pads which leave fuzz on lashes and skin. Clean as for sponges and use when dry.

CLEAN WHITE TISSUES To blot lipstick, hold under eye when using loose powder shadow, etc. Or, to save money, keep a roll of white toilet paper to hand.

COTTON BUDS For blending shadow, softening pencil lines, dotting foundation on face, removing smudges, etc.

SLANT-EDGED EYEBROW TWEEZERS These work closer to the skin than straight-edged tweezers.

For face

Buy brushes from art shops; ask for goat or sable hair. Clean by dusting off excess powder on tissue, and comb through hairs with a clean hair comb. Fill a glass with hot soapy water, swish brushes around and leave to soak for half an hour. Rinse well and pull into shape when wet. Dry in airing cupboard or top of warm stove. Do not be tempted to shorten the long handles of art brushes: you need the length to balance in crook of thumb and first finger for easiest application.

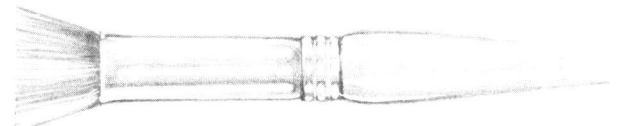

CONTOUR BRUSH Artist's brush with stubby bristles.

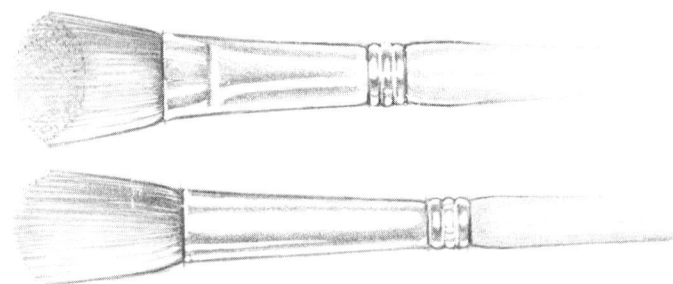

BLUSHER BRUSH Large, thick brush with long hairs and plenty of mobility: bristles should bend easily in palm of hand; ideal are Nos 5 or 8 artist's brushes (see above). Or use a fluffy blusher brush the make-up artists favour: designed for the Japanese kabuki theatre and available at ethnic shops here.

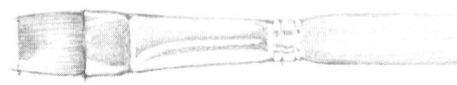

HIGHLIGHTER BRUSH As for blusher brush; optional: a small chisel-ended for highlighting smaller areas.

For eyes

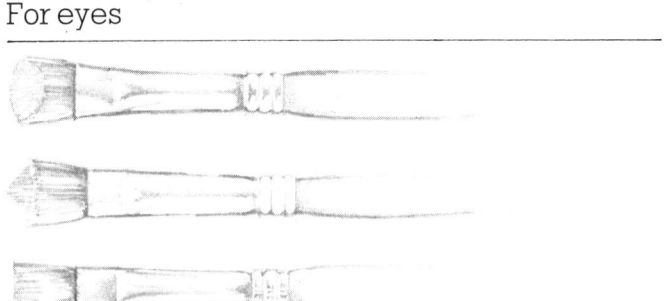

POWDER SHADOW BRUSHES Keep several, each one for a separate range of colours. Buy them from cosmetic counters or art shops. Brush width should be about 5cm. Choose from rounded, pointed or chisel-ended brushes; these last make sharper lines with edges of brush. Clean as for face brushes.

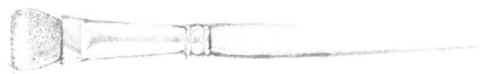

SPONGED-TIPPED APPLICATORS Useful for loose powder shadow to prevent it falling below, or into, eye. Clean by soaking for a short while before washing as above.
CREAM SHADOW BRUSHES As for powder shadow brushes. Clean by wiping off excess cream on to tissue, and rub in cleansing cream; wipe off on tissue till clean.

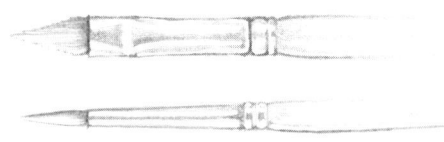

EYELINER BRUSH A small, fine brush with pointed tip; base of the brush can be flattened in appearance. Clean by washing in soap and water.

For lips

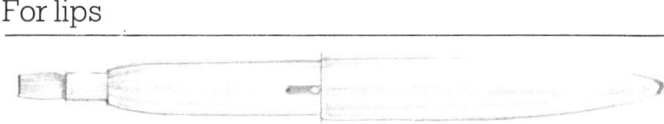

Use a cosmetic chisel-ended lip brush that is retractable, or has a protective lid. Clean as for cream shadow brushes.

Supplementary equipment

The following are used by many make-up artists and models; none is indispensable to the basic make-up kit but all are useful and inexpensive additions.

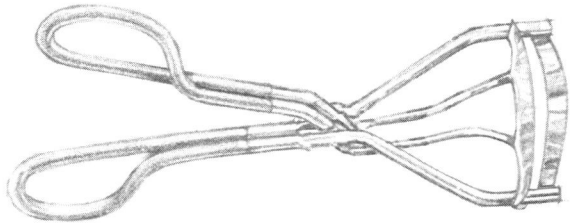

EYELASH CURLERS These lend a naturally curly look to lashes which has the effect of "opening up" the eye.
BRISTLE TOOTHBRUSH For sweeping brows into shape. Buy a travel toothbrush that snaps away in its own case to keep brush clean and in good shape. Wash the bristles regularly in soap and water.

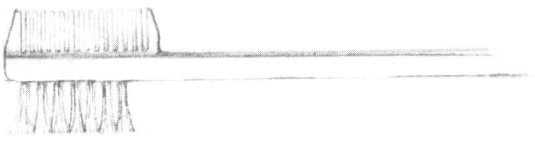

LASH BRUSH AND COMB Comb separates lashes after mascara application; brush makes them fluffier. Wash in soap and water.
PORTABLE HANG-UP MIRROR To place in suitable position for ideal lighting.

SMALL PLANT SPRAY OF DISTILLED WATER (OR SCENT ATOMISER) To set make-up so base stays looking fresh for hours.

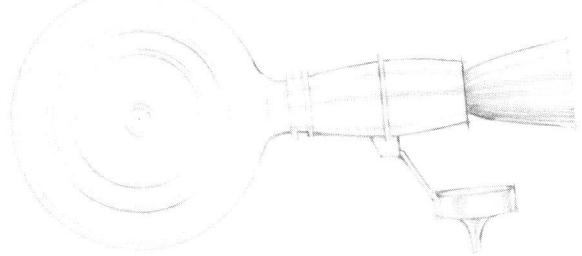

PHOTOGRAPHER'S LENS-CLEANING BRUSH For brushing and puffing off excess blusher or eyeshadow specks without smudging. Clean as for face brushes.

DOUBLE-HOLED PENCIL SHARPENER For use with all lip, cheek and eye pencils. Clean blade with surgical spirit and cotton-wool bud.

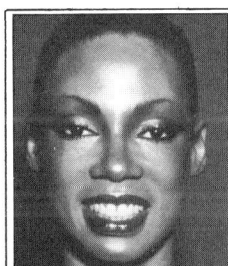

JAN STEVENSON, *model: "My basic make-up routine takes about half an hour. I spend most of that time emphasising my eyes. First I apply stick foundation over my skin to conceal large pores and tiny moles on my cheeks: I have several shades to wear at different times of the year, depending on how tanned I am! Over this base, I dust Christian Dior's Eau Sauvage beige talc, which looks better on me than conventional face powders. I think that highlighting is particularly important for dark skins, and looks best when it is not too subtle. I use a pink powder above my cheekbones, on the tip of my chin, just above my upper lip and on the centre of my browbone. I make my nose look narrow by highlighting it down the centre with gold powder. On my cheekbones I wear pinkish-brown blusher, extending the colour to my temples.*

"I shade the whole eye area except the lid: winging the colour outwards seems to make the eyes look larger and further apart. For this I use black eyebrow shadow over smudged black pencil, and a lighter tone, such as pink, below. Just under the inner corner of the eye I smudge bright blue or purple pencil, and brush pink powder highlighter over it to soften. My lower rim is defined with black kohl. I have few lashes so I apply six or seven coats of mascara, then separate the lashes with a pin. I have a large mouth and I make it look smaller by outlining with a lip brush, just inside my natural outline. Then I fill in with a strong colour. I use make-up to re-structure my face: without it you wouldn't recognise me!"

How to apply make-up as the professionals do

At first, the following make-up routine will take you a long time, but once you have mastered the principles, the process will speed up. In time, you will find that you can pare down, and adapt, the technique to suit your style.

Correct lighting

For day: Position yourself so you are facing natural light, with your mirror opposite. Do not sit in harsh sunlight, or you will tend to overcompensate with too heavy make-up.

For evening: Make up by electric light for accuracy, and then check for effect in a softer evening light, eg candlelight.

Preparation

1 Pin hair back so you can see your face shape clearly; cleanse face throughly.
2 Leave moisturiser on clean skin to settle.
3 Check brows for stragglers: remove from under, and between brows, only.
4 Line up cosmetics and applicators.
5 Wipe toner-soaked cotton wool swiftly over face to remove excess moisturiser.

Pre-base correction

Erase identations or shadows with white cream eye shadow or crayon stick; the consistency should be non-pearlised, thin and creamy. Stipple on cream and blend well with fingertips or sponge. Special watchpoints: lines running from nose to lip corners, pouches or shadows under eyes, and frown lines between brows.

Base

When you buy foundation, try it on your face, not on the back of your hand where skin tone is different. Never judge the colour of foundation by the artificial lights of a store: instead check outside, in natural daylight. Use a foundation that is beige/yellow toned, as close as possible to your skin colour. Even if you need a corrective make-up, note that two fine layers of light liquid base do a more effective cover-up job, and look more natural, than a thick cake foundation.

Apply foundation in swift, light strokes with clean fingers or a dampened sponge; blend immediately after applying to each area of skin, as it tends to dry quickly. Follow this order-of-application guide:

1 Across left cheekbone, under eye and across to temples; repeat on other side of face.
2 Along length of nose, blending up to forehead, and eyelids (this forms base for eye shadow).

3 Either side of jaw, blending away to neck.
4 Chin, gap between upper lip and nose.

Set base
Dip velours puff in translucent face powder, shake off surplus and apply to face in a press and roll motion; dust down afterwards with clean side of puff.

Contour face
With contour brush and peach/brown toned blusher, stipple on colour in a semi-circle around base of cheekbone. Contour applied to temples gives the face a more sculpted appearance; apply to any areas you wish to minimise or recede.

Colour face
Your blusher should be two shades deeper than skin; to choose correct tone, pinch cheeks: the natural flush that appears is the right colour for you. Save shocking pinks for dramatic evening make-ups. Dip blusher brush into rouge, dusting off excess on back of hand. Sweep lightly over cheekbones and temples and frame face softly around jaw and hairline. Wear blusher very high on the cheekbones to make your eyes look larger. Blusher should accentuate contoured areas. Powder face lightly to blend out any harsh edges.

Time saver: Use blusher to colour *and* contour; this needs practice to avoid a painted-doll look! Always remember to build up colour slowly and gradually — it is easier to add blusher than to remove it.

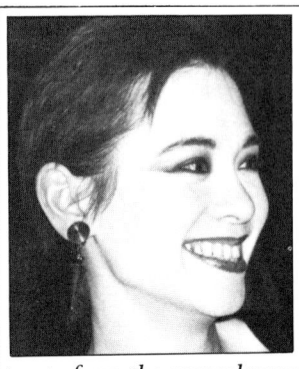

TINA CHOW, *Japanese/American ex-model and wife of restaurateur Michael Chow, says that many Oriental girls make the mistake of trying to westernise their features; cosmetics are designed to bring out the potential in a face, not to change it. "I accentuate my Oriental features by using very dark lip and eye tones, and an ivory foundation to contrast. Blusher is too much a part of the Western look and detracts from the monochromatic effect. I emphasise the elongated shape of my eyes with charcoal tones which I blend with a brush across my lids out towards my hairline; on the inside of my lids I use black kohl. I never use mascara — I know that's the ultimate sin for English girls — but it 'opens up' the eyes which is exactly the effect I do not want to achieve in my make-up. For special occasions I like a sparkly black, or dark mauve, eye shadow. I wear a bright lipstick: pillar-box red is a striking contrast against my pale skin. I find lip pencils tend to smudge, so I use a lip brush to outline, and then fill in with a brushful of colour."*

Highlight face
With highlighter brush and ivory (not white) powder, sweep over top of cheekbones and outer edge of eye. Centre highlighter on a low forehead to heighten, between eyebrows to create illusion of greater space between eyes, on a receding chin to strengthen.

Shade eyes

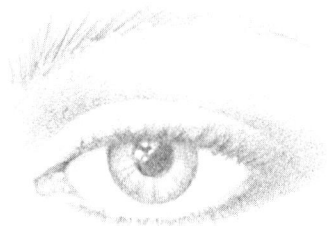

Always apply eye make-up before lip colour to avoid smudging lipstick. After every stroke of shadow, blend very well with fingertip or cotton bud to prevent any noticeable dividing lines or harsh effects.

Whether you choose colours or neutrals (and first-timers should experiment with neutrals as coloured shadows are trickier to apply), use three tones to define and contour eye: light, mid and dark. Apply in the following order, using appropriate brush:

Mid tone: In socket area, working out towards outer corner. If eyes are wide apart, shade inner corner of eye to create opposite effect; if close together, shade outer corner of lid.

Dark tone: Along base of top and bottom lashes to emphasis eye shape; to add depth to a weak socket, brush dark tone in socket so the lid appears larger.

Light tone: On inner corner of eye, on entire lid area, or middle of lid to highlight.

Fill in remaining areas with mid tone.

These are the three basic steps to follow; experiment until you find the most flattering effects, but always follow the lines and contours of your eyes; do not try to change them.

When you have mastered the eye-shading basics, try these two additional eye definers:

Eye pencil/kohl painted inside the lower lid — so that colour, not skin, is next to eye white — can be very striking. Even if you wear contact lenses you can try this effect; once you have the knack it is very simple. Use a toning, darker colour than eye shadow; kohl pencils are preferable to kohl, which needs a stick to apply and can be very fiddly. Hold bottom lid taut and slightly down with the left hand, and stroke pencil across on exposed skin from corner to corner. Soften a hard line by smudging gently with a cotton bud. You can paint on upper lid in the same way, but be careful — this could have the effect of making small eyes look smaller. For a fine line on upper lid, blink once slowly and a little of the lower lid colour will appear. Add touch of sparkle to eyes by using a coloured pencil on eyes shaded with neutrals; pale pink, peach or white pencils have the effect of "opening" the eye.

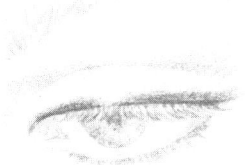

Eye liner accentuates eye shape. Always use a cake liner, so you can mix with water for the right shade. Liquid liners are too harsh. With eyeliner brush, paint liner from mid-eye to end on upper lid and, if it suits you, lower lid too. For a more cat-like effect, paint liner across entire length of lid. First-timers may find liner tricky to apply; to avoid wobbly lines, steady hand by resting elbow on solid surface. Shape eyes more subtly by dotting liner between lashes. To soften liner, brush same shade of powder shadow over line.

Shape brows

If brows are untidy, brush into shape with a dry toothbrush. Follow the natural curve, or brush upward for a wide-awake look that makes eyes appear larger. A little setting gel can be slicked on to keep them in shape. Use eyebrow pencil to supplement sparse hairs or compensate for overplucked patches. Avoid the darker shades of brown; the ideal tone is light brown with a touch of silver. Apply colour from middle of brow to end in light, feathery strokes to simulate hairs. Estée Lauder, the cosmetics queen, suggests using two toning shades of pencil for a very natural look. If the effect is too heavy, you could powder lashes and rebrush.

Mascara lashes

Apply eyelash curlers at this point, using several short, swift squeezes. You will find you need little mascara, as the curlier look gives an illusion of length and density. Make-up artists prefer cake mascara because you can control the consistency with water; wand mascaras are more convenient and some contain filaments to lengthen stubby lashes. Whichever type you prefer, follow this plan for mascara application so that lashes look natural and do not clog together:

1 Brush down from roots to tip of upper lashes, then brush upwards on both eyes.

2 Brush down from roots to tip of lower lashes; if they are long hold a rolled tissue underneath so mascara does not spot skin. If you do smudge mascara, remove with a cotton bud moistened with eye make-up remover.

3 Repeat step 1.

Make-up artists' and models' trick to separate lashes is to use a

Eight instant pick-up tricks

. . . to revive a jaded face — and morale

● Blue-tinted cosmetic eye drops make eye whites look brighter.

● Fake healthy freckles with a rust eye pencil across bridge of nose, fading out towards cheeks.

● Liven a sallow complexion with a rosy-tinted moisturiser; intensify colour on cheek "apples".

● Stroke sky-blue pencil on inside of lower lids; next to eye whites, adds a sparkle.

● Rosy blusher centred on browbone lifts tired eyes.

● Give your skin an instant tan — a great ego-booster — with a golden brown gel.

● Strategic use of blusher wakes up dull skin; dust along forehead, jawline and temples; Estée Lauder even advises a slick of blusher down the centre of nose — it works, but be sure to apply subtly!

● Desperate measure for a very apparent spot (Yvonne Gold confesses to this trick): cover spot with medicated cover-up before applying foundation and powder, then dot on dark brown or black pencil to convert to a *beauty* spot.

lash brush comb; wait until mascara has dried and comb through lashes, then brush upward to give lashes a fluffier appearance.

Define mouth

Foundation and powder should cover the edges of your mouth so an imperfect outline can be corrected. The lips should be defined with either a lip brush or a pencil. If you use a lip brush, do not overload with colour or line will smudge easily; if you prefer pencil, which is easier for beginners, keep the point sharp and choose one that tones with lip colour. First, define cupid's bow, then define upper lip from outer corners to centre, to avoid a downward droop. In the same way, define lower lip from corners to centre. If mouth tends to sink down at sides, bring lower lip line up slightly. Model Jerry Hall makes a sexy, pouty lower lip by outlining centre of lips just outside her natural lip line.

Upper and lower lips should be balanced in size: if top lip is smaller, paint just outside the natural lip line, and just inside the line of lower lip, and vice versa. An asymmetrical mouth can be evened out in the same way, with skilful corrective outlining. Add lip gloss if you wish; just a circle centred on lower lip is effective.

Final step

Assess the final effect by standing at least a metre away from the mirror — *that* is how people will see you!

HEALTH

How healthy are you? Do you take regular exercise, do you smoke or drink, do you eat balanced meals, are you around the right weight for your height? Being in good health involves all these things and more, and caring about it isn't just for the fanatics: it makes good sense for everyone because when your body and mind are working well you feel better, look better and generally get more out of life. In this chapter you will find all the facts about how your body works, what's good for it and what isn't, how to look after yourself, and where to get help and advice for the problems you can't cope with.

Cosmo women

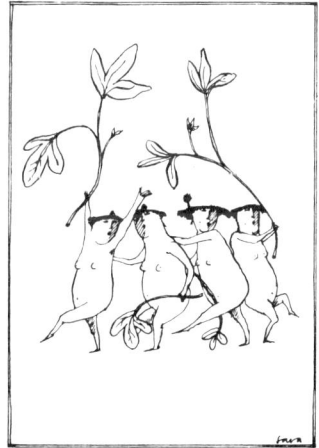

Women are highly skilled survivors, or so all the evidence has led us to believe. At all ages, almost fifty percent more men die from heart disease, cancer or accidents. Each year two percent of men under the age of sixty-five die compared with one percent of women.

It is generally accepted that women have a built-in physiological advantage over men. Clearly there must be some truth in this when we consider that even in the womb females are better survivors: more male embryos are miscarried. But be-

haviour and life-style also have much to do with death statistics. Male aggression leads to many more deaths, both among boys from adventurous play, and later from car smashes often associated with drink.

Women, on average, can still expect to live five to seven years longer than men, but it is time that the "women are better survivors" belief was, at least partially, debunked. The way in which women live may yet prove to be decisive.

They are fast acquiring male-initiated habits and stressful life-styles. It is too early to be sure what effect this will have on the incidence of heart disease and deaths during the prime of life. However, there are some pointers. Although more men than women still smoke, more men than women are giving up, and, very important, many more young women than men are starting to smoke. Deaths from lung cancer have increased more rapidly among women as they have taken up the habit.

Although the incidence of heart disease among younger women has crept up, as yet there is remarkably little research into what happens to women who work in demanding jobs, whether in factories, the professions or management. But one American study of women doctors shows that they are dying younger and from stress diseases.

Women have a strong influence on attitudes to health. Much television and magazine health advertising is aimed specifically at them, women see their doctors more often than men, and they arrange health care for their families. A man, if apart from his wife or mother, is said to behave in a way that puts him more at risk.

However, the women's movement towards equality on all fronts is causing a good deal of confusion with regard to health. We have created a society in which generally our life-style is hazardous to the health of men, and may also become so for women. Many are now acquiring the double stress of caring for a family *and* coping with a job. (Men rarely do both.) Many women manage magnificently but would also have to admit that some of their mental and physical well-being has been sacrificed. Instead, says an American report, the question we should perhaps be asking is, "Why can't men behave more like women?"

There are no easy answers. Health campaigns at present are primarily directed towards persuading people to change to a heathier life-style: smoke less, eat less, buy a pair of plimsolls and jog — your sex-life might also take a turn for the better. That is the message and the onus is on us to take more responsibility for ourselves. Being more conscious of the way we live won't actually create a generation of cheery centenarians,

but it might help more of us to keep the good health most have in our teens and twenties. Of course it is during this period, when we should actually be working out our life-style and developing good health habits, that most women abuse their bodies, laying up trouble which may be irreversible.

Some people resent exhortations to become healthier, but there seems little doubt that concern with health and well-being — and happiness, if you like — is becoming more than a passing fad. No one can force you to adopt a healthier way of life. It can only be personal decision based on your own assessment of what is known of the health risks.

Are you in good health?

Good health is difficult to define. Who possesses it? The person who cycles round the park each morning, the vegetarian, the thin person striding for the train to work or an apparently calm parent ferrying children around?

WOMEN			
Height without shoes metres	Small frame kilograms	Medium frame kilograms	Large frame kilograms
1.43	42 —44.5	43 —48.5	47 —55
1.45	42.5—46	44.5—50	48 —55.5
1.47	43 —47	46 —51.5	49.5—56.5
1.49	45 —48.5	47 —52.5	51 —57
1.52	46.5—50	48.5—54	52.5—59.5
1.54	47.5—51.5	50 —55.5	53.5—61
1.57	49 —52.5	51.5—57	55 —62.5
1.60	50.5—54	52.5—59	56.5—64.5
1.62	51.5—56	54.5—61.5	58.5—66
1.65	53.5—57.5	56 —63	60.5—68
1.67	55.5—59.5	57 —65	62 —70
1.70	57 —61.5	60 —66.5	64 —71.5
1.72	59 —63.5	62 —68.5	66 —74
1.75	61 —65.5	63.5—70.5	67.5—76
1.77	62.5—67	65.5—72	69.5—78.5
MEN			
1.54	51 —54.5	53.5—58.5	57 —64
1.57	52 —56	55 —60.5	58.5—65.5
1.60	53.5—57	56 —62	60 —67
1.62	55 —58.5	57.5—63	61.5—68
1.65	56 —60.5	59 —65	62.5—70.5
1.67	58 —62	61 —66.5	64.5—73
1.70	60 —64	62.5—69	66.5—75.5
1.72	61.5—66	64.5—70.5	68.5—77
1.75	63.5—68	66 —72.5	70.5—79.5
1.77	65.5—70	68 —75	72 —81
1.80	67 —71.5	70 —77	74.5—83.5
1.82	69 —73.5	71.5—79.5	76 —86.5
1.85	70.5—75.5	73.5—81.5	78.5—88
1.87	72.5—77.5	75.5—84	81 —90.5
1.90	74.5—79.5	78 —86	82.5—92.5

WOMEN					
Height without shoes ft in	Small frame st lb st lb		Medium frame st lb st lb		Large frame st lb st lb
4 8	6 8— 7 0		6 12— 7 9		7 6— 8 9
4 9	6 10— 7 3		7 0— 7 12		7 8— 8 10
4 10	6 12— 7 6		7 3— 8 1		7 11— 8 13
4 11	7 1— 7 9		7 6— 8 4		8 0— 9 2
5 0	7 4— 7 12		7 9— 8 7		8 3— 9 5
5 1	7 7— 8 1		7 12— 8 10		8 6— 9 8
5 2	7 10— 8 4		8 1— 9 0		8 9— 9 12
5 3	7 13— 8 7		8 4— 9 4		8 13—10 2
5 4	8 2— 8 11		8 8— 9 9		9 3—10 6
5 5	8 6— 9 1		8 12— 9 13		9 7—10 10
5 6	8 10— 9 5		9 2—10 3		9 11—11 0
5 7	9 0— 9 9		9 6—10 7		10 1—11 4
5 8	9 4—10 0		9 10—10 11		10 5—11 9
5 9	9 8—10 4		10 0—11 1		10 9—12 0
5 10	9 12—10 8		10 4—11 5		10 13—12 5
MEN					
5 1	8 0— 8 8		8 6— 9 3		9 0—10 1
5 2	8 3— 8 12		8 9— 9 7		9 3—10 4
5 3	8 6— 9 0		8 12— 9 10		9 6—10 8
5 4	8 9— 9 3		9 1— 9 13		9 9—10 12
5 5	8 12— 9 7		9 4—10 3		9 12—11 2
5 6	9 2— 9 11		9 8—10 7		10 2—11 7
5 7	9 6—10 1		9 12—10 12		10 7—11 12
5 8	9 10—10 5		10 2—11 2		10 11—12 2
5 9	10 0—10 10		10 6—11 6		11 1—12 6
5 10	10 4—11 0		10 10—11 11		11 5—12 11
5 11	10 8—11 4		11 0—12 2		11 10—13 2
6 0	10 12—11 8		11 4—12 7		12 0—13 7
6 1	11 2—11 13		11 8—12 12		12 5—14 3
6 2	11 6—12 3		11 13—13 3		12 10—14 3
6 3	11 10—12 7		12 4—13 8		13 0—14 8

We realise what it is to glow with health after a holiday and it is not difficult to analyse why this should be so. Apart from the stimulation of the change, it is probably a time when we take exercise, relax and sleep in a way that makes a health campaigner feel his message might be worth while after all. But in general many people, perhaps because of the pressure of circumstances, live life in permanent low health gear.

Your answers to the following questions form a broad guide to the quality of your health habits.

- Do you usually sleep between seven and eight hours a night?
- Is your weight between five percent under and 19.99 percent over desirable weight for height (see table)?
- Do you eat between meals only occasionally?
- Do you regularly engage in active sports, swim or take long walks, garden or do physical exercise?
- Do you drink no more than a few drinks at a time?
- Are you a non-smoker?

These questions were put to 7,000 Californians in a survey of good health practices. The results revealed that women with three or fewer good health habits are likely to die seven years earlier than those with six or seven good habits. The results were even more striking for men: life expectancy for those with three or fewer good health habits is eleven years less.

Regular breakfast and eating between meals did not seem to be quite so important for women as for men. But smoking and heavy drinking were significant risks, likewise with physical activity: the death rate was highest among those who never engaged in any regular exercise. Seven hours of sleep a night was the optimum.

Factors influencing health are very varied—heredity, stress, environmental pollution, occupational hazards may all play a part, so it is impossible to be dogmatic. Yet it is interesting that in the Californian survey the good health habits rule applied across income and living standards.

Cancer

Along with stopping smoking, action against cancer is a major preventive challenge for women, a message that may not yet have been pushed forcefully enough. For young women up to the age of thirty-four, cancer is the leading cause of death, ahead of car crashes and other accidents. It is a disease that women simply cannot ignore, nor can they assume that they need to take action only when older. Every woman should know what steps to take to avoid cancer or to make sure that it is diagnosed at the earliest possible moment.

Despite the fact that early action can save many lives, the cancer taboo is still strong. Many will not talk about the disease and they are fearful of taking advice about a suspicious symptom. Yet in the majority of cases you are likely to receive assurance that all is well, and end your anxiety. On the whole we — and this includes many doctors — tend to have a negative attitude towards cancer. There is a need for much more public health campaigning to promote the cancer awareness message. Experience in a number of other countries shows that "cure" rates for a variety of cancers are higher when there is more public understanding.

Cancer of the breast

There are about 30,000 operations for breast cancer a year and some 11,000 deaths. But cancer specialists emphasise the importance of early diagnosis: seventy-five percent of patients survive beyond five years compared with twenty-five percent of those with a late diagnosis and widespread cancer.

We do not as yet have a national screening programme for breast cancer. There is a handful of well-woman clinics throughout the country where breast-cancer screening is available, but largely the emphasis is on self-examination of the breasts about once a month, preferably after a period.

Check breast and up into armpits, by looking into a mirror, and by feeling with your hands when lying down or in the bath. Note any of the following:

Puckering or dimpling of the skin.
Changes in outline of the breast — a swelling, for instance.
Inversion or pulling in of a nipple if you have not had this before.
Bleeding or unusual discharge from the nipple.
Lumps or bumps — some people have naturally lumpy breasts, and after a while you will become accustomed to the natural feel of your breasts, and be able to appreciate any changes.

Remember that most changes have a harmless explanation — cyst, benign non-malignant lumps, scar tissue and so on. But in order to minimise risks, report any change immediately to your doctor.

For full details of self-examination a leaflet is available from your local health department or clinic, or from: Health Education Council, 78 New Oxford Street, London WC1 1AH. Mrs Betty Westgate, The Mastectomy Association, 1 Colworth Road, Croydon CR0 7AD, 01-654 8643, advises women who have had or are about to have a mastectomy — breast removal.

Cervical smears

Women most at risk of cervical cancer are those over thirty-five or younger women who have had three or more pregnancies. The disease is also linked with early sexual intercourse — nuns have the lowest risk of cervical cancer. If cancer is detected there is a very high chance of cure: try to have a cervical smear test annually, and don't delay if you have any unusual symptoms.

General cancer rules

- Don't be scared of cancer. Many common forms of cancer can be more easily cured than other serious illnesses.
- Report any of the following symptoms without delay:
  Persistent lumps or bumps.
  Changes in the appearance of any part of the body — don't forget skin and mouth.
  Development of a discharge or an ulcer.
  Impairment of movement.
  Sensory changes, including pain.
  Unusual bleeding.
- Any *persistent* symptoms, however trivial, should be reported. They might include: a cough which does not clear up; mild diarrhoea; mild indigestion; headache; unobtrusive, mild cystitis.

For further information about cancer, contact Women's National Cancer Control Campaign, 1 South Audley Street, London W1; 01-499 7532.

Smoking

Amazingly, in the next eight or nine years there may be more women who smoke than men. Although more men than women smoke now, they are giving it up in greater numbers, spurred on by anti-smoking publicity.

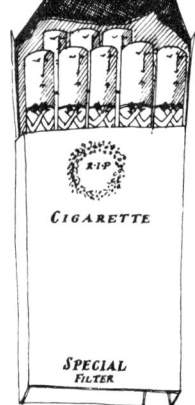

Overall, for men and women, some 60,000 deaths a year are thought to be attributed to cigarette smoking. Six thousand women a year die of cancer of the lung and respiratory passages. Smoking is probably one reason why the incidence of heart disease among women continues to increase. Among men it shows signs of levelling off. Recent reports on oral contraceptives suggest that smoking and taking the pill may increase the risk of heart disease. Bronchitis is another hazard, quite apart from the unpleasantness of smoker's cough, smoker's wrinkles and even earlier menopause. Doctors also say that smoking among pregnant women may account for the loss of 2,000 babies through miscarriages each year.

Apart from nicotine and tar, cigarettes also pump the poisonous gas carbon monoxide — present in car exhaust — into the body. This gas may replace oxygen in the blood by as much as twenty percent in heavy smokers, and it appears to increase the tendency to lay down fats in the blood vessels.

Because people may feel in good health when young they may be oblivious to the toll being exacted by cigarettes. Lungs and other organs are fantastically resilient to all types of onslaught when young (notice how skin heals more quickly, and several nights with very little sleep can, apparently, be written off). It may not be until there are symptoms of disease—breathlessness, chest pains, chronic coughs—that the damage has been inflicted, by which time it may be too late for a complete cure.

There is no doubt that giving up smoking is one of the most effective preventive health measures we can take, especially for women. If you plan to give up:
- Be absolutely certain that you do want to give up. There are no half measures if you smoke heavily. You are actually addicted to nicotine, and you are most unlikely to be satisfied with becoming an occasional smoker. You must stop altogether.
- Believe with all your might that it is possible to give up. Five million people in Britain have done so. It is torture, but it *can* be done.
- Work out a smoking strategy. You may have been smoking for years, and you will not give up a rooted addiction on a whim. One way is to set a date a few weeks ahead and work towards cutting down by de-conditioning yourself—not having favourite cigarettes in the morning, after dinner or whenever.
- Try the gadgets, acclaimed methods, chewing-gum and so on if you think they will help. Some people find they can manage better without. The graduated filters which slowly cut down the strength of your cigarettes are thought to be among the more useful aids. But none of the gadgets is a substitute for willpower.
- Don't despair if you fail. You may not have worked out your anti-smoking strategy well enough. Try another plan.
- Rewards are very important, say psychologists. Put money saved aside and buy a luxury with it. You'll feel healthier, too, once the hell of giving up has worn off.
- Women at home should plan extra activities. It is miserable giving up on your own and the temptation is to eat more.
- Give yourself a historical perspective. Smoking as a social habit is on the way out, especially among those in the higher income groups, where it began. You might as well be ahead of the game, and you are entitled to feel a little superior if you do give up.
- Be prepared for sudden cravings when you think cigarettes are a thing of the past. It may take about two years to be sure that you no longer need to smoke.
- Don't go on to cigars instead. You'll probably inhale them if you were a heavy cigarette smoker, and this is probably as dangerous as smoking cigarettes.
- Learn all about it. For further information about clinics, leaflets giving advice etc, contact ASH, 27 Mortimer Street, London W1.

Alcohol

It will probably surprise and perhaps warn most women to realise that there are as many female as male deaths from cirrhosis of the liver. Alcoholics Anonymous report an almost one to one ratio of men and women using their services.

Not only are more people drinking but more are drinking heavily than in the past. This is reflected in the growing number of people with "alcohol-related problems" — drunken driving resulting in accidents and deaths, poor performance at work, dropping out of education, broken marriage, liver and stomach disorders, and deaths from cirrhosis of the liver. "It's one long way to commit suicide," said one doctor. Possibly two to three million of the twenty million who drink regularly in this country fall into the heavy-drinker category. More than 10,000 are admitted to hospital each year with the diagnosis of alcoholism.

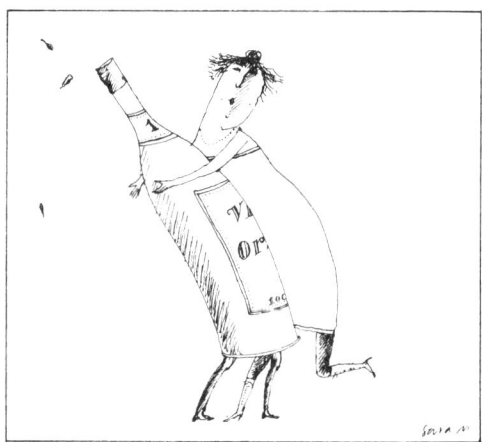

Some doctors believe that problem drinking may become so acute that it will replace smoking as the number one public health issue. Already some school-leavers and teenagers admit to anxiety about drinking. Removing the cause of the problem perhaps by reconciliation or a change of job might cure it.

As with other pleasures, moderation should be the aim. Few think we should become prohibitionists, but there is a view that we should be sterner with those who abuse drinking. One doctor maintains: "Threat of the sack might deter a problem drinker more than threats from wife or husband."

Keep drinking a pleasure:
- Check regularly that you are not gradually increasing the amount you drink.
- If you have a drink in the pub after work, don't have one at home in the evening.
- If you drink in the evening, don't drink at lunchtime.
- During the week, drink very little or not at all at weekends. Many whose jobs involve drinking adopt this approach.
- Try to eat when you drink.
- Drink small measures. Moving to large measures is a danger sign.
- Provide quality rather than quantity for your guests. Most would prefer to drink less of a better wine than too much cheap plonk.
- Don't drink to obliterate another problem. Women who drink heavily are frequently depressed, and are likely to reinforce their depression by drinking.

Facts about drinking

1 Heavy drinking means that you may still have more than the legal 80 mg per 100 ml of alcohol in your blood the following morning.

2 As little as 50 mg per 100 ml can impair judgement and driving ability. At 150 mg per 100 ml, social drinkers would feel unwell, and at 400 mg per 100 ml, they would probably be unconscious.

3 Food eaten when drinking slows down absorption of alcohol into the bloodstream, and the process of digestion speeds up its removal from the body.

4 Diluted rather than strong alcohol is less likely to irritate and inflame the stomach—hangover sickness is due to this. But dilute alcohol is absorbed more rapidly by the body and acts faster.

5 Some people can cope with high quantities of alcohol, but it is more likely that those who constantly drink heavily are not fulfilling their job potential. Most very successful people have strict drink rules.

6 There is no magic hangover cure.

Stress

One way of looking at stress is that of course it is an excellent thing, the spice of life, and that spurs us on to achieve our ambitions. The engineer has a precise definition: so much stress and his elegant tower will fall over in a high wind. Unfortunately we cannot subject humans to the same scientifically precise definitions. For one thing we are all constitutionally different, and for another we all live in different ways and in a wide variety of environments. Nevertheless, we do know that some people seem rejuvenated and appear to thrive on stress, whereas others become miserable under similar stresses and may even suffer mental or physical breakdown.

It seems as though it is not stress itself but excess of it that causes problems. A famous "life events" study showed that the stress-rating of people who suffered coronaries had increased sharply in the two years before an attack. Factors contributing to stress included such things as moving house, changing job or spouse and a bereavement, all crowded together.

As a handy definition we could say that the word "stress" summarises the balance between life-style and personality, all of which is influenced by background, childhood, sexual experiences, education, and our predisposition to illness such as coronaries, depression, high blood pressure and so on. Some experts maintain that we are becoming much too worried about stress, and that in fact such things as smoking, inactivity and being overweight are more important in the final analysis of what causes either ill-health or a feeling of living at marginally sub-healthy levels.

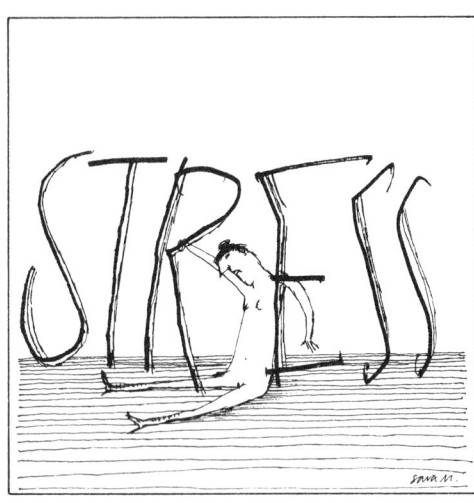

The body responds to a challenge of a stress with a primitive "fight" mechanism. Hormones pour out, blood pressure goes up, the heart pumps blood to the muscles, various fats are released into the bloodstream to provide energy, and the nervous system is finely tuned for a quick response. You may even look fierce, and possibly go to the lavatory to lose weight for the battle.

Primitive men and women, leading a much more physically demanding existence, used up the energy released, and calmed down naturally to wait for the next challenge. However, modern men and women are much less likely to use up the energy, and it may well become pent up. The fight "button" is pushed but no physical activity ensues. The fights are very often "bogies" — domestic or job worries, aggressive drivers, bureaucratic idiocy. Over the years, so the theory goes, the hormone levels get set high, blood pressure creeps up, fats are laid down and mental equilibrium is shunted towards breakdown or depression.

Coronary risk rating

Risk of heart diseases rises with smoking, high blood pressure, a family history of heart disease, overweight, high cholesterol levels in the blood, physical inactivity and age.

Without question, women are less at risk of heart disease than men. It is not until after the menopause that women begin to acquire a similar coronary risk rating. However, it is worth remembering that heart disease is still responsible for thirteen percent of deaths among women aged thirty-five to forty-four. Women should perhaps remind themselves occasionally that many are beginning to live the stressful life-styles that men have created for themselves with the present industrial society.

American research also has it that there are coronary prone personalities, so-called Type As, who are thrusting, aggressive, ever meeting deadlines and seemingly addicted to working under pressure. More organised Type Bs may actually be as successful in what they are doing but have a calmer, more thoughtful approach to life. They will take the jet a day or so before a crucial meeting. They also take a few days off afterwards instead of rushing for the homeward Concorde.

It is not a crazy idea, say the authors of this theory, for Type As to start lowering their heart risk by living like Type Bs, even to the more relaxed way they dress. They also say that although there is less coronary disease among American women they studied than among American men, there is nevertheless very much more among those falling into the Type A category.

The researchers suggest that there is less heart disease among women generally because as yet most of the Type As are less completely immersed in the type of environment that nourishes Type A personalities.

Stress equilibrium

Learn to recognise the symptoms of stress, and train yourself to take early action against the cause. Symptoms include: indecisiveness, panic, a sense of overwhelming urgency at a vast number of things to be done — women submerged by house and family may be prone to this — lack of enjoyment from usually pleasurable tasks, lowered resistance to infection, headaches, extreme tiredness, abdominal pains, loss of sex drive.

Look for causes of stress and acknowledge that they may be the cause of your problems — marital dispute, worry over children, personality clashes at work, ambition, lack of ability, money worries. You may not be able to banish them entirely but you can take avoiding action. You cannot sack the boss or hold up the bank, but you can train yourself not to react with fight hackles or a vicious circle of worry.

Know yourself and your limitations. Women are especially prone to feeling inadequate, often unnecessarily. Dwell on your good points. Talk to people. Bottling things up is a stress in itself.

If your problem is overwork, become more organised. Delegate if you can. Tackle the top-priority things to the best of your ability and leave the rest. You get more praise for producing first-rate work even if it's taken longer. There's more satisfaction in saying to hell with a household chore, and involving yourself in a creative activity.

Follow your instincts more often. Take time out regularly to ask yourself why you are doing something. Is it because you really choose to, or because it is generally recommended activity by someone else?

Don't take on more commitments if you are already at full stretch. If you do, you must drop something else.

Make rules about working late and stick to them.

Never give up something — a hobby or sport — that you enjoy for the demands of work. To some extent, stress is self-induced. If you are fit, and a reasonable weight, you are less likely to feel under pressure. Notice how top people frequent gyms and have a definite hobby.

Stress research shows that if you are so tired that you cannot solve a problem, it is better to take a swim than to sit around with your feet up. An evening out, too, is often more invigorating than collapsing in front of television.

Work out your personal philosophy, and get the rat race into perspective. Be your own woman.

Learn the art of relaxation

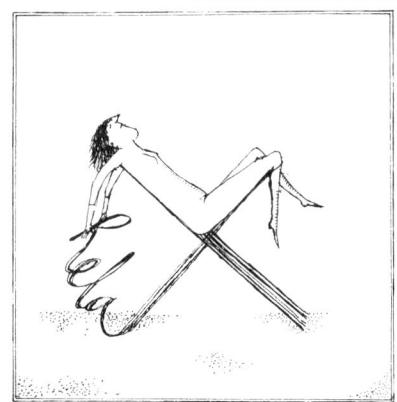

It doesn't matter how you relax. Yoga, meditation, exercises are mostly all harmless. It is what works for you that counts. There is no universal secret formula.

Deep relaxation may need to be taught. But all can practise relaxing by sitting comfortably in a chair and contracting and relaxing each muscle in turn. Learn the pleasure of a fully relaxed muscle. Concentrate particularly on muscles around the face — neck and eyes are muscle tension spots. You will gradually begin to know your muscles and pick up the signs of tension as they arise.

Relaxing is not eccentric or cranky behaviour. Don't wait for childbirth before acquiring the art. In fact, it is increasingly being taken up as an executive fashion: one management training school teaches it, and, in the City of London, relaxation classes for businessmen are a new trend.

Never rush frantically along corridors, vying with the tea trolley. Leave time to shop, so that you are not in a tense rush. Don't cook elaborate meals for guests if you are under pressure.

Learn to relax at certain moments — as you answer the telephone or look at your watch, for example. Stick a red spot on the telephone or watch to remind you.

Cat-nap if you can. This is the best way of quick relaxation.

If you feel a panicky, tense or fearful feeling starting to overwhelm you, breathe deeply and calmly, wait and allow the feeling to ride over you: do not fight it. Correct breathing is very important. One theory suggests that in moments of tension we may not breathe enough, hence we become slightly short of oxygen, and increase the tense anxious feeling.

Looking after your mind

Most people are lucky enough never to experience severe mental illness or breakdown. However, one in six women — and one in ten men — suffer each year from mental distress severe enough for them to be admitted to hospital. Further, it is likely that most people suffer to a greater or lesser degree, at some time, from anxieties, fears, depressions or nervous conditions. Or they may have a psychosomatic complaint, a chest or stomach pain, for instance, for which there is no apparent physical cause, and which may be masking a depression which in its turn is severely affecting relationships at home and at work.

People may be caught in chronic mild depression for a long time without realising it. They may even be subconsciously covering up their depression by, for example, drinking. This sort of suffering is distinct from despondence, gloom or "blues" which descend on us all from time to time. Drugs can help many types of mental disorder, but all too often the underlying problems remain.

First aid for the mind

● Take a more positive interest in mental well-being. It's more than likely your home has a book on physical illnesses but nothing about mental health, yet mind and body so influence each other that it is probably not possible to achieve good physical health without also being in reasonable mental trim.

● *Talk* about mental well-being, about relationships, your working environment, about different groups of people and how they react together. Try to understand what makes people or an organisation tick, and how inept handling of human relationships can lead to mental distress in yourself and people about you. Be constructively critical.

● Never sit on a problem threatening to damage a personal relationship even if you find it difficult to broach the topic.

● Is your environment conducive to depression? It may be time to change your job — after all, offices and organisations can have quite different characters.

● Three times more women than men visit their GPs with minor nervous disorders. Know the symptoms of depression so that you can forestall them. They include: feelings of isolation and inadequacy, lapses of concentration and memory, constant fatigue, overeating or undereating, crying, feelings of guilt and waking very early.

● Try to maintain your identity when married. Losing your sense of identity makes it harder to return to work or re-train later on if this is what you want.

● Don't overload yourself. Having a baby, getting back to work after a baby and, say, moving house all in one year can be emotionally shattering. Studies show that physical and mental breakdown occur when major life events are crowded together. Each can be enjoyable and rewarding if you allow yourself time to make the most of each.

● Try consciously not to be mentally stagnant. Ask yourself if you have changed your views on any subject in the past six months or so. It is probably a healthy sign if you have.

● Treat yourself to mental uplift. If you have never taken the office out for a drink on your birthday, now's the time to do it.

Fit for what?

Did you hear about the battery hens that escaped on to a busy road? They died not through being knocked down, but through heart attacks. Cooped up for so long, their hearts had scarcely any work to do and the sudden shock was too much for them. There is growing medical evidence that exercise is important for good health. A Swedish survey showed that those who had a reasonable amount of exercise had less heart disease. Most of modern life is geared to minimum exercise. An American professor maintains that most Californians would not be prepared to walk more than two blocks. But if you don't take your heart out for a walk occasionally, it scarcely ever has to make an effort. No wonder we become puffed on running for a bus.

Lack of challenge to the heart also means that we become tired easily, and collapse with exhaustion after a day's work.

Many people starting to exercise regularly for the first time often comment that they soon begin to feel less tired. A brisk walk, a game of squash, a swim, a cycle ride or a jog all help to dissipate the pent-up effects of the "fight" reaction, and keep the heart in trim. People worrying about feeling unhealthily overweight might reflect that if they were fit, their fat would

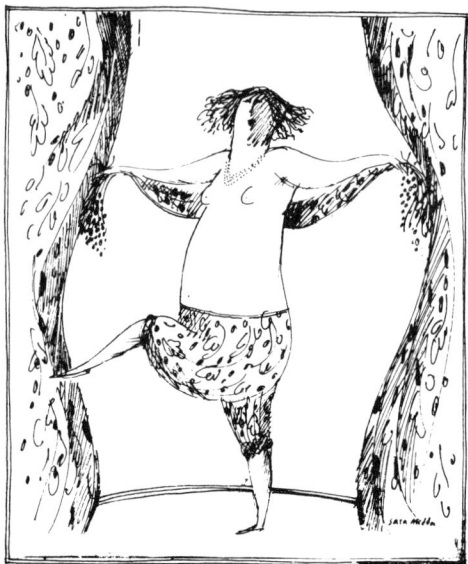

seem less like nasty flab and more like growing, healthy attractive flesh.

The big question is how to become fit. There's no doubt that women are discouraged by memories of gym and sports as presented at school. How many schoolgirls who wouldn't have been seen dead holding a hockey stick on the frozen pitch later display the kind of energy at a disco that would put Travolta to shame? And also how many who practically took their hockey stick to bed with them later use their cars for the shortest journey?

How to become fit

To become fit, that is, to keep your heart regularly overhauled, you have to raise the pulse rate consistently for about ten minutes three times a week. Skill at sports is quite unnecessary. You know that you are becoming fitter the more rapidly you recover from exercise and your heart rate returns to normal. Do not overdo things to begin with. Exercise should always be progressive.

● Brisk walking may do the trick but it has to be brisk. Al Murray, the former Olympic trainer who runs the City Gym in London, says that too often it is the dogs rather than the owners that become fit. Tennis may not be as effective as some imagine — you can actually play tennis quite slowly.

● Jogging may suit you. It certainly is one of the most efficient ways of becoming fit, yet some find it excruciatingly boring, and very unpleasant in the cold and snow. However, joggers' clubs and Sunday groups are drawing devotees.

● Essential to becoming fit is to develop a more active life generally. You cannot really be a "Sunday" exerciser only.

● *Walk* to the train, bus, school, pub, shop, doctor, friends, etc.

● Walk up stairs, down stairs and develop the habit of not groaning if required to walk half a mile down the road on an errand. Regard it as a bonus.

● Look on extra activity with regard to calories as well as fitness. If you can, build in a lot more activity. Keep an activity diary for a week, and see what extra you can manage.

In all sorts of small ways we have eliminated activity from our lives, and your aim should be to put it back. In calorie terms, as opposed to work for the heart, you utilise as many calories in walking a mile as running the same distance. You don't *have* to sweat to lose calories.

Note You should not engage in strenuous activity of any kind suddenly. It is always advisable to build up exercise gradually. If you think there may be a medical reason against exercise, consult your doctor.

The dangers of drugs

Around twelve percent of British women are thought to take tranquillizers daily for at least one month each year. While the "mind drugs" may help in the short term to get over the shock of a bereavement, broken relationship or disturbed sleep, they are likely to become largely ineffective if taken for longer periods.

They do little to get to the root cause of, say, mild depression or insomnia, and if taken for long periods, may simply be

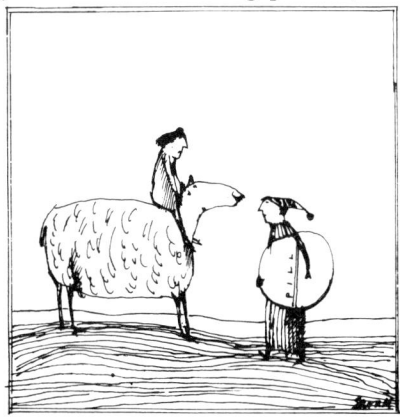

turning an anxious and basically clear-thinking person into a confused but still anxious person.

They also alter the nature of sleep so that when stopped, insomniacs should not be surprised if their sleep is disturbed as the body adjusts to normal.

Overdoses of the newer drugs such as Valium and Librium are less likely to cause death than the older barbiturates, yet there has been only a slight decrease in suicide and accidental deaths involving drugs according to an American report. The hazards of the newer drugs may not be appreciated, says the report. The active substances may linger in the body for much longer than has been realised.

We need not abandon the possibility of taking these drugs — they may, for instance, be helpful for severely depressed people. Yet we ought also to realise that mild depression, the anxiety of stress, and even insomnia are perhaps warnings of something wrong that we should react to and come to terms with rather than try to suppress with a pill. In that they are warning signs, mild depression and feelings of stress may actually be good for us.

Want your children

Given the range of modern birth-control methods and the information services and clinics available to advise on which method is most suitable, there are few excuses for any woman not availing herself of them. There need be few unwanted children: in the past twenty years development of contraceptives has given women virtually total control over their own fertility.

The chief question is which method to choose. Leaving aside the sheath — and no woman taking a responsible attitude towards birth control is likely to want to rely solely on that method — the main choice lies between oral contraceptives, intra-uterine devices and the diaphragm. Spermicide creams and foams are intended to be used as adjuncts to other methods, and not to be relied upon as safe on their own.

Ten years ago many women would have automatically chosen the pill for its virtual freedom from worry. However, there are now reservations over its use, following various medical reports in recent years. Informed women will need to weigh up the risks so far as they can be known, and make their own choice.

Balancing the contraceptive facts

For contraceptive reliability, the pill wins hands down: for 1,000 women on the pill, less than two will become pregnant each year, compared with an average of fifty for the diaphragm, and twenty for IUD users. However, when it comes to balancing the risk/benefit account, the pill does not score so highly.

Overall, there is an excess death rate of one for every 5,000 pill users, though it must be stressed that the chief risks are for those over the age of thirty-five *and who also smoke.*

More women are considering using the diaphragm as the most "natural" method, particularly if they are not too alarmed by the possibility of pregnancy. This might apply, for instance, to newly-marrieds, to couples about to get married or to women who are between children. Some doctors maintain that if the diaphragm is used with scrupulous attention to inserting it correctly, and with a spermicide, the failure rate could be at least as low as for IUDs.

The IUD has side-effects, which means that some women cannot tolerate it. However, many women who have completed their families find it an ideal method and it is gaining in popularity.

If you're considering going on the pill, or you already take it, the following guidelines may be helpful.

1 Find a good family planning clinic or doctor. Women who receive good advice appear to suffer fewer pill side-effects and are less likely to give up because of anxiety about side-effects.

2 Over the age of thirty-five: reappraise method of contraceptive. Continuous use of the pill appears to increase risks of major hazards in older women, especially if you smoke and have other heart disease risks such as overweight and high blood pressure.

3 Ages thirty to thirty-four: reconsider method with doctor if on the pill for a long time and if you smoke.

4 Under age of thirty: probably safe to continue, but cut out smoking.

5 Check that you are using the lowest-dose pill (low oestrogen content) that suits you. Check this with your doctor.

6 Make absolutely certain that family history is not a risky one — that is, immediate history of heart disease, high blood pressure and so on.

7 Make sure you have regular checks for blood pressure and general contraceptive advice.

8 If happy with method other than the pill, stay put.

Sterilisation

This is the fastest-growing contraceptive method. Up to 100,000 men a year are thought to be seeking vasectomies in this country. Because sterilisation for women is a more complicated procedure, there are fewer women than men who wish to be sterilised. The pattern for the future may be that if women have borne the responsibility for contraception early on, it will be the man's turn once families are complete, especially if, as seems the case, the pill holds extra hazards for older women.

Inform yourself

Ring or write to Family Planning Information Service for name of nearest family planning clinic, and for information about every aspect of birth control and VD. FPIS also has details of private vasectomy clinics.

GPs may carry out a family planning service, but if you are having an IUD fitted, make sure that your doctor has plenty of experience in doing so. Reports show that success with IUDs can have much to do with the skill of the person inserting it.

As much sex as you want

"Have as active a sex-life as you can," says one London GP. People who have happy, unfrustrating sex-lives are likely to be contented and fulfilled generally. An unhappy sex-life creates a stress that makes life difficult even if work and so on are satisfactory.

However, for all that is written about sex, many are still very inarticulate when it comes to communicating with their sexual partners. They are also filled with worries that to a large extent are foisted on them through sexual images and fantasies suggested by the media.

Sex help

● More GPs take an interest in psychosexual matters than in the past — many attend training courses. You'll probably know from your own doctor/patient relationship whether or not he or she will be helpful.

● National Health Service family planning clinics may run a session or so a week for psychosexual problems.

● The FPA run a number of psychosexual clinics.

● Ring the FPIS — anonymously — for information about these and sexual matters generally; 01-636 7866.

●The National Marriage Guidance Council may be able to help. See telephone book for nearest branch.

● The Association of Sexual and Marital Therapists will supply a list of private psychosexual therapists and centres. Fees may range up to £20 a session. Send large SAE to 79 Harley Street, London W1.

Gynaecological guide

Knowing your own body

Women spend far more time in their doctors' surgeries than men, not because they are neurotic, but because of the sheer physical consequences of possessing tubes, ovaries and genital organs that are buried deep within the body. Quite apart from babies, there are textbooks full of "women's conditions". By comparison, men, with their external reproductive organs, have much less to worry about.

In recent years there has been increasing emphasis on women becoming better acquainted with their own bodies. Some women's groups advise self-examination of the vagina and cervix. Why should the cervix be such a mysterious entity, they argue, with its presence confirmed only when bumped into during intercourse or when dilating to release a baby. It can actually be seen using a speculum — like a pair of scissors with broad blades — and a mirror. Not everyone will want to get involved in this kind of self-examination but for those who do, more information about this can be obtained from the *New Women's Health Handbook* (Virago, £1.95) which also has a useful list of women's health groups, and from *Our Bodies, Ourselves* (Penguin, £3.50).

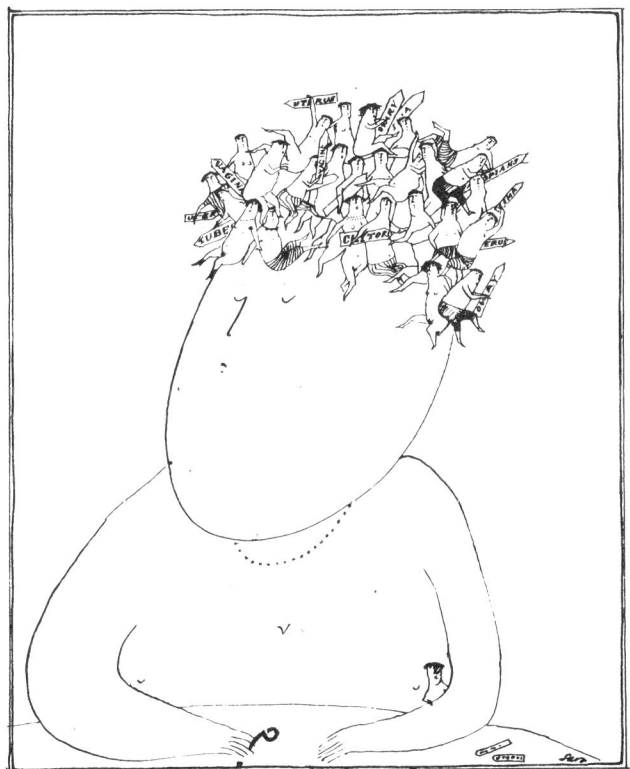

Knowing more will help women to spot the symptoms of trouble earlier, and also to react sensibly rather than fearfully. Even over such things as vaginal secretions, many women worry as to whether or not they are normal. Yet observations and comparing notes with others will reassure that there is a tremendous variation, both between women and individually, in the flow and consistency of these secretions. There is a monthly pattern, and around the time of ovulation the mucus becomes thin and stringy. Using this knowledge, some people are able to pinpoint their ovulation precisely.

With regard to monthly mood changes, while no one would want women to become preoccupied with the monthly ebb and flow of hormones, it may well be that with the pressures of jobs and running homes, women do not pay enough attention to their own body chemistry. There may be days in the month, usually around a period, when women learn from experience that it is best to avoid strenuous activity.

Symptoms to take to the doctor

Any unusual bleeding, from the external or internal genitals.

Abnormally heavy menstrual bleeding.

Missed periods.

Persistent pain, which you know from experience is not menstrual, in the abdomen or outer genitals.

Any lumps or bumps, or changes in genital anatomy.

Vaginal discharges that are clearly distinct from normal mucus. Usually obvious from offensive smell and colour.

Pain during intercourse.

Persistent vaginal itching, warts — usually white and feathery — or rashes.

Pain when urinating.

In most of these cases there will be a very simple explanation and remedy. However, a small proportion of these symptoms may have a serious cause, and would need further investigation. As with breast symptoms, do not delay seeing your doctor.

Premenstrual tension

It may well be legitimate criticism of doctors that because the majority are male, they have tended in the past to dismiss PMT, among other female complaints, as "something you'll have to put up with". There are indeed still a few around who decree that having a baby is the answer to a woman's gynaecological worries. However, the climate of opinion is changing, and while there are still doctors who think that we are over-sensitive to PMT, it has become accepted as a condition in its own right.

Chameleon-like, PMT may reveal itself as irrational outbursts of temper, and irritability alternating with lethargy and depression. Some suffer with migraines, breast tenderness, bloatedness, pains in the joints and even sinusitis and asthma. But whatever the symptoms, the classic indication of PMT is that you experience a time in the month when you feel normal, usually between the end of menstrual flow and mid-cycle ovulation.

Anti-depressants and tranquillizers may help if you feel acutely depressed. But although often prescribed these are not likely to have much lasting effect. If PMT affects you seriously — and the condition persists for years with some women — a course of the natural hormone progesterone may help. It may be worth suggesting this to your doctor if he or she does not do so to you.

Dr Katharina Dalton, a pioneer in PMT treatment, also suggests the following as a self-help guide to be followed during the build-up period.
- Limit fluid intake to four or so cups daily.
- Restrict salt in the diet.
- Relieve low blood-sugar levels — indicated by fatigue and feelings of exhaustion — with frequent high-protein snacks.
- Refrain from drastic dieting at this time.
- Avoid arduous appointments, long-distance driving and spring cleaning.
- Regular exercise — helps some people.

Cystitis

Four out of five women suffer from cystitis at some time, the chief symptoms of which are a burning sensation when passing urine and the urge to pass water frequently. If the symptoms occur soon after intercourse, there may be a gynaecological cause; bruising of the vagina, or anatomical closeness of the vagina and the opening through which urine passes may be a cause. Infection in the bladder is also a major cause, and accurate tests are necessary to identify the bacteria responsible, and thus to prescribe the most effective antibiotic.

Many people are treated successfully for cystitis and don't suffer from it again. But some women seem particularly prone to the disorder, and become recurrent sufferers. It was for such people that Angela Kilmartin founded her famous U and I Club. For people for whom cystitis is a major recurring problem, she advises the following:
- Ask your doctor to refer you to a urologist, in case you are suffering from a urinary infection that might lead to serious trouble.
- Ask to be referred to a gynaecologist to check if the cause is related to the state of the vagina or to some other gynaecological cause.
- Your doctor may be able to arrange accurate tests, but you may get a faster and more accurate check by going through a hospital "discharge" clinic, a special unit or a VD clinic (you do not need a doctor's referral). The Westminster Hospital in London runs a special "Housewives Clinic" simply for these complaints. Ring them on 01-828 9811 for an appointment.
- On the self-help front: if you have an attack, take a little bicarbonate of soda in water; drink masses of water and take pain-killers.
- On the preventive front: develop the habit of washing carefully after emptying bowels; drink three to five pints of water a day; limit alcohol, tea, coffee and spicy food intake; observe scrupulous sex hygiene and always use a lubricant.

For further information about self-help, write to Angela Kilmartin, U and I Club, 9e Compton Road, London N1, enclosing an SAE.

Discharge

Thrush We appear to be in the midst of an epidemic of this distressing complaint, which causes a thick and creamy discharge, often accompanied by irritation. The culprit is a fungus or yeast which thrives in the hothouse conditions of tight jeans and synthetic pants and tights. Probably eight out of ten women are affected at some time in their lives. And, as with cystitis, some become recurrent suffers. It is essential not to delay in seeking help: a course of anti-fungal pessaries and cream may clear up the problems. Remember not to use a tampon at the same time, as this absorbs the cream and reduces its effectiveness.

If a chronic sufferer, self-help may improve matters:
- Persist with the treatment. Ask your doctor for more if necessary: the usual two-week supply may not be enough.
- You may have a reservoir of infection in the intestine keeping the thrush going. Ask your doctor for oral anti-fungal tablets.
- About fifteen percent of husbands and lovers carry thrush too, so they may also need treatment to prevent re-infection.
- Avoid hot baths and tight pants. Cool and dry is the best advice, with showers and stand-up washes rather than baths. Wear skirts and cotton pants, stockings or crutchless tights and avoid skin-tight jeans and trousers. Boil pants: thrush is a tough survivor.
- Oral contraceptives may predispose you to thrush. If you absolutely cannot keep thrush at bay, changing your contraceptive may be a last resort.
- Antibiotics also predispose the vagina to conditions in which thrush thrives, so you may need an anti-fungal pessary at the same time.
- Keep off sugary foods — diabetes predisposes to thrush.
- Avoid perfumes, talcs and vaginal deodorants. They may, in some cases, provoke an attack.
- If thrush resurges after a period, use an anti-thrush pessary at end of period. A build-up of sugary glycogen in the vaginal wall may provide the trigger.

Trichomoniasis is caused by a small living organism. It is nearly always transmitted sexually but can be caught from contaminated clothing or lavatory seats. Some people may exhibit few symptoms but it may cause a profuse watery discharge, which is intensely irritating and inflaming to the thighs.

The standard treatment is a course of Flagyl pills—(not to be taken early in pregnancy). Partners must take the medicine too, as the infection may alternate between sexual partners. Scrupulous attention to hygiene is necessary.

Cervical erosions are very common, particularly after pregnancy and after taking the pill. Delicate mucus cells creep out of the canal of the womb to form shiny red plaques on the neck of the womb. They may come and go, occasionally causing pain on intercourse. But they may also become infected with bacteria, giving rise to a virulent discharge. Cervical erosions can be cauterised — chemically or electrically. The infection can be treated with antibiotics but beware the well-known side-effects of thrush.

Non-specific vaginitis includes a variety of low-grade infections or local infection flare-ups at the site of a bruise or tear in the sensitive vaginal lining. Oral antibiotics may be the answer, or local application of a mercury salt or sulphonamide cream.

Foreign bodies. Forgotten tampons can cause unpleasant-smelling discharges which clear up as soon as the cause is removed.

Vaginal deodorants irritate some people, causing soreness and discharge: they are unnecessary. Save the money and buy a pair of sexy pants.

Menopausal changes Hormonal changes around the menopause may alter vaginal ecology, making some women more prone to dryness, irritation or infection: hormone creams may help to soften and moisten the vaginal area. If the vaginal or vulval irritation persists for many months, the skin should be examined to rule out more serious changes.

Your doctor

Before you sign on with a doctor it is worth asking around to get some impression of what local doctors are like and what sort of reputation they have. You can visit the surgery — examine the queues and so on. Once you have made your choice, try to establish some sort of relationship. Talk to the doctor. Good GPs should record something about their patients — their job, for instance — as well as their medical history.

Always ask the doctor to explain something if you are not sure about it. Take notes if you want to. It's amazing how much you forget once outside the surgery.

Don't be frightened to ask for a second opinion. You are perfectly entitled to one if not happy with what your doctor has told you, though, naturally, you will not be popular if you make this request every time you visit a GP. Likewise in hospital: if, say, a gynaecologist recommends a major operation, and you feel uncertain about it, ask for a second opinion from a colleague. There are pros and cons for all sorts of medical conditions, so you won't be considered an idiot for wanting reassurance.

We make sure cars are regularly checked, and very likely feel quite nervous if this is not done. We are exhorted to see a dentist at six-monthly intervals — though for some people this

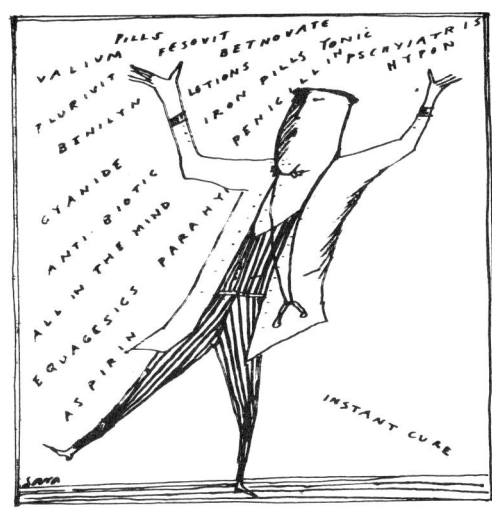

may be too frequent. But when it comes to body checks, our GPs are unlikely to be sending out reminder cards. Naturally, the full screening service available at private clinics, like those offered by BUPA, would be very costly for the health service. But there are doctors who believe that it should be possible for an occasional general check coupled with good advice. For women it is, of course, important that they have regular cervical smears — which your GP will take — and examine their breasts (see p 153).

However, many experts say that in addition everyone should know their own blood pressure. This may be an indication of state of health if it starts to go up. GPs do not measure blood pressure as a matter of course but will usually do so if asked. You would also get to know your blood pressure if you became a blood donor.

Are you breaking your back?

Not everyone who suffers from back trouble could necessarily have avoided it. Yet there are many ways in which we can care for our backs and perhaps save ourselves trouble later on. Many women suffer from bad backs, and find the problem very difficult to banish. Prevention is well worth while.

● Always sit comfortably. Straight-backed chairs that support the spine are essential if in a sedentary job. It is also important to have your chair at the correct height for your desk, with your feet on the ground too, of course.

● Banish soft beds. There is less backache in Scandinavian countries where they use boards instead of springs.

● Lift correctly. Don't twist as you're lifting. Lift with knees bent and use arms and legs to lift, not back and tummy muscles.

- Carry comfortably by splitting large parcels into two.
- Get up and walk about if sitting for a long time.
- Sudden strenuous activity, when your body is unaccustomed to it, can result in back trouble. Avoid this by exercising regularly (see p 75 of Exercise chapter).

Time off

The time people take off work through illness ranges from nineteen in every 1,000 days at work for professional workers to as many as 122 per 1,000 for unskilled manual workers. Sickness absence of more than six weeks or so a year, when not related to actual serious illness, may tell you more about the nature of a job and its monotony than the person taking the time off. At the other end of the scale, some people may be suffering from what one doctor calls "delusions of indispensability".

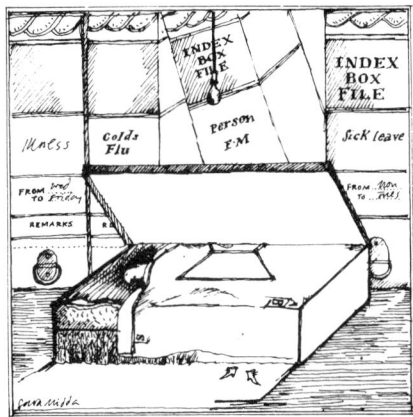

There is a happy medium. There's no point in infecting an entire office with a cold or flu. There is no need to feel guilty about being ill.

TEETH

A confident smile revealing white, even teeth is something to be envied. If you're the proud possessor of a set of gleaming, healthy teeth, don't turn the page: read how to keep them that way. And if you've been neglectful in the past, or need a little improvement, find out here what the options are.

Preventive dentistry

There is more to looking after your teeth than cleaning them twice a day. If you want your teeth to last a lifetime, follow Elaine Dutka's advice: start looking after your teeth now!

The statistics are frightening. Twenty-nine percent of adults over sixteen have no natural teeth at all. Some teeth, of course, are lost through accidents, but by far the greatest cause of tooth loss is gum disease. What is most remarkable about these statistics is the fact that gum (or periodontal) disease can so easily be avoided. By spending a few extra minutes each day on caring for your teeth, there's every chance that you can keep them healthy throughout your life.

What causes gum disease?

The chief culprit is plaque, a sticky film of harmful bacteria that's constantly forming inside your mouth. While not harmful in themselves, these bacteria, if allowed to remain on tooth surfaces and in spaces along the edges of your gums for more than twenty-four hours, organise into colonies where they begin to produce irritating poisons and enzymes. Result: gum inflammation, or gingivitis. Meanwhile, the plaque begins to harden, building up layer by layer as it turns into a deposit called calculus or tartar. This deposit causes further irritation until finally a more serious form of gum disease — periodontitis — sets in. At this stage, gums begin to withdraw from teeth, leaving hollow pockets which become filled with bacteria and food residue.

Eventually, fast-multiplying bacteria attack not just gums but also supporting bone structure, so that teeth become loose and they may eventually even be lost. Deadly as plaque is, though, it can't take all the blame.

Potential accomplices include badly decayed teeth, worn-out fillings or crowns, and bridges or partial dentures that no longer fit well because of changes in your mouth. Poor tooth alignment can also cause problems, as can a number of bad habits such as holding pins between your teeth, grinding or clenching teeth, or using toothpicks improperly. So be careful. If plaque doesn't get your gums, one of these still might.

How do you know if you have gum disease?

Most people don't — at least not in the disease's early stages. Often, gingivitis causes so little discomfort and develops so slowly that its victims simply accept the situation as normal. Some cases may even be completely asymptomatic (except to the trained eye of your dentist). In any event, the condition often goes undetected until real trouble begins — and sometimes that's too late. To avert problems, have dental check-ups regularly — or *immediately* if you notice any of these symptoms:

● *Bleeding gums during flossing and brushing.* "Pink toothbrush" — the most common sign of gingivitis, means that calculus has invaded below the gum (when you brush, inflamed gums bleed).

● *Persistent bad breath.* Whether or not you "cover up" with mouthwash, chronic halitosis may indicate gum infection and/or decayed teeth. (If bad breath persists after your dentist has given you a clean bill of health, consult your doctor.)

● *Swollen, loose, flabby gums.* Inflammation, plus spaces or pockets between teeth and gums, is another important danger signal. Often, nothing more than prophylaxis, or simple cleaning at your dental surgery, is needed to scrape away the irritating calculus and halt the condition. But postponing treatment virtually guarantees that more extensive work will be needed later on.

● *Loose teeth*. If teeth have begun to wander out of line or shift position you've probably been ignoring all the symptoms above: don't overlook this one! Loose teeth are a sign that gum tissue and bony support structure are being destroyed, but as long as fifty percent of the bone still remains intact, your teeth can probably be saved.

So, what steps should I take now to avoid gum disease?

The key to preventive dentistry is plaque removal. As long as plaque is broken up and removed every twenty-four hours, the disease process never gets started. Alas, though, removal isn't quite as simple as it sounds. We have as many as thirty-two teeth, each with five surfaces that need cleaning. To clean thoroughly takes time . . . and a little patience. And regular use of dental floss.

While brushing removes plaque and food particles from teeth's easy-to-reach surfaces, it *can't* reach the other fifteen percent of the mouth — between teeth and along the gum-line — where eighty-five percent of all dental disease starts. To get at these areas, dental floss is vital. A nuisance, yes. Flossing is more time-consuming than brushing and lacks the immediate pay-offs — fresh breath and a clean-tasting mouth. Also, it can't halt destruction that's already begun deep in the perio-dontal pockets; only a dentist can do that. But if you're faithful about daily flossing, in addition to brushing, you can look forward to one-third less gum inflammation and bone-loss than if you didn't regularly use floss.

What's the right way to floss?

You can do it either before or after brushing, though some people prefer to floss first so they can brush away dislodged particles. The technique may seem a little complicated at first, but you'll soon be doing it without even looking. Here's how: tear off twelve to eighteen inches of dental floss (waxed or unwaxed) and wrap the two ends around your middle fingers. To floss upper teeth, stretch the floss taut across your thumb and the opposite index finger, fingertips about a half-inch apart; for lower teeth, use both index fingers. Once you're holding the floss properly, work it gently back and forth between two teeth until it slides past the tight spot. (Don't force it or you'll cut the gums.) Next, wrapping floss around the side of each tooth in a curving "C" shape, move it up and down in a scraping motion — down to the gumline, but not *into* the gum — to remove plaque and polish the tooth surface. Repeat on each tooth until all have been thoroughly cleaned. If you've been using the unwaxed variety of floss, you can check up on your work with the "squeak test": when you hear a squeak, you've done enough flossing. Though a little bleeding is natural at the beginning — especially if gums are tender or inflamed (rinsing with salt water helps them heal) — a few days of proper flossing should put an end to it, and should

make a big difference in the appearance of your gums.

How often should I brush?

While a few dentists suggest brushing after each meal, most feel once a day is enough to prevent plaque colonies from building up and releasing toxins. Some, in fact, believe brushing more than that may be harmful. There's a very common problem called "toothbrush abrasion" to which women between the ages of about eighteen and twenty-eight seem particularly prone. They are so determined to have fresh breath they brush their teeth three, four, five times a day — often with a stiff brush and abrasive toothpastes. Then they complain that their mouths are full of cavities . . . that their teeth are sensitive to sweets and cold.

"What they've been doing," explains one dentist, "is brushing away their whole periodontal structure. Around the thirtieth birthday, things really start to break down, and by the time they're forty, their entire mouth is ready for crowns. I tell my patients who are concerned about having a clean mouth and fresh breath to brush not more than twice a day with a soft toothbrush and a non-abrasive toothpaste, and the rest of the time just to rinse after eating. That really is enough."

So what else should I know about brushing?

● *Toothbrushes*. To avoid abrasion damage, dentists recommend using a flat-surfaced brush with soft bristles. Since loose or bent bristles make cleaning that much harder, replace the brush as soon as it shows signs of wear. Rubber tips on toothbrushes are fine for removing food debris, but have no effect if used improperly (ask your dentist to demonstrate correct rubber-tip technique). As for electric toothbrushes, their powered strokes remove debris some human brushers might miss but they won't do all the work . . . you really do still need to floss!

● *Toothpastes*. Nearly all products now remove stains and freshen the mouth, though claims made for chemical additives such as hexachlorophene and chlorophyll are so far unsubstantiated. Still, fluoride toothpastes have been shown to cut down on decay.

● *Water piks*. Many people swear by this oral irrigating device which directs a strong pulsating stream of water to between-teeth spaces. Just remember that the water pik is intended only as an *aid* to, not a substitute for, other methods. Two possible drawbacks: excess water pressure may damage gum tissue or drive food particles deeper into the gum (especially with advanced periodontal disease), and/or dissolve the cement seal of poorly made inlays and crowns. For best results "pik" just before flossing and brushing — and only use this technique if you're sure your gums are reasonably healthy.

● *Toothbrush technique*. So you think you know how to brush? According to dentists, as many as eighty-five percent of us do it wrongly. This is one method they recommend: place brush at a forty-five degree angle towards the gum-line, gently sliding some of the bristles under the edge of the gum. Move brush back and forth over two or three teeth at a time, using short strokes and a *gentle*, circular "scrubbing" motion. After brushing the outer surfaces of each tooth — about ten strokes per section — do the same for inner surfaces, chewing surfaces (brush flat against the teeth), as well as gums and tongue . . . they've got bacteria-catching grooves in them just as teeth have. With a little practice the entire flossing/brushing programme should take no more than six or seven minutes.

To check on how you're doing, scrape your nail over the teeth from time to time. If any film comes off, your mouth isn't clean. Blood, too, could indicate problems: if "pink toothbrush" (or floss) persists, your plaque-removal technique probably needs improving. For the ultimate test, though, ask your dentist or chemist for some inexpensive "disclosing tablets", pills containing a harmless food colouring which stains plaque red. Bite down once, then swish the pill around in your mouth to reveal areas that need more attention. One last point: no matter now good your technique, you probably won't get *all* the plaque, so have teeth cleaned professionally every six months to keep calculus from accumulating.

What about sugar — is it really so bad for teeth?
Yes, because combined with certain strains of plaque bacteria called streptococci, sugar forms dextran, a sticky substance that attaches plaque to teeth. It also reacts with "strep" to produce acids which eat away at teeth and gums. If you need convincing, just consider that Alaskan Eskimos had little or no tooth decay until taking up the average American diet, loaded with sugar. Now they have the same rate of decay as the rest of us have.

If you're an average consumer, you devour an impressive 16.72kg (36.79lb) of pure sugar each year. And that's *before* you attack all those other sources, such as sugar-coated cereals, cakes, mayonnaise, even some frozen vegetables. (To avoid "hidden" intake, read labels before buying.) More important than the amount consumed, though, is the *form* in which you eat your sugar. Sticky foods — including glazed doughnuts, toffees and popcorn — are the worst offenders, since they cling and have more time to erode gums and tooth enamel. Equally crucial is how *often* you indulge a sweet tooth. Each time the plaque on your teeth is exposed to sugar, tooth-destroying acid is produced for twenty to thirty minutes. While gulping five boiled sweets one after another produces just thirty minutes of acid, eating them twenty minutes apart results in 100 minutes — or three times as much destruction! Moral: if you must eat sweet things, it's best to choose a few specific times to indulge — only at meals, for instance.

Why is a balanced diet so important?
Because your eating habits affect teeth and gums just as they do every other part of the body. First, of course, you need adequate protein, which is essential to the formation and maintenance of healthy tissue; nutritionists speculate that protein not only increases our resistance to gum problems, but reduces the severity of the disease if it does strike. Vitamins and minerals are also essential. Lack of calcium can weaken tooth enamel, while vitamin deficiencies can often lead to gum disease.

Besides a diet rich in protein, calcium, vitamins B and C, dentists advise eating foods that require a lot of chewing, since chewing increases saliva production (saliva restores vital calcium and phosphorus that plaque has demineralised from teeth). Crunchy, firm fruits and vegetables are recommended, too, since they help clean teeth and gums. Keep in mind, though, that no food can take the place of dental floss and a good toothbrush!

What if I've already got gum disease — how is it treated?
In the earlier stages, "curettage" — which involves scraping under the gum margins to remove plaque, calculus and inflamed tissue in the pockets — is all that's needed to allow gums to re-attach to the teeth. Later on, though, treatment becomes more complex. If deep pockets remain after scraping, some dentists will suggest gingivectomy to cut away diseased gum tissue and reduce pocket areas. This procedure can be done under local anaesthetic in a dentist's surgery. Sometimes, too, in severe conditions where supporting bone structure has begun to melt away, "flap surgery" may be performed — after gum tissue is lifted away from the teeth and infected tissue and calculus are removed, the gums are sutured into place just below the new bone level. Other tooth-saving methods, which may be used in addition to flap surgery, are splints to attach weakened teeth to stronger adjacent ones, plastic surgery to graft gum from one tooth to another.

So now you know . . . gum disease is expensive, ugly, and as common as the cold. But you can avoid problems by eating well and spending just a few minutes each day flossing and brushing. You should also ask your dentist for advice on up-to-date preventive dentistry techniques. Think about it. You've got nothing to lose — but your teeth!

Countdown to healthy, beautiful teeth and gums

1 Always brush teeth twice daily but note that brushing once a day correctly is more valuable than brushing twice incorrectly.
2 Change your toothbrush at least every two months.
3 Use dental floss every day. It should become a habit.

4 Avoid harsh, abrasive tooth polishes, pastes and powders.

5 You *must* visit your dentist twice a year.

6 Have teeth scaled and polished every six months whether you smoke or not.

7 Diet for healthy teeth and gums should be high in protein and calcium found in meat, eggs and dairy products; vitamins A & B contained in offal, yogurt, whole grains, greens; and vitamin C from citrus fruits, bananas, shellfish.

8 Invest in a water pik for gum massage. Only use if gums are healthy.

9 Always be gentle when using tooth piks, dental floss, etc. Tearing the gum can cause infection and is painful.

10 Once teeth are in good shape, keep smiling at yourself in the mirror to remind yourself that they really are worth looking after!

Cosmetic dentistry

Whether you've neglected your teeth and they need cosmetic treatment, or you want healthy but yellowing teeth capped toothpaste-ad white, read Joan Burnie's low-down on the way to a winning smile.

Cosmetic dentistry to most people used to mean rows of Osmond-like teeth, with no imperfections, milk-white and gleaming, expensive and totally uniform, and only to be contemplated by those with bank balances to match their egos. But these days most of us know someone who's had the commonest of all treatments — *capping* or *crowning*. This is simply the filing down of natural teeth to a narrow point and covering the point with a cemented hollow porcelain substitute. Crowning can be done on the National Health for a small cost, but unless the disfigurement is extremely severe or the psychological trauma great, it is usual for the treatment to be done privately for between £80 and £120 a tooth.

Implants are more complex, and more expensive. They are necessary when there is no tooth at all to be capped! Implantation can be painful, looks natural and is extremely expensive.

Most gaps can be filled by bridging. The teeth on either side of the space are strengthened and capped and a false tooth is cemented between them. Bridging work again is not cheap — count on about £500 as the average cost to fill the average gap.

The art of orthodontics is now so skilful that nothing seems to be beyond its capabilities. It can both improve and imitate nature, but no responsible practitioner will begin any expensive treatment on teeth or gums which are not completely disease- and plaque-free. And never forget that those crowned and capped teeth still have roots, which food particles attack whether the teeth are natural or porcelain. For a dentist to do an expensive bridging or crowning treatment on top of unhealthy gums is like taking the pill when you're pregnant: silly, useless and far too late.

Some people, instead of having too few or too big teeth, have too many, and in the wrong place. An NHS dentist will probably simply remove a tooth, usually a back molar, and either let the teeth sort themselves out in the new space or brace the teeth with metal bands to force them into place. It looks ugly, though you may only have to wear the brace at night, and it takes time, but the end result, especially in children, is perfectly satisfactory. However, the whole operation can be carried out differently and more aesthetically if you are willing to pay.

It would be a mistake to think that the only patients the orthodontist deals with are the well-known and the would-be-well-known: a large percentage of the private patients of dentists live very normal lives; housewives, salesgirls, mechanics, bank managers, many of whom have saved for years or given up holidays to bridge unsightly gaps, to cap protruding teeth and to be able to laugh again or for the first time without embarrassment. But it should be said here that not every mouth can take implants for all sorts of technical and medical reasons, so remember, prevention is better than cure.

Why can't it all be done on the National Health for which we all pay every week? Dentists say (and can produce the laboratory fees from their mechanics to prove it) that even if the work is deemed necessary (and if more than two adult teeth need to be crowned, a dentist requires the authority of the local health board before he can proceed), the NHS fees awarded for these highly technical and skilful operations do not even begin to

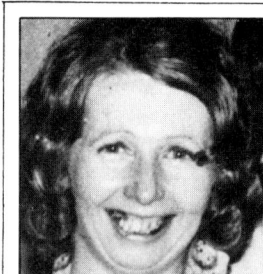
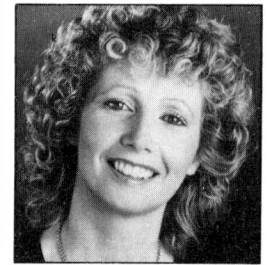

JOAN BURNIE, *journalist and writer of this article: "I'm the unproud possessor of a half set of implanted teeth. Look after your teeth* now *— don't end up like me! But having had the operation, I must admit it's the best investment I've ever made, better than gold, much better than diamonds — I think that orthodontists ought to be canonised!"*

cover their cost. On top of this, dentists' salaries have fallen behind those of other professions, although this has been remedied to some extent. This should go some way towards easing the move to private practice, since the payment per job which forms a dentist's salary has now gone up and makes treatment like crowning worthwhile once more.

Not all specialist work can be carried out by any dentist, but most of them will not mind saying, "I can't do what you want myself, but I can recommend Mr X." And don't be afraid to ask for second opinions. The days of tooth extraction at the first sign of trouble are indeed over. They are, after all, your teeth, and you are entitled to ask for all the help that modern technology offers — but don't forget, you *are* going to have to pay for it.

People who have teeth problems discuss them endlessly and someone somewhere will be willing and able to recommend their dentist or their orthodontist to you. Like good gynaecologists, good dentists are passed around . . . which is just as well because, as yet, they are forbidden by law to advertise their skills. Not every dentist can or will do complicated bridging and/or implant treatment. The possibility of complicated work being paid for by the NHS is a far-off dream. So you will have to pay. It is impossible to say how much, simply because every mouth is different. It is also unrealistic to expect a whole set of teeth, lost years ago, to be replaced completely by implants. Finding a dentist who will do orthodontics (restructuring of teeth) is not easy. The dental profession is so keen to prevent advertising that its members are almost invisible. There *is* an Orthodontists' Association but they are not allowed to send you members' names and addresses. If you have a dental hospital in your area it should be possible to get an expert opinion on whether your mouth and gums are suitable cases for treatment. Or get a list of National Health dentists in your area from your local post office, or look under "Dentist" in the Yellow Pages; then work through the list asking every dentist if he does implant or bridging work and if he will consider you as a patient, and on what terms, NHS or private. Remember that the whole point of modern cosmetic dentistry is that it is individual and not production-line work — and most dentists are willing to give estimates before they begin. If all else fails, try writing to The Secretary, The British Society for Restorative Dentistry, London Hospital Medical College Dental School, Turner Street, London E1, or The Secretary, The British (Endosseous) Pin-Implant Society, 39 Carlton Hill, St Johns Wood, London NW8, who may be able to help you.

COSMETIC SURGERY

Most women have considered, at some time in their lives, braving the surgeon's knife to improve their faces or bodies; many women have done so. But is it worth the cost, time and trouble? Can a new nose or large breasts change your life for the better? Whether the idea of cosmetic surgery appeals or repels, you'll be interested to read the extent to which it changed four girls' lives. And if you're seriously considering cosmetic surgery, we explain what's involved, and offer sound advice on where to go for best results.

The four most popular cosmetic surgery operations

If you've ever considered having a nose job, face-lift, breast alteration or an eye-lift, you'll find all the questions you've ever wanted to ask a top surgeon answered here.

The face lift

Q What's the best age for a face-lift?
A Most patients are in their late forties to late fifties — but lifts can be done well before and after that, too. Some actresses and public figures will choose to have lifts while still in their thirties. These lifts are not "preventive" — there *is* no such thing — but the benefits are fairly minimal, since there isn't usually very much excess skin to remove in a woman under forty. For the average woman, it's generally wise to wait until your face has noticeably "fallen" before having it lifted!

Q I've heard it's a clever move to have a lift before you really need it. Is this true?
A No — cosmetic plastic surgery is corrective, *not* preventive! A face-lift should be done only after the skin has sagged enough to justify the operation; if you do it before there's loose skin to "lift", you're wasting your money.

Q Does a face-lift last for the rest of your life?
A Yes and no. A lift can tighten your skin so that you look five to ten years younger, but you'll carry on ageing at the normal rate. In ten years or so, your skin will be sagging again, and you may opt for a *second* lift. But once a lift is done it is permanent in the sense that it never "lets go".

Q What is the actual procedure during a face-lift?
A There are variations in technique and in the patient's individual needs, but this is the basic routine: incision is made in hair-line from temple to top of ear, then around in front of ear (scar will be hidden in natural fold there), under earlobe, and up into hair-line at back of neck (a). The skin is then undermined — separated from the underlying tissue and fat — so it hangs free, like a loose flap of fabric (b). As the surgeon cuts and undermines, the severed blood vessels are electro-cauterised to stop the bleeding. How much undermining is done depends on where the face is sagging; it can be *very* extensive — almost to the corners of the mouth and far down into the throat. The loose flap of skin is then pulled up into its new (tighter) position, sutured into place, and the excess skin snipped off (c). Some doctors insert drains in the incision in case bleeding under the skin occurs later. The eyelids may be done either last or first. This is a matter of individual preference among surgeons.

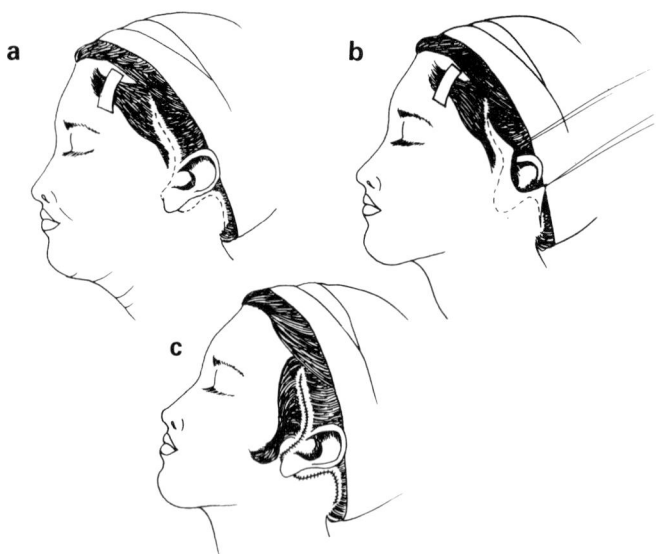

Q How much pain is there?

A Doctors say a face-lift involves very little pain; patients, however, vary in their reactions. Some find the recovery period really quite painful; others get by with a few aspirin.

Q What kind of anaesthetic is used?

A The vast majority of plastic surgeons use a local anaesthetic mixed with adrenalin to reduce bleeding. You would also be given a tranquillising shot of Valium to make you groggy. (Many patients fall asleep during the operation.) Some surgeons prefer to use a general anaesthetic, even though the risks are greater than with a local. (From the patient's point of view, a local is almost always to be preferred. It's not only safer, but you'll feel better post-operatively: no anaesthesia hangover, and no sore throat from tubes having been inserted during surgery.)

Q How long does the operation take?

A A complete lift, including eyes, usually takes about five hours on the operating table which indicates that this is no minor operation — and not to be undertaken lightly!

Q Will my head be shaved?

A Probably not. Most doctors merely pin the hair back. You will be able to wash your hair a few days after the operation, but you shouldn't colour it for at least a month.

Q Will my face be bandaged after the surgery?

A Almost certainly. Most doctors use a face pressure bandage with holes cut in it for the eyes, nose and mouth. Some doctors prefer not to bandage at all, but this is a highly controversial point. The purpose of the pressure bandage is to prevent bleeding (some doctors also insert drains), and it is usually removed after twenty-four hours or so. After that, you will wear a small turban bandage for a few days.

Q Will the scars show?

A The only visible scars will be in front of the ears. Suture line starts above temple, where it's hidden in hair-line, then emerges at ear, loops back under and behind ear to end in hair-line at nape of neck.

Q How long before I can go out in public?

A Recovery time is variable and unpredictable, but the majority of patients can go out socially in about three weeks. There will still be some bruising then, but it can be camouflaged with make-up.

Q Can I have my eyes done at the same time as the face-lift?

A Yes, eyes are generally considered an integral part of a total face-lift. (Very few women would need the lift and not need the skin around the eye tightened . . . although the reverse is also often true.)

Q Can a sagging, crepey neck be improved with a face-lift?

A Yes. In addition to the usual tightening of the skin on the throat, the doctor can reposition the platysma muscle, which will then act as a little interior "girdle" for the neck. The platysma muscle runs vertically down the throat. By freeing the lower end, pulling it upward to the side, and suturing it in place there, the entire chin and throat area will be tightened and firmed.

Q A friend is planning a partical face-lift, so no scars will show. Is this possible?

A Yes, in a temporal lift the suture line stops at the top of the ear, so scar is entirely hidden behind hair-line. This half-way measure is fine for the top half of the face — smooths out crow's feet and saggy skin around temples and eyes — but does nothing for the lower half of the face. If you have sagging cheeks, droopy jowls, or a crepey throat, you'd be wise to opt for a total lift in spite of the scars — which are usually tiny and fade completely with time, anyway.

Q What can go wrong with a face-lift?

A The commonest complication is hematoma — bleeding under the skin from a blood vessel that wasn't completely cauterised, or which opened up after the incision was closed. This can be a minor problem (treated with simple aspiration to suction off the blood) or it can be quite major, in which case it requires reopening the incision. If they feel there's a danger of hematoma, some surgeons place surgical drains in the incision when they suture it. While the problem of post-surgical infection is almost non-existent after a face-lift, there is a possibility of skin "slough". If the skin is redraped too tightly, circulation can be impaired, and the skin — deprived of its blood supply — will die, and slough off. (This can be repaired — but it's a good reason not to urge your doctor to make your new face as tight as he possibly can!)

Q Is there anything you can do to prepare for a face-lift, in order to get optimum results?
A Lose weight if you need to. Get down to your ideal size (or even a bit below) so skin will not be plumped out with extra fat and the doctor can take up the maximum slack.

The nose job

Q Can a nose be radically altered by surgery?
A Yes — with plastic surgery a nose can be shortened, narrowed, straightened, or built up.

Q Does the surgeon have pictures of noses I can choose from — or do I tell him what I'd like?
A You must let the surgeon decide what is necessary. He will not give you the nose you'd necessarily choose for yourself; a little *retroussé* nose would not suit a broad face, an aquiline nose is not suited to a rounded face. The surgeon decides on the "new" nose by considering many factors, including your height, build and dimensions of your face — even your personality! He will take "before" pictures of your nose for reference during the operation, too.

Q Is there any special age at which a nose job is preferable?
A No, you can have a nose job at any age.

Q Is it true that my new nose will need time to take on its new shape?
A You will have a rough idea of how your new nose will look directly after the plaster cast is removed, but the nose carries on slimming down for several months afterwards, so the final effect cannot be judged until then.

Q Are nose jobs always successful?
A Aesthetically speaking, most patients are delighted with results. Women who are disappointed usually expected more drastic alterations, but these may not be surgically possible. The most successful nose job is one that looks natural, and complements your other features. Nose jobs are the trickiest and most delicate of the common plastic surgery operations, and the result is totally dependent on the skill of the surgeon: another case for choosing the best!

Q How long does the operation take?
A About two hours.

Q Is there any scarring?
A There is no visible scarring at all.

Q Which type of anaesthetic is used for the operation?
A Usually a general anaesthetic is preferred; sometimes local anaesthetics are used, but not many patients care to see what's happening!

Q What does the operation involve?
A Procedure is the same — cartilage and bone are removed or altered — but method varies slightly depending on alterations needed. The diagrams below illustrate procedure for straightening a humped nose (the most usual problem). Incision (a) is made inside nose. Vertical saw cuts (b) — dotted lines at right — score bone at both sides of nose. This is the fracture line, where bone will later be broken. The bony hump, sawn off in sideways slicing motion, is reduced to desired contour. (Sawn-off fragment is withdrawn with forceps through nostril.) With hump gone (c), apex of nasal arch gapes open. Surgeon applies pressure, usually with thumbs, at saw-cut fracture line, breaks the bones and pushes them together over the open space. (Bone also fractures high up on bridge of nose, resulting in post-op black eyes!) Incision is then closed, nose packed with sterile gauze, and plaster cast applied. New nose (d) — with new straight profile — eventually emerges after swelling and bruising have disappeared.

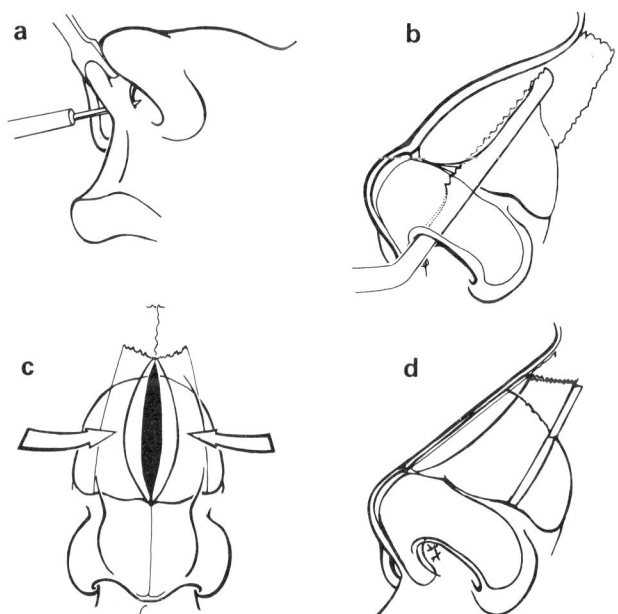

Q Is there much pain involved?
A There is discomfort rather than pain; initially after the operation you have to breathe through your mouth, and your throat will be very dry.

Q I've heard bruising after the operation is awful and lasts for ages. How long is it before I can walk around without looking as if I've been in a fight?

A Initial bruising looks alarming — black and blue marks around the eyes — but disappears after a few days. After the operation, you have to keep the plaster cast on for a week before the surgeon removes it; some people don't mind being seen with plaster across their nose! It is important during this healing period that your nose is not knocked — and you are asked to *try* not to sneeze or blow your nose!

Breast reduction and augmentation

Q Can I choose the size of breasts I wish to have?

A Your surgeon will advise you which size is most suited to your height and body type. If you have been flat-chested all your life, you may fancy having large breasts, but on a small frame, they could look ridiculous! Note that neither breast reduction nor augmentation are simple operations and you should only consider them if you have a very small or very large bust to begin with.

Q What does the operation for breast augmentation involve?

A Envelope-like sacs filled with silicone gel are inserted into the breasts. No reputable plastic surgeon uses liquid silicone to plump up breasts; it is dangerous. Implants are available in different sizes, depending on size of breast required. See diagram below for method used in breast augmentation: Incision (a) is made under the bottom curve of the breast. Implant (b) is slid up through incision and manoeuvered into position. Side view (c) shows implant in place behind the mammary wall, next to chest wall. Mesh backing of implant attaches itself to chest wall.

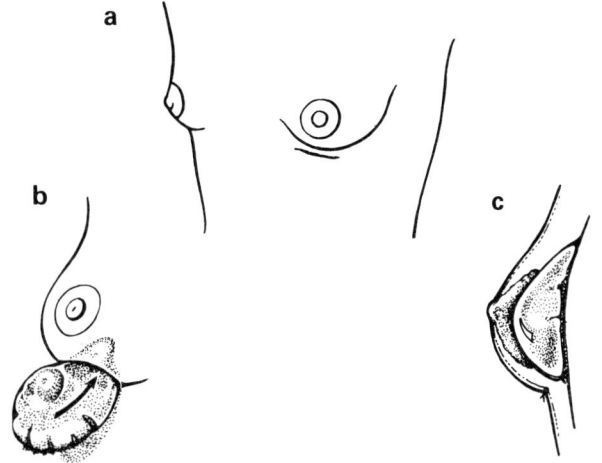

Q What does the operation for breast reduction involve?

A The most common method of breast reduction is for an incision to be made just below each nipple and under the breasts. Tissue is removed from the area between incisions, then skin is folded up like a flap and resewn. In a similar method the nipple is re-sited, but it remains intact.

Q Which kind of anaesthetic is used?

A A general anaesthetic for both operations.

Q How long do the operations last?

A Depending on the operation, from two to three hours.

Q Is there much pain involved?

A As with most plastic surgery operations, the worst you should feel is discomfort, mostly due to the after-effects of a general anaesthetic! You will probably experience stiffness in the breasts for about two weeks.

Q How long before my breasts look normal?

A Bandages are wrapped around the chest after the operation, and have to stay there for several days. Swelling and bruising should clear up after a fortnight; stitches are removed from five to ten days after the operation. There is a little scarring under the breasts after augmentation, but this fades after a few months and is in a position where it is not likely to be noticed. Scarring below each nipple, and under breast, where incisions have been made for breast reduction are minimal and will fade after a time.

Q Can anything go wrong?

A If you are having breasts reduced, you should be told by your surgeon before the operation that breast feeding will not be possible. The greatest hazard of breast surgery is the aesthetic one of uneven breasts or badly repositioned nipples; again a good plastic surgeon lessens the likelihood of these occurrences. In rare cases nipples lose their sensitivity, but in some cases where breasts are reduced, sensitivity is increased.

The eye-lift

Q What's the average age for an eye-lift?

A Most patients are in their forties, but the age range is wide — partly because different ethnic types seem to sag at varying rates. A fair, thin-skinned blonde might require a lift in her early thirties; a thick-skinned Mediterranean type might not droop until fifty or so. Some young women in their twenties need to have bags under the eyes removed, but these pouches aren't necessarily a sign of age. They're usually the result of a congenital (inherited) condition, in which fat deposits push against the muscle wall and cause the lower lids to bulge outward, causing pouches.

Q Are both upper and lower lids done at the same time?
A Usually. In about ten percent of cases, the lower lid is still firm and unlined, in which case only the droopy upper lid is tightened.

Q How much loose skin should you have before surgery?
A That's entirely a matter of subjective opinion. Some women rush off to the surgeon at the first sign of sagging (though reputable doctors won't operate unless it's really needed), whereas other women will put it off until the redundant skin hangs down to the lash-line (or even beyond), obscuring vision and making it hard to keep the eyes open! Generally, the right time for surgery is when the amount of droop is aesthetically offensive to you.

Q Can the operation be done again?
A Yes, but only a small percentage of patients want or need a repeat. (The procedure for fat removal under the eye is always permanent, as the body doesn't produce more fat.) A lift for sagging skin is usually good for ten years or so.

Q What are the dangers, if any, of eye-lift surgery?
A Hematoma — bleeding under the skin — is possible, though rarer than in a complete face-lift. (One purpose of the iced compresses is to constrict blood vessels and minimise bleeding.) If hematoma occurs, it is drained, and the bleeding vessel coagulated with electrocautery. A fairly common eye-lift complication (in about twenty-five percent of cases) is the formation of milia — cysts — along the incision line. Sebaceous material and cellular debris collect in tiny pockets of scar tissue and must be excised. Milia usually appear two to three months after surgery; it's a simple matter to get rid of them. The worst complication of an eye-lift is ectropion — in which the lower lid is pulled down and outward. This can happen when the surgeon goes too far and overtightens the under-eye area. (It can be corrected with skin grafts, usually taken from behind the ear.) Ectropion is rare, fortunately; but it's a good reason to choose a conservative doctor who, if he errs at all, will take too little loose skin rather than too much.

Q What anaesthetic is used for the operation?
A Most doctors prefer to use a local. The typical anaesthetic is a mild sedative, often with a little adrenalin — to lessen bleeding — added. Many doctors prohibit the use of aspirin for a week or two prior to (and after) surgery, in a further effort to discourage bleeding.

Q How long does the operation take?
A About an hour.

Q What exactly is done to the eyelids in the operation?
A An incision is made in natural fold of upper lid (a) and just under lash-line in lower one, and excess skin is snipped away

(b). This is the tricky part: deciding just how much skin to eliminate. The incision is then closed, often with a long continuous suture (c), running under the skin from one end to the other. The eyes are not usually bandaged, but ice gauze packs — frequently changed — are put over them right away and remain for one or two days. Vision is poor right after the operation, as gooey salve is applied along the incision line. Stitches are removed between the second and fourth days. (The longer the stitches stay in, the more external scar tissue is formed, so doctors try to get them out as soon as possible.)

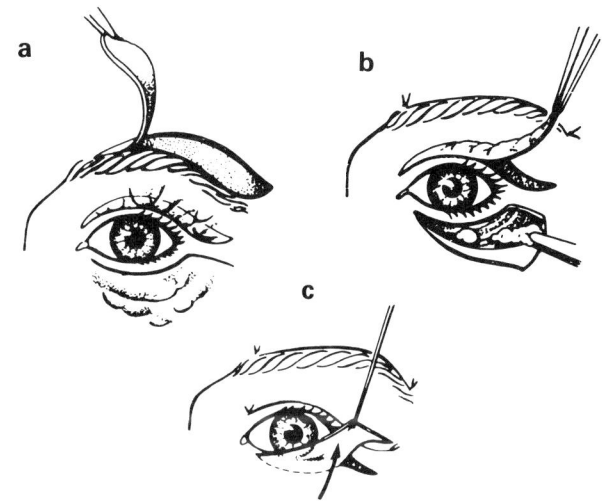

Q What are the scars like?
A Minimal. You can see a fine red line just under lower lashes (it extends out laterally into a crow's foot) for two or three months; then it fades, and after a year or so you can't see anything at all. The upper lid's scar is hidden in the skin fold.

Q What about make-up?
A You can resume using eye make-up about a week after surgery, but you should stay out of the sun for at least two months. A scar "matures" over a period of six months to a year, and you don't want to stress the scar as it matures. Even a mild sunburn can cause swelling to which the scar tissue might react badly.

Q How soon can you go out in public after surgery?
A Swelling and bruising vary greatly, but the recovery time ranges from three to eight days. Many patients are out and about — although in sunglasses, to be sure — in three days, and it is not unusual to be back in the office on Monday morning after a weekend's recuperation. While you may still have some faint bruising after a week, you can by then cover it with make-up.

Lesser-known operations

Stomach reduction. For stretch marks due to pregnancy or sudden weight loss or for scars. Can remove slack skin, but not solid fat. Major operation in which a vast amount of skin is undermined (detached from underlying tissues) and repositioned. Incision made along pubic hair-line leaves scar that is hidden by bikini!

Chin augmentation. For building up "weak" chin. This operation is often performed at the same time as nose is corrected. Silicone sac is implanted into chin. No scarring.

Ear correction. For large, protruding ears. Comparatively simple operation which makes ears smaller and causes them to lie flatter against head. Patient is required to wear bandages for several days. Hearing is not affected. No visible scarring.

Body reshape surgery. Still in infancy stages in this country. Fatty tissue is removed from thighs, buttocks, upper arms. Operations are complicated and scarring is inevitable, so think carefully before going ahead: perhaps diet and exercise classes would be safer — and cheaper!

When it's worth having cosmetic surgery

Four girls, who made the big decision, talk to Irma Kurtz.
A riddle: what is it that nobody else is closer to than you yet others might see clearer? What is it that you look at every day but it never looks back at you? The answer, of course, is yourself: your face, your body. And even when you look at yourself, you do not really see yourself, you see a reflection in the mirror or an appraisal in the eyes of another person. Most women are more or less comfortable inside their containers, they apply a fresh coat of paint every morning and scrub it off every night, they adorn themselves in a fashionable way and they get on with living from the inside out, aware of their physical imperfections only when circumstances like a new bikini or a new man make them aware.

Others, however, carry their hooked noses or crows' feet like a burden that is only just bearable, a burden so heavy it can in fact suffocate pride and joy. "We love you anyway," their friends say, but that just doesn't help the woman who wants to be loved every way, not "anyway", the woman who cannot love herself with such a nose, such a jaw, such bags under her eyes, in such an unaesthetic container.

"I never considered myself a pretty child. People would say, 'Look at so-and-so, she's worse off than you,' but that didn't help because as far as I was concerned you only live once and I know it's more important to have something up there, something inside your head, but . . . I used to buy all these clothes and make-up but then I'd look at myself in the mirror and be unhappy. I remember times when I was very young when I would sob and say, 'Why me?' Not a day of my life went by when I wasn't conscious of my nose; if I was watching TV and there was a joke about somebody with a big nose I'd be conscious of it, or if I was sitting on a bus I'd always try to sit where I wasn't in profile to anybody."

Sandy McGee is a dainty blonde who now turns an interested male head or two or three on a sunny day in London. Her eyes are large and beautiful, her make-up is subtle over delicate bones and her nose is a perfectly nice nose; people who see her don't say, "My, what a lovely nose!" although they probably say, "My, what a pretty girl." Sandy is twenty-three and just under a year ago she had cosmetic surgery. Until relatively recently, cosmetic surgery was considered to lie half-way between Hollywood and voodoo. There are still plenty of people who think we should put up with our God-given packages no matter how flawed they may be, and there are also those, especially among the American affluent, who think of cosmetic surgery as a small step up from Elizabeth Arden. These attitudes about elective cosmetic surgery, however, have nothing much to do with people like Sandy who used to be afraid to go to parties and suffered even during visits to a favourite aunt. For Sandy, cosmetic surgery was, in a way, life-saving.

If Sandy opted for life-saving surgery, then Dee Taylor chose what could fairly be called face-saving surgery. Dee's reasons were not as radical as Sandy's, perhaps, or as fraught with misery, but they were just as valid. Dee, who now looks ten years younger than her thirty-seven, is an exercise teacher; she is lithe, and has a bubbling personality.

"The kind of bags I had under my eyes were hereditary; they usually are. I thought about having them done and having the puffy fat removed from my upper lids ten years before I

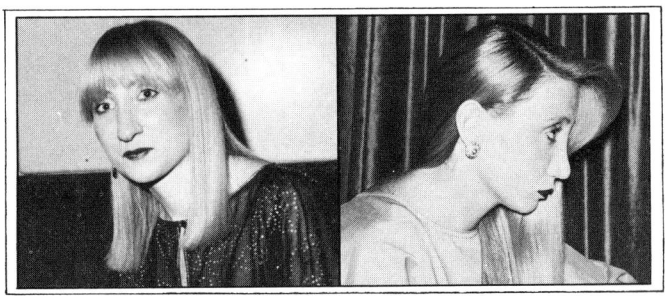

Sandy: before   *After*

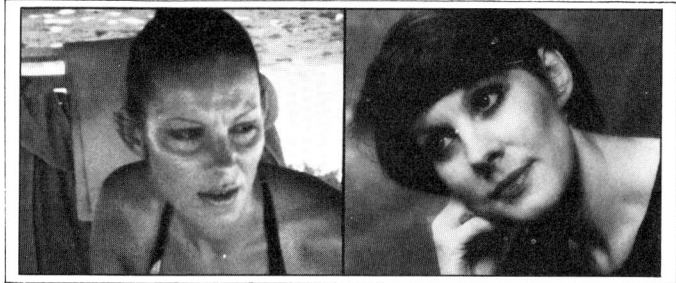

Dee: before   *After*

actually did it. It started worrying me when people said, 'You look tired', and I wasn't in the least tired.

The more people said it to me, the more I looked at myself and realised it was my eyes. And then the business I'm in is so physically demanding that within one hour — I do five hours sometimes — I looked knocked out although I didn't feel it. And people kept saying, 'Are you all right?' So in the end I thought I just had to do something about it. I had a very good friend and he said to me, 'I love the bags under your eyes.' But I said, 'It's not enough. I've got to love myself.'"

Both Dee and Sandy could have survived without surgical intervention; for both of them surgery was a matter of operating on the quality of life, not the fibre of life. For Denise Barnes however, cosmetic surgery was a necessity and the cosmetic advantage, she says, came as a bonus. Denise had a pugnacious jaw with an out-thrust chin that gave her a severe underbite; her dentist told her that in a short time she was destined to lose her teeth, a grim prognosis when you're still young.

Denny, whose operation was technically more complicated than Sandy's or Dee's, retains the forthrightness suggested by her pre-surgical appearance, but her face now is sweet, feminine, the chin more madonna than Hapsburg, and those school chums who used to call her Bob Hope would be surprised to see her — though, as it should be with all successful cosmetic surgery, they would not know precisely why she looked so great or precisely what had changed.

"After the swelling was nearly down I met a guy I'd known for about eight years. I'd worked with him, sitting at the next desk, for two years. And I said, 'Hello Nick,' and he said, 'Who are you?' And I said, 'It's Denny,' and he said, 'It is not!' I cried then. It was like losing my identity a little."

Since Denny's operation did not take place primarily for cosmetic reasons, she cried where Dee or Sandy might have laughed. Denny's appearance had never bothered her, she says, and she hadn't found it at odds with her personality, while Dee's ebullience was betrayed by nature, and Sandy's gentle charm was belied by what she calls "a nose that made me look mean". The purpose of cosmetic surgery is to bring a woman's appearance into harmony with the person she knows herself to be, the person who lives inside.

Alas, we know ourselves imperfectly but we know our surgeons even less. It is as well for any patient undergoing any surgery to be confident in the surgeon, but if the surgery is elective, then that confidence must be nearly perfect. It is not coincidence that Dee, Denny and Sandy all speak of their surgeons with the kind of love patients formerly reserved for their psychiatrists. The cosmetic operation is deeper than a mere rearrangement of tissue, it is an operation performed on the body but simultaneously on an image, the image in the mirror and the one which each person carries inside himself or herself.

"My first impression when the plaster came off was, 'That's me. It's great!' " Sandy said. "My surgeon actually drew the curtain back and there was a mirror behind it. The funny thing was, the night before I'd seen the old Joan Crawford movie, *A Woman's Face*. I didn't shout or scream or kiss the surgeon," she said with a touch of regret, "because I felt too reserved. I wanted to, but I'll always be shy."

Dr J is a celebrated plastic surgeon and, it so happens, an articulate man, a sort of medical philosopher, interested in the ethics and the aesthetics of his work. "Beware the plastic surgeon who says, 'Yes, what do you want done? Let's have a look at you. When do you want it done? See my secretary on the way out for an appointment.' Nothing is that simple. First of all, when they come here to see me, they are complaining of some inadequacy or other. They don't accept their own visual or body image.

"Why not? That's the first thing I have to find out. Whether he likes it or not, the plastic surgeon must play psychiatrist. He wants a well-motivated, goal-orientated patient with emotional stability. It is never a question of operating on wallets or doing surgical exercises. The best surgeon knows when not to use the knife. He studies points about his patients, how they approach, what they do, how they sit, how they walk, body language. Everything. Then he decides if this person is really going to be happier as a result of surgical intervention. If not, it's not on."

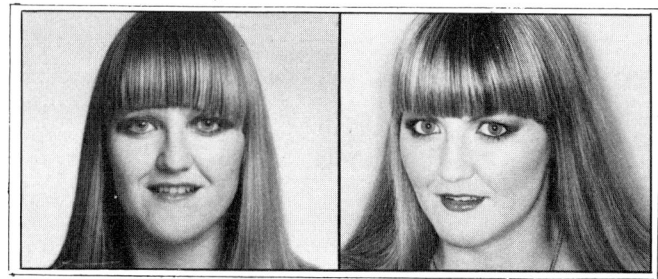

Denny: before   *After*

Dr J sometimes sends patients for psychiatric assessment, not because he thinks they must be mad to want to modify their appearance but because he wants no shadow clouding his rapport with the man or woman upon whom he is going to exercise his skill and judgement. He is wary of patients who postpone appointments or who pace his waiting-room like tigers, who are rude to his staff or who want written guarantees of perfection. "The only guarantee a surgeon should give is for one hundred per cent of his effort. When people talk about perfection or pull out a photograph of Elizabeth Taylor, I say, 'Forget it'."

Dr J is aware, as any man in his profession must be, that people can project emotional problems on to their bodies, and when this is the case, no surgery will ever satisfy and no improvement in appearance ever change the essential self. It is significant that Dee, Sandy and Denny agree that surgery made no change in their personalities — Dee is still an enthusiast, Sandy is still shy and Denny will always be capable and outspoken — but surgery added the one ingredient each lacked to some degree: confidence in the women each of them was and had always been.

"My local butcher said it to me first," Dee said. "One morning after my operation I went in to buy some meat and he said, 'My God! You look blooming today,' and I knew it, I knew it!"

Of course a new dress gives a woman confidence, too, or a new hair-style or make-up; surgery is a pretty extreme booster. No matter how eagerly Brazilian millionairesses go under the cosmetic knife, it is a wise woman who considers the perils of surgery, any surgery. "There is a hazard in having surgery," Dr J said. "There is a hazard in having an anaesthetic, there is a hazard in having an injection."

Dee and Sandy suffered degrees of discomfort from their operations. Denny, who had the surgical equivalent of a seamstress's dart taken in each side of her lower jaw, awoke to seventeen gruelling hours in an intensive care unit. Dee said she didn't so much as leave her house for a full week after her operation; even though she had been a nurse and knew what to expect, the extent of the swelling and temporary disfigurement was shocking. Denny caught sight of her face in a bedpan and mistook it for a reflection of her bottom, and Sandy still had a numb place on her nose six months after the plaster came off.

"There was a suction machine all the time by the side of my bed," Denny remembered. "And the nurses were instructed that if I was about to be sick they should cut the wire binding my jaws together. My face was as swollen as the moon. When I went home after ten days, I felt so tired, absolutely knackered! After seven weeks they unlocked my jaws and I just had the braces on my teeth, so I thought, 'Right, now I eat steak!' but I couldn't. I'd expected to lose two stone but in fact I put on weight because I got so hungry I was liquidising potatoes. It was six months before the swelling went and I felt really good."

Admittedly, Denny's recuperation was longest and hardest because her operation was the most extensive of the three, but any elective surgery and its after-effects demand — deserve — great determination.

All three women say they cannot imagine undergoing body surgery, but then all three have good, firm bodies. Oddly enough, Joy Slater, who had silicone implants in her breasts and cosmetic surgery to her stomach, cannot imagine undergoing facial surgery. Joy is a petite brunette who bears a slight resemblance to Elizabeth Taylor — a name that arises constantly in cosmetic surgery circles.

In her early thirties, Joy carried the ugly scars of two Caesarean sections done in the outmoded transversal way. (Whenever it is feasible, surgeons now use the "bikini" or "Hollywood" cut which is horizontal and leaves virtually no visible scar.) After childbirth her breasts had sagged and dropped. To her husband, anyway, she was no longer the girl he had married.

"I knew at the time my husband was being unfaithful. It was his idea to have my breasts done. I wanted my stomach done and I wasn't too worried about my breasts, but he said he thought it would help our marriage. A woman trying to save her marriage will do anything. I suppose it failed to save my marriage. My husband says he still loves me but he doesn't want to come back only to let me down again. I couldn't care less. You can't spend all your time in mourning. But now I'm going to be on my own, the surgery has given me added confidence and if I hadn't done it three years ago, I'd have done it now. I think if one can improve oneself, why not? My husband still says it was the best investment he ever made."

Surgeons and patients agree that body surgery is a more highly-charged area than facial surgery. A woman's face is the face of a person, it is the face of all she is as well as being female; her body, however, is feminity, it is a woman's body. To judge

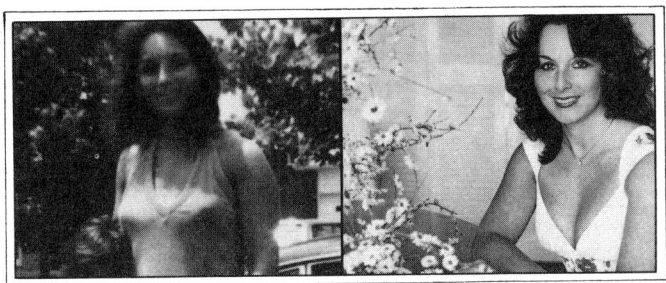

Joy: before   *After*

from the letters in Dr J's file, the motivation for cosmetic breast surgery is quite often an attempt to save a marriage, and once in a while it succeeds, or perhaps it is the added confidence of the restored woman that helps the marriage. Breast surgery, particularly breast augmentation with implants, can entail complications for patient and surgeon.

"A patient will come in whose boobs you've done and it has made no difference to her marriage so she complains that one breast is half a millimetre lower that the other. Why? Because the surgery failed to save the marriage and the surgeon is the fall-guy. If you have acute appendicitis, you always thank God for the surgeon who saves your life, but elective surgery is not the same thing."

Dr J always details the physiological risks of breast augmentation to his patients and asks them to sign a form saying they have understood these risks before surgery. It would be a foolhardy patient who did not want to know the perils of any operation and particularly one that implants man-made material — in this case something resembling half a grapefruit — into the body.

Vanity is a fair motivation for any cosmetic surgery, and why should it not be? Vanity is a component of all healthy personalities, although it is one some people find difficult to confess to, a demurrant which is in itself vanity. Those who have had cosmetic surgery and are happy with the results confess to vanity more easily than many others would, perhaps because they understand the pleasure of giving into it better than most. Dee Taylor, who had been under analysis for two years before her operation, could not make even her sage psychoanalyst understand why her natural motivation was stronger than his logical arguments. "He said to me, 'So now you want to go and butcher yourself,' but he was totally wrong. He said I was going for different reasons and not for vanity. I went for vanity. It wasn't a mental problem, it was vanity. That, I don't think he could ever understand. I'm happy with the results and I'd do it again. I will do it again if I have to when I'm sixty or sixty-five."

Dr J, who encounters naked vanity more often than most, does not have contempt for it. "What do you owe yourself? That's the question. Vanity is a healthy commodity. It's right and proper for people to be vain. If surgery is sought for ulterior motives — to please a husband or to save a business — then the patient should be studied meticulously."

If a patient says she is having surgery to please her husband and then it fails to please him, or she is having it done to preserve her business as, say, a boutique owner, and then the business fails, it means the surgery must be seen as a failure. If the patient honestly says she is doing it to please her own vanity, then the surgery has a far greater chance of succeeding.

Dee had a divorce already under way when she decided on surgery; Sandy was very happily married to a man who loved her with the nose she had and loves her with the new nose; Denny met a new boyfriend two weeks before her operation but would have had it done whether or not he thought it necessary; only Joy's surgery failed in terms of holding her marriage together, but Joy is a well-balanced woman, tempered by pain and, as she says, she would have her surgery done again anyway for herself. She admits to human vanity and she is not in the least embarrassed about having had silicone implants and a scar correction. "I told all my friends, and whenever I'd visit, they'd say, 'Come in and strip so we can see you.' One of my friends was so impressed she said, 'Can my husband come and have a look?'"

Physical vanity does not always depart with age, and moralising about that is futile as far as people with lined faces who still feel young inside themselves are concerned. If a woman of seventy wants her face lifted, as Dr J has known it to happen, why should her motives not be examined precisely as a younger person's would be and, if the surgeon assesses her positively, why should she not have the surgery she wants? Vanity can lie in different areas and if an intellectual woman would consider submission to the cosmetic knife an absurdity, it only means her personal resources are always of a different and more enduring kind than those of her sisters . . . and brothers, too, for men are not immune to vanity. In one week recently, for example, Dr J lifted four male faces against the ravages of time.

"If you tell a woman of thirty-nine who wants a face-lift to wait until she is forty-nine, you are saying, 'Go away and live with it for the next ten years'; why should you do that? By what right? The age to do cosmetic surgery is at whatever age the patient happens to be when he or she turns up in the surgery because that is just the time when the patient is actually being bothered."

A candidate for cosmetic surgery should try first to assess for herself whether she is blaming a defect of her body for some subtler handicap no surgeon's knife can repair. If her feelings about herself are unclear, chances are her motivation will not be strong enough to carry her through the preliminary stages or even into the surgeon's consulting room. If she is honest about herself, however, nothing will stop her. Sandy, for example, although she is by nature agreeable and acquiescent, ignored the disapproval of friends and even turned down her father's offer of £1,000 to spend on clothes if only she would forgo surgery. Dee didn't listen to her trusted psychoanalyst. If a woman gets as far as the surgery carrying mixed and complicated emotions with her, the surgeon, if he is a good one, should see to it that she is clear about herself and her motives before he actually agrees to take her as a patient.

Any prospective patient owes it to herself, moreover, to put to the surgeon every possible question or doubt that she may have and to demand straight answers. The only shock that Denny had was waking up in the glare of the intensive care unit, even though she was told that that would happen; the only surprise Dee had was the extent of swelling and no doctor could have forseen that because it varies from person to person. The only surprise Joy had was the pleasant one of added sensitivity in her breasts, and Sandy, who had dreamed about having her nose done from the time she was twelve, and had read everything she could find on the topic, was surprised only by the extra confidence the operation gave her.

Unless a woman has a lot of money, her motivation will be sorely tested by her need to find the fee. Sandy and Dee spent approximately £600 for surgery and after-care, Joy spent £770 six years ago and would need considerably more now; Denny had her operation on the National Health because the imminent threat of losing her teeth gave her priority. Anyone planning cosmetic surgery privately can count on spending into four figures; it is impossible to say precisely how much because no two operations are ever the same. Elective surgery is available on the National Health and in more affluent days it was done quite frequently; now, however, burn cases and road accidents take up the limited money available and the wait for elective surgery can last for two years or more.

"All doctors want to help their patients and none of us believes anyone is willing to undergo surgery just for the hell of it," one frantically busy GP said. "But extreme things must be done first. When money pinches, it's hard to get elective cosmetic surgery and it is going to get harder. You must realise that when a doctor starts taking grit out of a young girl's face (the victim of a road accident), it means twenty or thirty operations with *petit-point* stitching. More and more work is being perfected on disfiguring skin diseases and burns; that means more essential plastics and less to spare for elective surgery. If your doctor seems brusque it could be because he is frustrated by his inability to help.

"Of course, it is true that any GP who had just diagnosed a bronchial carcinoma might be abrupt with a man who wants an old tattoo removed, or a nose job, but that is understandable. The fact remains, if a candidate for elective surgery can afford to go privately, her GP will have the name of a plastic surgeon — we all do — and if he doesn't give her the name, he's a pig."

Before anyone wastes any doctor's time, or her own, she should try to be sure in herself that the surgery she is seeking is to correct a genuine physical flaw in the container, not in its contents; and that the outcome of plastic surgery will not be a disguise but will reveal the real person inside.

How to choose a cosmetic surgeon

The success or failure of a cosmetic surgery operation depends largely on the skill of the surgeon. Medical expert Christine Doyle advises you on the right — and wrong — ways of finding the very best.

Demand for cosmetic surgery is growing rapidly in Britain, and a face — or tummy — lift is no longer the preserve of the idle rich or those whose jobs depend upon their beauty.

Entrepreneurs, eager to latch on to the boom, have opened private clinics, whose services are frequently advertised in the "small ads" in newspapers and magazines.

Yet care and commonsense should be the approach, say both the British Medical Association and the British Association of Plastic Surgery. Both associations warn of possibly "appalling mistakes" if cosmetic surgery is carried out by surgeons who are not properly qualified.

Some time ago, a Sunday newspaper paid for a young woman to have reconstructive surgery after being what the paper described as "butchered" by a surgeon who was untrained in plastic surgery.

The worry is over the mushrooming growth of the private clinics. These may offer tempting cosmetic surgery "package deals" but their surgeons may not be properly qualified. They may have letters after their name, but these may indicate only that they are general surgeons. They are not necessarily skilled at carrying out delicate plastic surgery. To be sure of skilled surgery, cosmetic operations should be carried out by surgeons who are members of BAPS. The association is at present monitoring complaints from people who are dissatisfied with their operations. It is also holding talks with the BMA's ethical committee. There may be, it is thought, some justification for insisting on minimum standards of care and qualifications for cosmetic surgery clinics and the surgeons who operate them. An analogy might be with abortion clinics which have been brought under strict licensing controls.

Meanwhile, ask your GP for a letter of introduction to a plastic surgeon. You may feel embarrassed about going through your GP, or fear he may not refer you to the best face-lift surgeons locally. However, GPs are more used to such requests than is imagined. If not familiar with a suitable surgeon, they can find out to whom to refer you from BAPS or from their professional association. Patients themselves cannot ask the medical organisations for names as this would infringe the advertising ethics.

Most reputable plastic surgeons will ask for a referral letter.

This helps them assess the reasons for the breast increase or reduction, nose "job" or ironed out "bags". Many people have high expectations and are disappointed afterwards. They are perhaps seeking personality changes that might save their marriages or relationships, or get them a better job, only to find that underneath it all they remain the same after an expensive operation.

Some surgeons actually insist on a second opinion from a psychiatrist. Surgeons must also weigh up the symmetry of the face — some patients demand a shape that may not be possible, or would be incongruous. One of the concerns about private clinics is that new noses, say, are chosen out of a series of photographs or a magazine without due regard for the face to which they are attached.

If it is beauty you are after, you will probably have to go privately. NHS waiting lists are very long, and you are unlikely to be placed on one, unless you are scarred after an accident or suffering from severe psychological stress as a result of deformity.

Once you have a referral letter, you should ask for an initial consultation which may cost anything from £10 to £25. Quiz the surgeon's secretary a little. Ask how often he or she carries out the operation you are seeking. If it is only infrequently, it may be better to look for another surgeon. If you wish, you may look up the credentials of the surgeon in The Medical Directory — there should be a copy in your local library. You should also ask the secretary at this stage for some idea of the fees for the operation in question.

If, despite the warnings, you are tempted to pursue a "small ad" private clinic, be certain to ask *who* would be carrying out the operation. Check his — or her — credentials and experience. You could ask your GP if he would check the clinic. A reputable clinic should ask for a referral letter.

Fees for cosmetic surgery vary throughout the country. In London the fees for the nursing home or hospital bed will be roughly twice those outside the area. The following is an approximate guide to fees outside London. They include the surgeon, anaesthetist and hospital bed fee. Add about £50 a day for London. Most procedures take two to five days.

Nose reconstruction: around £700. Face-lift with reduction of upper and lower eyelids: £800 to £1,000. Face-lift alone tailored to needs, not necessarily with eyelid reductions: £750 to £800. Upper and lower eyelids alone: about £500. Upper or lower eyelids: £450. Breast augmentation: £600 to £700. Breast reduction: £800. Abdominal reduction — the "tummy" lift, becoming popular once childbearing is over: £800.

REFERENCE SECTION

If you want to know where to go in your area for a salon facial, a week at a health farm or a good haircut, you'll find the answer in our comprehensive guide below.

Your Health and Beauty Address Book

LONDON
Beauty salons

Blanche Kramer & Helena Harnik, 25 Welbeck St, W1; 01-935 1754. Specialists in problem skin: treatments and facials for acne, blackheads, open pores, red veins, etc; chemical deep-peeling treatment; electrolysis. They make all their products, which you can buy; mail order service.

Brownies, 32 Fouberts Place, W1; 01-434 3401. Sun-tan parlour: Solartone UVA sunbeds with curved UVA canopies for even tanning; each session lasts 45 minutes.

Clinical Cosmetic Centre, 33 New Cavendish St, W1; 01-486 9761. Acne treatments, cosmetic camouflage, capillary treatments, facials, electrolysis, solarium, aromatherapy, faradic and galvanic slimming treatments; make-up lessons using Jerome Alexander products.

Cosmetics à la Carte, 16 Motcomb St, SW1; 01-235 0596. Wide range of make-up made on premises; specialises in unusual colours. Advisory service; can experiment with no obligation to buy. Make-up lessons; facials, manicure and pedicure, lash-dyeing.

Elizabeth Arden, 20 New Bond St, W1; 01-629 1200. Facials, body massage, fibro-therapy, steam cabinet, wax bath, solarium, manicure, pedicure and chiropody; fake tanning; Red Door Beauty Workshop: make-up and skin care lessons.

ESSANELLE SALONS IN STORES
Facials including deep pore cleanse, Bio-cellular treatment, Sea Spa facials, all using Adrien Arpel products; electrolysis; liquid organic waxing for hair removal, manicure and pedicure; hair salon.

Army & Navy Stores, Victoria St, SW1; 01-834 1234.
Barkers, Kensington High St, W8; 01-937 5432.
Bournes, Oxford St, W1; 01-636 1515.
Fenwicks, Brent Cross; 01-202 8200.
Harrods, Knightsbridge, SW1; 01-730 1234. Treatments at Harrod's Hair & Beauty Salon include body massage, sauna and treatment for cellulite.
Selfridges, Oxford St, W1; 01-629 1234.

GLEMBY INTERNATIONAL SALONS IN STORES
Facials using Orlane products, lash-dyeing, manicure and pedicure; ear-piercing; hair salon.
Harvey Nichols, Knightsbridge, SW1; 01-235 5000.
Hawkins Clinic, 42 Beauchamp Place, SW3; 01-589 1853. Electrolysis, facials including Cathiodermie and Bio-peel, galvanic and faradic slimming treatments, aromatherapy, sunbeds, body massage and specialised cellulite treatments.
Headlines, 33 Thurloe St, SW7; 01-584 9900. Wide range of body, facial and hair conditioning treatments, including paraffin wax, fake tanning.
Joan Price's Face Place, 33 Cadogan St, SW3; 01-589 9062 and 31 Connaught St, W2; 01-723 6671. Wide range of body and facial treatments including solarium. Good ranges of cosmetics to experiment with; no obligation to buy.
Joan Price's Top Place, Horseshoe Yard, W1; 01-493 3955. As above; make-up lessons.
Katherine Corbett, 21 South Molton St, W1; 01-493 5905. Specialities are removal of thread veins, moles, superfluous hair and leg vein treatment.
Molton Brown, 58 South Molton St, W1; 01-629 1872. Facials; make-up lessons using their own range of cosmetics (on sale).

Morlé Slimming & Beauty Centre, 176 Kensington High St, W8; 01-937 9501.
Cellulite and stretch mark treatments, aromatherapy, supervised gym, sauna, solarium, massage, facials.
Marguerite Maury aromatherapy by Daniele Ryman, Suite 101, Park Lane Hotel, W1; 01-493 6630.
Facial and body massage using the Marguerite Maury aromatherapy method with essential oils mixed to suit individual needs.
Owen Owen, Finchley, N12; 01-445 3366.

LONDON
Gyms, dance and exercise studios
Granny's Beautiful Bodies, 2 Albert Gate Court, 124 Knightsbridge, SW1; 01-930 6301.
Yoga-based isometric exercises; disco dancing classes; also solarium.
Gym 'N' Tonic, 4 Welbeck St, W1; 01-584 4556.
Gym, sauna, whirlpool, health bar; half-hour work-out classes at lunchtime and after work hours.
London School of Contemporary Dance, The Place, 17 Dukes Rd, WC1; 01-387 0161.
Classes in contemporary dance and exercise.
The Body Control Studio; address and telephone as above.
Individually tailored programmes by physiotherapists to suit specific needs for exercise and postural correction.
Lotte Berk, 29 Manchester St, W1; 01-935 8905.
Classes of very strenuous ballet movements, bar and floor work.
Pineapple Dance Centre, 7 Langley St, WC2; 01-836 4004.
Every type of dance and exercise class from classic Indian to disco; for beginners and professionals. Classes all day and after work hours.
Westside International Health Centre, 201/207 Kensington High St, W8; 01-937 5386.
Well-equipped gym, sauna, exercise and dance classes.
YMCA, 112 Gt Russell St, WC1; 01-637 8131.
Exercise classes, classical ballet, mime classes; Arlene Phillips of Hot Gossip teaches disco classes. Also swimming pool, sports facilities, sauna, solarium.

LONDON
Hair salons
Colombe, 8 Motcomb St, W1; 01-235 3286.
Cutting & Co, 186 Castelnau, SW13; 01-748 9221. Beauty salon too.
Daniel Galvin Colour Salon, 59 George St, W1; 01-486 8601/2.
Specialises in hair colour, conditioning and perming; own products.
Ellishelen, 75 Walton St, SW3; 01-589 8519.
Specialises in short hair cuts, perming.
John Frieda, 75 New Cavendish St, W1; 01-636 1401.
Joseph Kendall, 69 York St, W1; 01-723 7553.
Leonard, 6 Upper Grosvenor St, W1; 01-629 5757.
Mane Line, 22 Weighhouse St, W1; 01-493 4952 and 25 Savile Row, W1; 01-734 2242.
Specialises in colouring and perming.
Michaeljohn, 23a Albemarle St, W1; 01-629 6969.
Molton Brown, 58 South Molton St, W1; 01-629 1872.
Specialises in styling for long hair; own products. Beauty salon too.

Neville Daniel, 15/17 New Cavendish St, W1; 01-487 5634.
Specialises in colouring; beauty salon.
Ricci Burns, 94 George St, W1; 01-935 3657 and 151 Kings Rd, SW3; 01-351 1235.
Schumi, 8 Yeoman's Row, SW3; 01-584 4070 and 16 Pont St, SW1; 01-235 3888.
Specialises in avant-garde cutting, styling and colouring.
Teal's, 5 Pond Place, SW3; 01-584 0105.
Vidal Sassoon, 44 Sloane St, SW1; 01-235 7791; 130 Sloane St, SW1; 01-730 7288 and 60 South Molton St, W1; 01-491 8848.
Specialises in precision cutting.

BEAUTY FARMS AND HEALTH HYDROS
Champneys, Tring, Herts; Berkhamsted 73155.
Faradic and galvanic slimming treatments, diet plan, gym, yoga, relaxation classes, sauna, heat treatments, jacuzzi, beauty and hair treatments.
Forest Mere, Liphook, Hampshire; Liphook 722051.
Underwater massage, physiotherapy, osteopathy, faradic and galvanic slimming treatments, swimming pools, beauty treatments, including Cathiodermie.
Grayshott Hall, Grayshott, Nr Hindhead, Surrey; Hindhead 4331.
Faradic and galvanic slimming treatments, underwater massage, games room, gym, solarium, osteopathy, yoga, skin conditioning treatments, including Cathiodermie, Bio-peel and Vapozone.
Henlow Grange, Henlow, Beds; Henlow 811111.
Exercise classes, paraffin wax treatments, solarium, Swedish massage, hydrotherapy, sports facilities, beauty and hairdressing.
Ragdale Hall, Ragdale, Nr Melton Mowbray, Leics; Melton Mowbray 75831.
Faradic, galvanic and mud slimming treatments, wax baths, calisthenics, gym, underwater massage, sauna, aromatherapy, Infra-red treatment, beauty treatments including Cathiodermie and Bio-peel.
Shrublands, Coddenham, Nr Ipswich, Suffolk; Ipswich 830404.
Hydrotherapy, sauna, yoga, physiotherapy, colonic irrigation, sports facilities, pot reducing treatments, facials.
Stobo Castle, Peebleshire, Scotland, EH45 8NY; Peebleshire 249.
Exceptional grounds, sports facilities, massage, aromatherapy, faradic and galvanic slimming treatments, sauna, steam baths, wax and mud treatments, yoga, extensive beauty treatments, including Cathiodermie, air conditioning and leg waxing.
Tyringham Naturopathic Clinic, Nr Newport Pagnell, Bucks; Newport Pagnell 610450.
Stringent vegetarian diet plans and fasting, therapeutic hydrotherapy, acupuncture, osteopathy, yoga, sauna, sports facilities.

REGIONAL
Hair and beauty salons, gyms, dance and exercise studios
Figures appearing directly after addresses are telephone numbers.
ABERDEEN
Essanelle Salon in Arnotts Ltd, 143 George St; 27222.
Hair salon; lash-dyeing, waxing, electrolysis.
Glemby Salon in Esslement & McIntosh, Union St; 27983.

Hair salon.
ALDERSHOT
Essanelle Salon in Army & Navy Stores, High St; 20255.
Hair salon.
BANGOR
Essanelle Salon in Debenhams, High St; 2491.
Hair salon; lash-dyeing, waxing, electrolysis.
BATH
The Beauty Connection, 15 John St; 331237.
Facials include Bio-peel, Cathiodermie; make-up lessons.
Opposite, 8 George St; 310445.
Facials, manicure, Kwik-slim, electrolysis; hair salon.
BELFAST
Norman Frederick, 18 Howard St; 42203.
Hair salon.
BIRMINGHAM
Outline Figure & Fitness Club, 41 Smallbrook, Queensway; 643 8712.
Gym, sauna, exercise classes, Slendertone; beauty salon.
Essanelle Salon in Rackhams, Corporation St; 236 3333.
Hair salon; Adrien Arpel facials; UV treatment, lash-dyeing, waxing, manicure and pedicure, electrolysis.
BLACKPOOL
Essanelle Salon in Binns Ltd, Bank Hey St; 21464.
Hair salon; lash-dyeing, waxing.
Glemby Salon in Lewis Ltd, 50 Promenade; 25272.
Hair salon.
BOLTON
Glemby Salon in Whitehead & Sons, Deansgate & Crown St; 32555.
Hair salon; Orlane facials, lash-dyeing, manicure and pedicure, ear-piercing.
BOURNEMOUTH
Outline Figure & Fitness Club, 215a Old Christchurch Rd; 28755.
Gym, sauna, exercise classes, Slendertone; beauty salon.
Essanelle Salon in Beales, Old Christchurch Rd; 22022.
Hair salon; Adrien Arpel facials, lash-dyeing, waxing, manicure.
BRADFORD
Glemby Salon in Rackhams, 26 Market St; 23434.
Hair salon; Orlane facials, UV treatment, lash-dyeing, manicure and pedicure, ear-piercing.
BRIGHTON
Hawkins Clinic, 194 Church Rd, Hove; 775341.
Facials including mini-face lift, Cathiodermie; aromatherapy, UV treatment, massage, slimming treatments including Kwik-slim.
Hair by Michael, 10 Market St; 28608.
Hair salon.
Salon 22, 22a East St; 23871.
Hair salon.
BRISTOL
Glemby Salon in Dingles, 45 Queen Rd; 291471.
Hair salon; Orlane facials, lash-dyeing, manicure and pedicure, ear-piercing.
BROMLEY
Glemby Salon in Medhursts, High St; (01) 464 6533.
Hair salon; Orlane facials, lash-dyeing, manicure and pedicure,

ear-piercing.
CAMBRIDGE
Sally King, 102a Cherry Hinton Rd; 47016.
Hair salon.
Cambridge Health and Beauty Salon, 27 King St; 356600.
Facials, cosmetic camouflage, lash-dyeing, waxing, massage, solarium, electrolysis, manicure and pedicure.
CANTERBURY
Essanelle Salon in Ricemans, St George's Lane, Canterbury; 66866.
Hair salon; Adrien Arpel facials, waxing, manicure, electrolysis.
CARDIFF
Tao Clinic, 18 Queen St; 26276.
Electrolysis, waxing, lash-dyeing.
CHELMSFORD
"Hairworks" in Miss Selfridge, 1 High Chelmer; 83094.
Hair salon.
CHELTENHAM
Glemby Salon in Cavendish House, Promenade; 21300.
Hair salon; Orlane facials, lash-dyeing, manicure and pedicure, ear-piercing.
CHESTER
Essanelle Salon in Browns of Chester, Eastgate Row; 20001.
Hair salon; Adrien Arpel facials, lash-dyeing, waxing, electrolysis.
CHICHESTER
Cammack, 13 St Pancras; 780863.
Hair salon.
Emiles, 66 South St; 782440.
Facials, lash-dyeing, waxing, manicure and pedicure.
The Herb Garden, Little London, Chichester; 783653.
Facials; body massage, aromatherapy, slimming treatments, electrolysis, lash-dyeing, waxing, manicure and pedicure; produce own skin care range using natural ingredients.
CIRENCESTER
Glemby Salon in Rackhams, 29 Market Place; 2391.
Hair salon; Orlane facials, lash-dyeing, manicure and pedicure, ear-piercing, Kwik-slim.
COLCHESTER
Glemby Salon in William & Griffin, High St; 71212.
Hair salon.
CORK
Essanelle Salon in Cash & Co, St Patrick St; 26774.
Hair salon; waxing, electrolysis.
COVENTRY
Essanelle Salon in Owen Owen, Broadgate; 25566.
Hair salon; lash-dyeing, waxing, electrolysis.
DERBY
Glemby Salon in Brindleys, 4 Babington Lane; 364817.
Hair salon; Orlane facials, lash-dyeing, manicure and pedicure, ear-piercing.
Shair, 33 Pentland Rd, Dronfield, Woodhouse, North Derbyshire; (Dronfield) 417208.
Hair salon.
DONCASTER
Essanelle Salon in Binns, Baxtergate; 25001.

Hair salon, lash-dyeing, waxing, manicure, electrolysis.
DUBLIN
Essanelle Salon in Switzer & Co, Grafton St; 776821.
Hair salon; lash-dyeing, waxing, manicure, electrolysis.
DUNDEE
Essanelle Salon in Arnotts, 80 High St; 24022.
Hair salon; lash-dyeing, manicure, waxing, electrolysis.
DURHAM
John Gerard, 16 Claypath; 66428.
Hair salon.
EDINBURGH
Mary Reid, Frederick St; 225 3167.
Body massage, steam baths, camouflage make-up, slimming treatments.
The Edinburgh Club, 2 Hillside Crescent; 556 8845.
Gym with exercise classes, massage, squash courts, sauna, judo, karate; sauna, UV treatment.
Brian Drumm, 37a & 58 George St; 226 5885; 225 2760.
Hair salons.
Cheynes, 37a Dalry Rd, Haymarket; 346 0000 and 57 South Bridge; 556 0108.
Hair salons.
EXETER
Glemby Salon in Dingles, High St; 36938.
Hair salon; Orlane facials, lash-dyeing, manicure and pedicure, ear-piercing.
GALWAY
Glemby Salon in Moons, Eglinton Buildings, Shop St; 68602.
Hair salon.
GLASGOW
Essanelle Salon in Arnotts, Argyle St; 248 2951.
Hair salon.
Glemby Salon in Lewis Ltd, Argyle St; 221 9820.
Hair salon; Orlane facials, lash-dyeing, manicure and pedicure, ear-piercing.
GLOUCESTER
Ian Wallace, 35 Clarence St; 35926.
Hair salon.
GRIMSBY
Essanelle Salon at Binns, Victoria St; 59581.
Hair salon; lash-dyeing, waxing, electrolysis.
GUILDFORD
Essanelle Salon in Army & Navy Stores, High St; 68171.
Hair salon; Adrien Arpel facials, manicure, waxing, lash-dyeing, electrolysis.
HARROGATE
Essanelle Salon at Binns, James St; 55174.
Hair salon.
HARTLEPOOL
Essanelle Salon in Binns, Victoria Rd; 65301.
Hair salon; lash-dyeing, waxing, manicure and pedicure, electrolysis.
HULL
Glemby Salon in Binns, Paragon Square; 26951.
Hair salon.
ILKLEY

Headline, 126 Bolling Rd. Ben Rhydding; 609809.
Hair salon; sauna, facials, waxing, massage, Slendertone, manicure.
IPSWICH
Woottons, 10a Queen St; 52002.
Hair salon.
KINGSTON-UPON-THAMES
Essanelle Hair & Beauty Centre, 12 Fife Rd; (01) 549 5196.
Hair salon; Adrien Arpel facials; lash-dyeing, waxing, manicure and pedicure, electrolysis.
LEAMINGTON SPA
Essanelle Salon in Rackhams, The Parade; 27900.
Hair salon; Adrien Arpel facials; lash-dyeing, waxing, manicure and pedicure, electrolysis.
LEEDS
Vidal Sassoon, 63 Albion St, West Riding House; 448813.
Hair salon.
Essanelle Salon in Schofields Ltd, The Headrow; 35235.
Hair salon; lash-dyeing, waxing, electrolysis.
LEICESTER
Essanelle Salon in Fenwick, Market St; 50144.
Hair salon; lash-dyeing, waxing, manicure, electrolysis.
Glemby Salon in Rackhams, Hotel St; 29004.
Hair salon.
LIMERICK
Essanelle Salon in Todds, O'Connell St; 47222.
Hair salon; Adrien Arpel facials, lash-dyeing, waxing, manicure, electrolysis.
LINCOLN
Jane Hair Stylist, 445 High St; 21733.
Hair salon.
Watson's Face Place, 6a Bailgate; 36487.
Facials including Cathiodermie and Bio-peel; massage, waxing, manicure and pedicure.
LIVERPOOL
Essanelle Salon in Owen Owen, Clayton Square; 709 6060.
Hair salon; Adrien Arpel facials; lash-dyeing, waxing, manicure, electrolysis.
Glemby Salon in Lewis's, 40 Ranelagh St; 709 7000.
Hair salon.
MANCHESTER
Vidal Sassoon, 19 King St; 833 0376.
Hair salon.
Outline Figure & Fitness Club, 21/31 Oldham St; 832 2555.
Gym, sauna, exercise classes, Slendertone; beauty salon.
Essanelle Salon in Kendal Milne, Deansgate; 832 3414.
Hair salon; Adrien Arpel facials; UV treatment, lash-dyeing, waxing, manicure, electrolysis.
MIDDLESBOROUGH
Essanelle Salon in Binns, Linthorpe Rd; 246371.
Hair salon; lash-dyeing, waxing, electrolysis.
NEWCASTLE-UPON-TYNE
Anne Hesselberth, 11 Bank Chambers, 51 Grainger St; 610166.
Facials, waxing, manicure and pedicure.
Newbegin Dance Centre, 36 Grainger Park Rd; 739987.

Dance and exercise classes.
Intrim Exercise Studio, 4 Waterloo St; 26184.
Gym and exercise equipment; sauna, solarium.
Europa, 20 Saville Row; 22288.
Hair salon.
Jap, 8 Princess Square; 27572.
Hair salon.
NORTHAMPTON
Debenhams, The Drapery; 34391.
Hair salon; facials, electrolysis, waxing, lash-dyeing, Kwik-slim, make-ups.
NORWICH
Glemby Salon in Bonds of Norwich, All Saints Green; 60021.
Hair salon; Orlane facials, lash-dyeing, UV treatment, manicure and pedicure, ear-piercing.
NOTTINGHAM
"Hairworks", Miss Selfridge, 107/110 Victoria Centre; 44058.
Hair salon.
OLDHAM
Outline Figure & Fitness Club, Rhodes Bank, Union St; 652 7418.
Gym, sauna, exercise classes, Slendertone; beauty salon.
OXFORD
Glemby Salon in Fenwick, St Ebbes St; 47158.
Hair salon.
Glemby Salon in Selfridges, 27 Westgate; 46237.
PLYMOUTH
Glemby Salon in Dingles, Royal Parade; 266611.
Hair salon; Orlane facials, lash-dyeing, manicure and pedicure, ear-piercing.
PORTSMOUTH
Landports, Commercial Rd; 21221.
Hair salon.
READING
Robert Seligman, Debenhams, Broad Street; 51210.
Hair salon.
Saunapines Health and Beauty Clinic, 230 Peppard Rd, Emmer Green; 473731.
Facials, group therapy slimming, solarium, massage, sauna, waxing, electrolysis, manicure and pedicure.
RICHMOND
Glemby Salon in Owen Owen, George St; (01) 940 0458.
Hair salon; Orlane facials, lash-dyeing, manicure and pedicure, ear-piercing.
ROMFORD
"Hairworks", Miss Selfridge, 1/3 Liberty; 27751.
Hair salon.
ST HELENS
Outline Figure & Fitness Club, 26 Barrow St, St Helens; 32535.
Gym, sauna, exercise classes.
SHEFFIELD
Headlines, 42/46 Fargate; 738661.
Hair salon.
Essanelle Salon in Rackhams, High St; 28121.
Hair salon; Adrien Arpel facials, lash-dyeing, waxing, electrolysis.

SHREWSBURY
Essanelle Salon in Rackhams, High St; 4678.
Hair salon; Adrien Arpel facials, lash-dyeing, waxing, electrolysis.
SKIPTON
Glemby Salon in Rackhams, High St; 2363.
Hair salon.
SOUTHAMPTON
Essanelle Salon in Owen Owen, Bargate; 23891.
Hair salon; electrolysis.
"Hairworks", Miss Selfridge, 111 Above Bar; 31433.
STOCKPORT
Outline Figure & Fitness Club, Mersey Square; 477 0160.
Gym, sauna, exercise classes; beauty salon.
STOKE-ON-TRENT
Glemby Salon in Lewis Ltd, Lamb St; Hanley; 261331.
Hair salon.
STOURBRIDGE
The Beauty Centre, 126 Hagley Rd, Old Swinford; 4047.
Electrolysis, steam baths, massage, facials, make-up lessons, waxing, UV treatment, slimming treatments, hair salon.
SUNDERLAND
Glemby Salon in Joplings, John St; 57601.
Hair salon.
SURBITON
Kaye T Urwin Beauty Clinic, 10 St Mary's Rd; (01) 399 2658.
Electrolysis, sauna, facials including Bio-peel and acne treatment, Slendertone.
SWANSEA
Glemby Salon in David Evans, Princess Way; 51525.
Hair salon.
TAUNTON
Hatcher & Sons, High St; 2277.
Hair salon.
TUNBRIDGE WELLS
Glemby Salon in Mary Lee Ltd, Mount Pleasant; 25222.
Hair salon.
WALSALL
Outline Figure & Fitness Club, 9/10a The Bridge; 37225.
Gym, sauna, exercise classes, solarium.
WHITLEY BAY
Ocean Boulevard, 2 Park Rd; 522555.
Hair salon.
WIGAN
Outline Figure & Fitness Club, Library St; 31439.
Gym, sauna, exercise classes, solarium.
WOLVERHAMPTON
Outline Figure & Fitness Club, 3 Woolpack St; 772356.
Gym, sauna, exercise classes, solarium.
WORTHING
Glemby Salon in Bentalls, South St; 31801.
Hair salon.
YORK
Glemby Int, Cresta House, Davygate; 56644.
Hair salon.

INDEX

Acne, 26–27
Alcohol, 17, 155
Anorexia nervosa, 42
Antiperspirants, 105
Aromatherapy, 110
Astringent, 18

Back, 163
  exercises for, 75
  problems, 73, 74
Bath additives, how to make your own, 98
Bath treatments, 99
Bathroom, 95, 96
Beauty therapist, 24
Bicycling, 69
Birthmarks, 25
Blackheads, 21
Body, 95–124
Bodywrap, 121
Bras, 112
Breakfast, 3, 50, 51
Breasts, 110, 112, 174
Brewer's yeast, 135

Caffeine, 3
Calisthenics, 69
Calories, 44, 45, 46, 47, 48
Cancer, 153, 154
Carbohydrates, 64, 65
Cellulite, 37, 100
Children, 159
Chocolate, 4, 15
Cleansers, skin, 17
  for removing make-up, 20
Coffee, 3
Cold sores, 26
Contraception, 159
Cosmetics, 16
Cosmetic surgery, 112, 171–181
Crudités, 4
Cystitis, 162

Dentistry, cosmetic, 168
  preventive, 165
Deodorants, 105
Dermatologist, 25
Diets, 3, 16, 19, 33–66, 123
Discharge, vaginal, 162, 163
Diuretics, 42
Drugs, 42, 159

Eczema, 26

Eggs, 5
Exercise, 42, 67–94
Eye-lift, 174

Face-lift, 171
Face masks, how to make them, 18, 24
Facials, how to do them yourself, 21, 22
Facial sauna, 16
Fasting, 9, 41, 60
Feet, 116–117
Fish, 6
Fitness, 158, 159
Food, 3–14, 40
Forbidden foods, 59
Foundation, 15
Fruit, 5, 60

Gynaecologist, 160

Hair, 102, 125–143
  blow-dry, 134
  colouring, 139–143
  equipment, 125–127
  home-care treatments, 130–131
  how to cut, 132–133
  how to shampoo, 129
  perming, 139
  problems, 135
  products and how to make them, 130–131
  removal of superfluous, 102–104
  scalp massage, 133
  tips, 138, 139
  types, 127
  waves, 136, 137
Hands, 117–121
Health, 151–164
Health farms, 122, 123, 124, 184
Health foods, 15, 41
Hives, 26
Honey, 61
Humidity, 16
Hydrotherapy, 112

Jogging, 67, 68

Liver spots, 25
Legs, 113–115

Make-up, 145, 149
  equipment, 145, 146, 147
  how to apply, 147–149
Massage, 106–110, 112
  different kinds of, 106
  how to, 107

Meat, 6
Moisturiser, 15, 16, 18
Moles, 25
Monosodium glutamate, 4

Night cream, 18
Nose job, 173
Nourishing cream, 18
Nutrition, 3–14

Oils, how to make, 105

Pasta, 57
Pill (the), 17
Pimples, 25
PMT, 161
Pollution, 16
Posture, 73
Psoriasis, 26

Red veins, 25
Relaxation, 157

Sauna, 101
Shingles, 26
Skin, 15–28, 96
  peeling, 26
  problems, 25
  types, 18
Skin-care products, 17
  how to make them, 22
Skipping, 70
Sleep, 16
Slimming, 33–66
  foods, 36
  clubs, 41
Smoking, 17, 154
Snacks, 3
Soap, 15, 17, 97
Solarium, 122
Soups, 56
Sport, 67
Spots, 24
Steambaths, 101, 122
Stress, 16, 155
Sun, 29–32
Sunburn, 31
Swimming, 68

Tanning, 29–32
  artificial, 31, 32
  preparations, 30
Tea, herbal, 3
Teeth, 165–169

gums, 165, 166
Trichologist, 135

Ultra-violet rays, 17

Vacuum suction, 121
Vegetables, 5, 60
Vegetarians, 10
Vitamins, 7, 15

Walking, 68
Warts, 25
Water retention, 38
Water therapy, 100, 101
Weight loss, 16, 33–66
Whiteheads, 25
Wholefoods, 6
Wrinkles, 15

Yoga, 70, 91, 92
Yogurt, 8